Uveitis

E. Mitchel Opremcak

Uveitis
A Clinical Manual for ·
Ocular Inflammation

With Line Illustrations by Kendra Kachelein

With 140 Illustrations, 78 in Full Color

Springer-Verlag
New York Berlin Heidelberg London Paris
Tokyo Hong Kong Barcelona Budapest

E. Mitchel Opremcak, M.D.
Associate Professor of Ophthalmology
The Ohio State University
465 West Tenth Street
Columbus, OH 43210
USA

Cover illustration by Kendra Kachelein. *Background:* Posterior synechiae in an eye with uveitis. *Foreground:* Normal eye.

Library of Congress Cataloging-in-Publication Data
Opremcak, E. Mitchel.
    Uveitis : a clinical manual for ocular inflammation / E. Mitchel
Opremcak.
        p.   cm.
    Includes bibliographical references and index.
    ISBN 0-387-94247-5. — ISBN 3-540-94247-5
    1. Uveitis.   I. Title.
    [DNLM: 1. Uveitis.   WW 240 062u 1994]
RE351.067 1994
617.7′2—dc20
DNLM/DLC
for Library of Congress   94-13826
                                                                   CIP

Printed on acid-free paper.

Production managed by Terry Kornak; manufacturing supervised by Jacqui Ashri.
Typeset by Asco Trade Typesetting, Hong Kong.
Printed and bound by Walsworth Publishing Co., Marceline, MO.
Printed in the United States of America.

9 8 7 6 5 4 3 2 1

ISBN 0-387-94247-5 Springer-Verlag New York Berlin Heidelberg
ISBN 3-540-94247-5 Springer-Verlag Berlin Heidelberg New York

*This book is dedicated to Shelley Ann and Jessica Lee,
and to Colleen Marie, their mother, whom I have loved
with all my heart*

Preface

As a garden is to a gardener, so a book is to its author. Nurtured out of love, both are a source of pride and hope. Microbiology, immunology, infectious diseases, rheumatology, and ophthalmology are the seeds of this textbook on uveitis. Over the years, these branches of medicine have been cultivated and garnered to care for patients with inflammatory diseases of the eye, a most hardy species in the family of ocular maladies.

The aim of this clinical manual is to give both a serviceable framework and practical information on ocular inflammatory disease. The first section is devoted to general principles and commonly held suppositions in the field of uveitis. A system of diagnosis, based on the differential, is also offered. Traumatic uveitis is addressed in the second section. The third part examines infectious diseases that have been identified with uveitis. These are frequently curable forms of ocular inflammation caused by replicating foreign antigens. The fourth section of this textbook considers inflammatory diseases of the eye with a presumed autoimmune mechanism. A disobedient, autoreactive immune response is postulated to play a role in these forms of uveitis. Masquerade and idiopathic conditions are discussed in the final chapters. Etiology, epidemiology, pathogenesis, clinical presentation, diagnosis, differential diagnosis, treatment, and prognosis are provided for each disease syndrome.

As with most gardens, there are many styles and delightful entrances to the field of uveitis. The writings and fruition of other authors including Alan C. Woods, Theodore F. Schlaegel, G. Richard O'Conner, Ronald E. Smith, Robert A. Nozik, Robert B. Nussenblatt, Alan G. Palestine, Ellen Kraus-Mackiw, Jack K. Kanski, and William J. Dinning should be accessed and are well worth the journey.

Time transforms all vistas. Closely held ideas and concepts in the field of uveitis will without a doubt change as we gain more understanding of these challenging diseases. Forthwith, I offer one such path, a single season, an evanescent view of the realm; flowers amid weeds, mosses upon stone.

> *Asagao no*   *Above the fence,*
> *matamata taranu*   *a morning glory stretches*
> *kakine kana.*   *still unsatisfied.*

Shukyo, Haiku Poet, 1826 A.D.

E. Mitchel Opremcak

Acknowledgments

It would require a separate text to encompass the profound influence and teaching of my many mentors. I must acknowledge, however, the instruction, kindness, and support of the following individuals:

Drs. Robbins and Angell, Drs. DeGowin and DeGowin, Dr. Earl N. Metz, Dr. Ronald L. Whisler, Dr. William H. Havener, Dr. Torrence A. Makley Jr., Dr. Elson L. Craig, Dr. Paul A. Weber, Dr. Frederick H. Davidorf, Dr. Charles D. Regan, Dr. Evangelos S. Gragoudas, Dr. Donald J. D'Amico, Dr. Carmen A. Pulliafito, Dr. Johanna M. Seddon, and Dr. Lloyd M. Aiello.

Medical students, residents, and fellows with whom I have worked including Dr. Michael B. Raizman, Dr. Ramzi Hemady, Drs. Neil M. and Susan B. Bressler, Dr. David K. Scales, and Dr. Ivo Kocur.

Nancy A. Kelso, Beth A. Ferguson, Holly N. Dotin, and Diane M. Combs for their boundless energy, enthusiasm, and valued friendship.

Kendra E. Kachelein and Esther T. Silverman for their skillful medical illustration and thoughtful editing.

All of my patients and their referring ophthalmologists for their trust and for allowing me to participate in their care.

Most of all, to Dr. C. Stephen Foster—without whose philosophy, expertise, discipline, and instruction the cogent and viable aspects of this endeavor would be but ephemeral. I bid both my gratitude and heartfelt admiration.

Contents

Ocular Inflammation Associated with Immunologic Diseases

Ocular Inflammations Associated with Masquerade Syndromes

General Principles

1
Introduction

General Information

The uveal tract is the highly vascularized middle layer of the eye. Situated between the scleral coat and the neurosensory epithelium, its major function is to provide nourishment for the intraocular tissues including the retina, lens, and cornea.[1]

The uveal tract is composed of the iris, ciliary body, and choroid (Fig. 1.1). Uveitis is the inflammatory process involving these structures. Clinically, however, the practice of uveitis has evolved to encompass inflammation of virtually any structure within the eye including the lens, vitreous, retina, retinal pigment epithelium, cornea, and sclera.

With its complex organization and delicate structure, the eye has low tolerance for inflammation. Approximately 10% of all blindness in the United States is due to the complications of uveitis.[2] Corneal scarring, cataract, glaucoma, vitreous opacification, macular edema, retinal detachment, and periretinal fibrosis are common sequelae of uveitis that can impair visual function. All forms of ocular inflammation, therefore, are potentially sight-threatening.

Until recently, uveitis had been approached as a single-disease entity, and treatment was either supportive or limited to corticosteroids. Our understanding of uveitis has improved considerably because of advances in microbiology, immunology, and immunohistology and through the development of animal models of uveitis.

Today we know that uveitis is not one condition, but a group of disorders initiated and maintained by trauma, infectious microorganisms, autoimmune responses, and neoplastic or degenerative diseases. Consequently, caring for the patient with uveitis is both challenging and rewarding.

The presence of ocular inflammation often denotes an underlying systemic or even life-threatening condition. The practitioner, therefore, needs to be familiar with the principles and practice of general internal medicine, infectious diseases, and rheumatology. Many diseases, including syphilis, ankylosing spondylitis, juvenile rheumatoid arthritis (JRA), multiple sclerosis, and sarcoidosis, may present in the eye well before other systemic manifestations become evident. Moreover, ocular findings are frequently key diagnostic features in disorders such as Reiter's syndrome, cytomegalovirus (CMV) retinitis and acquired immunodeficiency syndrome (AIDS), Behçet's disease, and Vogt–Koyanagi–Harada (VKH) syndrome. As such, the ophthalmologist is often in a position to assist in the diagnosis and treatment of a wide variety of diseases.

Definitions

The following basic terms and definitions are used throughout the text.

Cell and flare: Cell implies the presence of

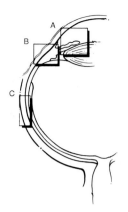

Figure 1.1. The uveal tract. The uveal tract can be divided anatomically into the iris (*A*), ciliary body (*B*), and choroid (*C*). Uveitis is the inflammatory process involving these structures.

leukocytes within the anterior, posterior, or vitreous chambers. Flare results from a breakdown of the normal blood–eye barrier and represents increased serum proteins in the intraocular fluids.

Choroiditis/chorioretinitis: Inflammation involving the choroid (choroiditis) or secondarily the contiguous retina (chorioretinitis).

Hypopyon: An accumulation and layering of inflammatory cells within the anterior chamber.

Iritis/cyclitis/iridocyclitis: Inflammation of the iris (iritis), ciliary body (cyclitis), or both (iridocyclitis).

Keratic precipitates (KP): Collections of inflammatory cells on the corneal endothelium. The iris (IP), lens (LP), vitreous (VP), and retina (RP) also may form inflammatory precipitates.

Retinitis/retinochoroiditis: Inflammation of the retina (retinitis) or secondarily the contiguous choroid (retinochoroiditis).

Synechiae (anterior and posterior): Inflammatory adhesions between the iris and cornea (anterior synechiae) or the iris and lens (posterior synechiae).

Vitritis: Inflammation within the vitreous cavity.

Uveitis: Inflammation of the uveal tract proper (iris, ciliary body, choroid).

Vasculitis: Primary or secondary inflammation of the retinal arterioles, capillaries, or venules.

Epidemiology

Uveitis affects an estimated 1.2 million Americans, with 45,000 new cases reported each year.[2] Although anterior uveitis (8–12 per 100,000 population) is more common than posterior uveitis (3 per 100,000 population), most published studies on the epidemiology of uveitis report a preponderance of posterior forms.[3,4] These reviews are often based on large referral or tertiary practices and reflect a greater respect for the deeper forms of ocular inflammation.

Uveitis can occur at any age. In a series of 854 consecutive patients with uveitis referred to The Ohio State University College of Medicine between 1989 and 1992, 494 (58%) were females and 360 (42%) were males. The mean age of these patients was 43, with a range of 3 to 91 years.

Several important associations between tissue type [human leukocyte antigens (HLA)] and uveitis syndromes are helpful, both from an epidemiologic standpoint and in understanding the pathogenesis of certain diseases. These associations also provide a genetic basis for susceptibility. The strongest HLA association is that of HLA-A29 in patients with birdshot retinochoroidopathy: 97% of these patients have this tissue type, with a calculated relative risk of 50 to 224.[5,6]

In addition, HLA typing often supports a clinical impression and may help establish a specific diagnosis. For example, 90% of patients with ankylosing spondylitis and 75% of patients with Reiter's syndrome exhibit the HLA-B27 haplotype.[7] Both these disorders can be accompanied by an iridocyclitis. More than 50% of patients with idiopathic, acute anterior iridocyclitis have this same tissue type.[8] Single-antigen testing can be obtained to support the clinical

Table 1.1. HLA and disease associations.

Antigen	Disease	Relative Risk
HLA-A1	Sarcoidosis	—
HLA-A11	Sympathetic ophthal-mia	—
HLA-A29	Birdshot retinochoroid-opathy (>97%)	50–224
HLA-B51	Behçet's disease	4–6
HLA-B7,DR2	Presumed ocular histo-plasmosis syndrome and disciform macu-lar scar	12
HLA-B8	Anterior uveitis	5
HLA-B12	Behçet's disease (oral), ocular cicatricial pemphigoid	3–4
HLA-B27	Ankylosing spondylitis (90%)	100
	Reiter's syndrome (76%)	40
	Acute anterior uveitis (55%)	10
	Inflammatory bowel disease	—
	Psoriatic arthritis	—
	Behçet's disease	—
HLA-B53	VKH syndrome	75
	Glaucomatocyclitic uveitis	75

HLA, human leukocyte antigen; VKH, Vogt-Koyanagi-Harada.

diagnosis. Other important HLA associations are listed in Table 1.1.

Several mechanisms have been proposed to explain the relationship between HLA and disease.[9,10] For example, individual HLA antigens may serve as a cell surface receptor for infectious agents. The presence of a specific HLA protein would allow a microorganism to bind to the cell, thereby predisposing the host to disease. Alternatively, HLA surface antigens may become "modified," allowing the development of an autoimmune response. These new cell surface antigens would be recognized as foreign to the host's immune system and would provoke an immune response directed toward the altered self-proteins. Chemicals, viral antigens, and other agents may initiate an autoimmune response

through this mechanism. Finally, foreign proteins (yeast histones) may possess a structure similar to HLA antigens, which may make them capable of triggering an overlapping inflammatory response ("molecular mimicry").

Pathology/Pathophysiology

The effect of inflammation on the ocular tissues depends to a certain degree on the pathophysiologic mechanisms responsible for the disease and the layer of the eye involved. Each form of uveitis has a characteristic clinical course and unique set of complications. The known pathologic effects of each disease are discussed in subsequent sections.

Clinically, it is often helpful to determine whether the inflammatory process is *granulomatous* or *nongranulomatous*. These terms refer to the biomicroscopic appearance of the inflammatory precipitates within the eye. These precipitates can occur anywhere within the eye: on the corneal endothelium (KP), trabecular meshwork (TP), iris stroma (IP), vitreous (VP), vitreous face, retinal vessels, and sensory retina (RP) (Fig. 1.2).

Granulomatous precipitates are large and yellowish white. They often have a

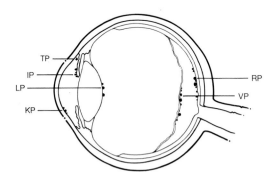

Figure 1.2. Inflammatory precipitates. Inflammatory precipitates may be found on the corneal endothelium (*KP*), iris (*IP*), trabecular meshwork (*TP*), lens (*LP*), vitreous (*VP*), and retina (*RP*). Precipitates may be granulomatous or nongranulomatous in appearance.

"greasy" appearance. On the cornea, they are called "mutton-fat" KP. Koeppe and Busacca nodules are granulomatous iris precipitates that occur in the pupillary margin or iris stroma, respectively. Clinically, large vitreous "snowballs" and retinal vascular "candle wax drippings" are characteristic of a granulomatous inflammation as well. Some forms of uveitis may begin with nongranulomatous findings and over time develop granulomatous features. Diseases such as sarcoidosis, toxoplasmosis, tuberculosis, syphilis, VKH syndrome, and sympathetic ophthalmia will often have granulomatous-appearing precipitates during the disease course. Nongranulomatous precipitates are small, fine, and whiter in color. Conditions such as Fuchs's heterochromic iridocyclitis, JRA, ankylosing spondylitis, and Reiter's syndrome have a nongranulomatous appearance on biomicroscopic examination.

Classification

Uveitis has been classified in several ways. It can be grouped by age of onset, sex, or race of the patient; by the type of inflammation present (granulomatous vs. nongranulomatous); and by whether the disease is acute, recurrent, or chronic.[11] Each of these approaches has merit and addresses unique aspects of individual diseases. For example, JRA occurs predominantly in girls during childhood and is a nongranulomatous, chronic disease. In contrast, ankylosing spondylitis–associated uveitis often occurs in young men as an acute iritis. Certain disorders have racial predilection as well. Sarcoidosis is more common among black patients; VKH syndrome occurs in American Indians and Asian patients more frequently than in whites.

The most useful classification organizes uveitis into four predominant pathophysiologic mechanisms responsible for initiating or maintaining the disease process[12] (Table 1.2): traumatic, infectious, immunologic,

Table 1.2. Classification of uveitis by the pathophysiologic mechanism.

Trauma
  Surgical
  Nonsurgical
Infection
  Viral
  Bacterial
  Fungal
  Protozoal
  Helminthic
  Insect
  Animal
Immunologic disorders
  Type I hypersensitivity (IgE mediated)
  Type II hypersensitivity (ADCC)
  Type III hypersensitivity (IC)
  Type IV hypersensitivity (CMI)
Masquerade
  Vascular
  Infectious
  Congenital
  Metabolic/degenerative
  Neoplastic

IgE, immunoglobulin E; ADCC, antibody-dependent cellular cytotoxicity; IC, immune complex; CMI, cell-mediated immune response.

and masquerade diseases.[7] Although the mechanism of inflammation may be established more firmly for certain diseases such as syphilis, CMV retinitis, and herpes zoster infections, the exact pathophysiology is less apparent for other conditions. The "theoretic" categorization of an individual disorder to a specific disease mechanism often requires significant poetic freedom. This is illustrated in the naming of diseases such as the presumed ocular histoplasmosis syndrome and in the frequent use of colorful, yet descriptive, terms such as birdshot retinochoroidopathy.

Several diseases may have multiple and/or overlapping mechanisms. For example, tuberculosis may cause disease directly as a result of bacterial replication; in addition, cell wall proteins of the dead organism (Freund's adjuvant) are a potent stimulus for the immune system. These proteins, as shown in animal models, may promote both an adjuvant uveitis and a true autoimmune response toward ocular self-proteins.[13] Thus, the predominant mechanism may often be difficult to ascertain.

This classification system will be used throughout the textbook. Efforts have been made to place distinct uveitis syndromes into one of these categories. The rationale for placing an individual syndrome within one of these pathophysiologic groups is discussed in each section. As we gain more knowledge about these diseases, many will undoubtedly be reassigned. Nevertheless, this framework is useful to permit the design of rational therapies, whether specific antibiotic treatment, anti-inflammatory agents, or immunosuppressive regimens.

Ocular Inflammation Associated with Trauma

Trauma may cause severe inflammation within the eye. Both surgical and nonsurgical injuries produce tissue damage that lead to a breakdown of the blood–eye barrier. The release of potent inflammatory mediators including arachidonic acid, prostaglandins, and leukotrienes increases vascular permeability and causes the recruitment of inflammatory cells into the eye. If the noxious stimuli are transient, the eye is often able to reestablish the normal physiologic milieu. Continual injury such as occurs from retained intraocular foreign bodies or ill-fitting intraocular lenses may cause chronic inflammation.

Ocular Inflammation Associated with Infectious Diseases

The infectious forms of uveitis can be divided into viral, bacterial, and protozoal diseases and into macroscopic organisms including helminthic, insect, and animal mediated disorders. Each has been associated with distinct types of ocular inflammation.

Microorganisms can cause injury by several mechanisms including direct cell lysis, endotoxin and exotoxin damage, and re-

lease of destructive enzymes. The host's inflammatory and immune responses often contribute to tissue injury through the recruitment of other inflammatory cells and the release of oxygen-free radicals and various cytokines designed to eradicate the invading organism. Macroscopic organisms may cause direct mechanical trauma or injury through the release of complex proteins after death.

Ocular Inflammation Associated with Immunologic Diseases

Immunologic disorders can cause ocular inflammation and, similar to infectious forms, can be divided into four distinct hypersensitivity types[14] (Fig. 1.3).

Type I hypersensitivity disorders are immunoglobulin E (IgE)-mediated. IgE is an antibody produced by antigen-committed B cells. This class of immunoglobulin binds to mast cells via the Fc receptor. When specific antigen comes in contact with the membrane-bound IgE, the immunoglobulin cross-links on the surface of the mast cell. This surface event signals the mast cell to degranulate, releasing multiple vasoactive amines, including histamine and bradykinin. The release of these agents produces the itching, vasodilation, vascular leakage, and tissue edema characteristic of type I hypersensitivity reaction. Although most HT-1 disorders affect the ocular surface (hay fever and atopic keratoconjunctivitis), mast cells are found within the choroid and may play a role in other forms of intraocular inflammation.

Type II hypersensitivity diseases are mediated by antibodies with a specificity for self-proteins. These autoantibodies bind to cellular antigens and can result in the activation of complement, macrophage phagocytosis, or killer cell (K cell) functions. The complement cascade, in turn, can promote further injury through enhanced chemotaxis and cytolysis. The result of a type II hypersensitivity reaction is specific, antibody-directed immunologic damage of the

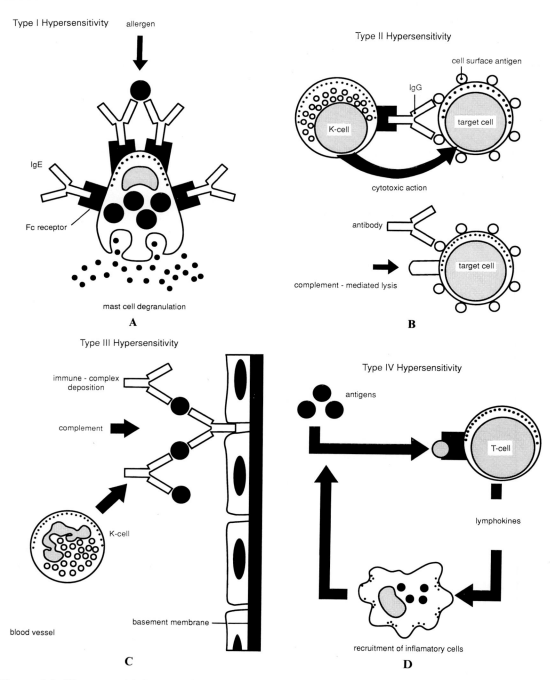

Figure 1.3. Hypersensitivity reactions. Hypersensitivity reactions can be divided into four types. **A:** Type I hypersensitivity is mediated by IgE. Contact with specific allergens results in the release of vasoactive amines from IgE-primed mast cells. **B:** Type II hypersensitivity reactions are mediated by antibodies binding to cell-associated autoantigens. Subsequent activation of complement, macrophage, or killer cell functions results in an antibody-dependent cellular cyto-toxicity and tissue damage. **C:** Type III hypersensitivity responses are mediated by IC formation and activation of complement within blood vessels or tissues. **D:** Type IV hypersensitivity occurs when autoreactive T cells promote a cell-mediated immune response directed against certain tissues. Damage may occur with the release of cytokines and the recruitment of other inflammatory cells.

target tissue or cells. Ocular cicatricial pemphigoid and lens-induced uveitis appear to have an important type II reaction, with anti-conjunctival basement membrane and anti-lens antibodies participating in the autoimmune response.[15–18]

Type III hypersensitivity reactions are a result of immune complex (IC) formation and deposition. Immune complexes may be deposited within the wall of the blood vessels or may form in the tissues (Arthus reaction), depending on their size and antigen specificity. Certain ICs can fix and activate complement. Vasculitis results when the IC remains within the lumen or walls of the blood vessels. Nutritional compromise, tissue ischemia, and hemorrhagic necrosis may result from such vascular injury and occlusion. Type III mechanisms appear to play a role in systemic lupus erythematosus (SLE), Behçet's disease, polyarteritis nodosa (PAN), Wegener's granulomatosis, and other collagen-vascular diseases.[19,20]

Type IV hypersensitivity is the only cell-mediated autoimmune mechanism. Autoreactive T cells, which are capable of recognizing self-antigens, promote a cell-mediated immune (CMI) response via the secretion of several potent cytokines called *interleukins* (IL-1 through IL-13).[9,21] Each interleukin has pleiotropic and multifaceted effects on the recruitment of inflammatory cells to the site of injury. Examples of ocular diseases that may have a predominant type IV autoimmune mechanism include sympathetic ophthalmia, VKH syndrome, and birdshot retinochoroidopathy.[22–25]

Ocular Inflammation Associated with Masquerade Syndromes

The masquerade syndromes are a collection of disorders in which inflammation is secondary to another process other than trauma, infections or immunologic diseases. Vascular tumors, congenital anomalies, degenerations (amyloidosis, retinitis pigmentosa), and neoplastic diseases (lymphoma, leukemia) can all result in a break-

down of the blood–eye barrier. This breakdown often results in the presence of inflammatory cells within the eye. Retained intraocular foreign bodies and endophthalmitis are also considered masquerade syndromes.

Etiology and Diagnostic Considerations

Because individual diseases affect distinct regions, layers, or tissues within the eye, it is useful diagnostically to divide ocular inflammation anatomically into anterior, intermediate, posterior, and diffuse forms (Table 1.3).[26,27] In anterior uveitis, inflammatory cells are primarily within the anterior and posterior chambers, with minimal "spillover" into the anterior vitreous (Fig. 1.4). Intermediate uveitis, also called chronic cyclitis or peripheral uveitis, is characterized by inflammatory cells within the vitreous cavity. The cells may be more numerous in the anterior vitreous or may be distributed diffusely throughout the vitreous gel. Vitreous "snowballs" and "snowbanks" may be noted, but are not the sine qua non of intermediate uveitis. Posterior uveitis is defined as inflammation predominantly involving the retina or cho-

Table 1.3. Distinct ocular regions involved in uveitis.

Conjunctival, corneal, and scleral layers: Inflammation involving the conjunctiva, cornea, or sclera
Anterior uveitis: Inflammation involving iris and/or ciliary body with cells predominantly within the anterior or posterior chamber and minimal "spillover" into the anterior vitreous cavity
Intermediate uveitis: Inflammation involving the ciliary body or peripheral retina, with cells predominantly within the anterior vitreous cavity
Posterior uveitis: Inflammation involving the retina and/or choroid, with cellular infiltration of the choroid, retina, or posterior vitreous cavity
Diffuse uveitis: Inflammation involving the entire eye with inflammatory cells distributed diffusely throughout all chambers and layers of the eye

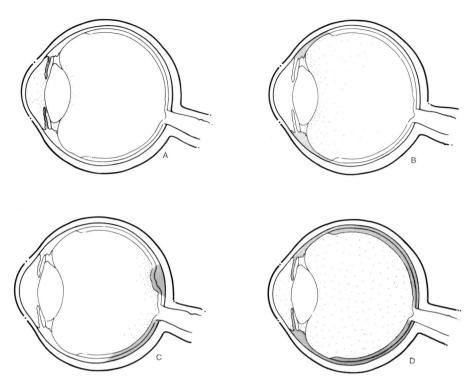

Figure 1.4. Location of intraocular inflammation. Individual diseases affect distinct regions or tissues of the eye in uveitis. Location of the ocular inflammation should be determined as primarily anterior (**A**), intermediate (**B**), posterior (**C**), or diffuse (**D**).

Table 1.4. Uveitis series: location of inflammation.

Author	No. of patients	Year	Geographic location	Anterior (%)	Intermediate (%)	Posterior (%)	Diffuse (%)
Perkins[28]	172	1984	Iowa	59	5	21	16
Henderly[3]	600	1984–87	California	28	15	38	18
Weiner[4]	400	1982–88	Israel	46	15	15	25
Opremcak	854	1989–92	Ohio	36	17	28	19

roid. In diffuse or panuveitis, all layers or regions of the eye are affected equally (Table 1.4).

By categorizing ocular inflammation into these regions, the physician begins to construct a differential diagnosis. Rheumatoid arthritis characteristically involves the conjunctiva, episclera, and sclera, without significant intraocular inflammation. Juvenile rheumatoid arthritis, Fuchs's heterochromic iridocyclitis, ankylosing spondylitis, and Reiter's syndrome affect the anterior structures. Intermediate uveitis is noted in pars planitis, sarcoidosis, multiple sclerosis, and Lyme disease. Toxoplasmosis, histoplasmosis, Toxocarasis serpiginous chorioretinitis, and birdshot retinochoroidopathy affect primarily the retina and choroid. Sympathetic

Table 1.5. Common entities associated with ocular inflammation.[a]

Disease	1984 Perkins[28] (%) (n = 178)	1987 Henderly[3] (%) (n = 600)	1991 Weiner[4] (%) (n = 400)	1992 Opremcak (%) (n = 854)
Sarcoidosis	5	4	1	10
Pars planitis	6	15	15	8
Fuchs' heterochromic iridocyclitis	6	2	2	7
Idiopathic iritis	33	12	—	7
Toxoplasmosis	9	7	4	6
Histoplasmosis	—	4	—	6
Reiter's syndrome	5	1	1	4
Scleritis	—	—	—	4
Traumatic	—	1	8	4
HLA-B27 iritis	—	3	3	3
HSV	—	2	—	3
Tuberculosis	—	<1	<1	3
Lens induced	—	<1	1	2
Endophthalmitis	—	—	—	2
Cicatricial pemphigoid	—	—	—	2
Herpes zoster	—	<1	—	2
Idiopathic diffuse uveitis	3	8	—	2
CMV	—	2	1	2
JRA	5	3	5	2
Ankylosing spondylitis	6	2	—	2
VKH syndrome	—	3	—	1
Beçhet's syndrome	3	2	3	1
Retinal vasculitis	5	7	—	—
Serpiginous	—	2	1	<1
Idiopathic posterior	7	4	—	<1
Toxocara	3	3	1	<1
Inflammatory bowel disease	3	<1	1	<1
Sympathetic ophthalmia	—	<1	4	—

[a] Reported at >2% in the Series.
HSV, herpes simplex virus; CMV, cytomegalovirus; JRA, juvenile rheumatoid arthritis; VKH, Vogt-Koyanaga-Harada; HLA, human leukocyte antigen.

ophthalmia, VKH syndrome, and Behçet's disease often cause a diffuse uveitis.

Several authors have reviewed the etiology for the ocular inflammation in these regions of the eye. Table 1.5 summarizes four recent studies of patients with uveitis.[3,4,28,29] Listed in the table are 28 diseases that were found in more than 2% of patients. Other syndromes such as birdshot retinochoroiditis, syphilis, acute retinal necrosis syndrome, PAN, and SLE accounted for less than 2% of all cases and are not included in this table. The differences in disease incidence in these studies reflect not only geographic considerations but also the nature of the tertiary referral center.

In a series of 854 consecutive uveitis patients referred to the Uveitis Service at The Ohio State University College of Medicine between 1989 and 1992, 97% of all patients fit into 1 of 81 separate syndrome diagnoses; 3% could not be classified further.[29] 38% of patients had underlying systemic illness that was responsible for the ocular inflammation.

Uveitis is a challenging area of ophthalmology. A wide variety of systemic and local ocular disorders can result in ocular inflammation. Efforts to establish a diagnosis that is as specific as possible and to determine the predominant mechanism of inflammation are required to design rational therapies and by that minimize visual impairment in these patients.

References

1. Scales DK, Fryczykowski AW, Opremcak EM. The choroid. In: Albert DM, Jakobiec FA, eds. *Principles and Practice of Ophthalmology*. Philadelphia: WB Saunders; 1994;2:252.
2. The 1983 Report of the National Advisory Eye Council, Vision Research—A National Plan. Summary panel reports on retinal and choroidal disease. Bethesda: National Eye Institute; 1983:23.
3. Henderly DE, Genstler AJ, Smith RE, Rao NA. Changing pattern of uveitis. *Am J Ophthalmol.* 1987;103:131.
4. Weiner A, Benezra D. Clinical patterns and associated conditions in chronic uveitis. *Am J Ophthalmol.* 1991;112:151.
5. Nussenblatt RB, Mittal KK, Ryan S, et al. Birdshot retinochoroidopathy associated with HLA-A29 antigen and immune responsiveness to retinal S-antigen. *Am J Ophthalmol.* 1982;94:147.
6. Priem HA, Kijlstra A, Noens L, et al. HLA typing in birdshot chorioretinopathy. *Am J Ophthalmol.* 1988;105:182.
7. Calin A. Ankylosing spondylitis. In: Kelley WN, Harris ED, Ruddy S, Sledge CB, eds. *Textbook of Rheumatology.* 2 ed. Philadelphia: WB Saunders, 1985:993.
8. Brewerton DA, Caffrey M, Nicholls A, et al. Acute anterior uveitis and HL-A27. *Lancet.* 1973;2:994.
9. Opremcak EM. Cellular cooperation. In: Albert DM, Jakobiec FA, eds. *Principles and Practice of Ophthalmology.* Philadelphia: WB Saunders, 1994;2:770.
10. Bottazzo GF, Pujol-Borrell R, Hanafusa T, et al. Role of aberrant HLA-DR expression and antigen presentation in induction of endocrine autoimmunity. *Lancet.* 1983;2:1115.
11. Duke-Elder WS, Perkins ES, eds. *System of Ophthalmology, Vol. IX: Diseases of the Uveal Tract.* St. Louis: CV Mosby, 1966:41.
12. Intraocular inflammation and uveitis. In: *Basic and Clinical Science Course (1986–1987).*

Section 3: Intraocular Inflammation, Uveitis, and Ocular Tumors. San Francisco: American Academy of Ophthalmology, 1986:70.
13. Wacker WB, Donoso LA, Kalsow CM, et al. Experimental allergic uveitis: isolation characterization and localization of asoluble uveitis-pathogenic antigen from bovine retina. *J Immunol.* 1977;119:1949.
14. Roitt IM, Brostoff J, Male DK. *Immunology.* 3 ed. St. Louis: CV Mosby, 1987:191.
15. Furey N, West C, Andress T, et al. Immunofluorescent studies of ocular cicatricial pemphigoid. *Am J Ophthalmol* 1975;80:825.
16. Mondino BJ, Ross AN, Rabin BS, Brown SI. Autoimmune phenomena in ocular cicatricial pemphigoid. *Am J Ophthalmol.* 1977; 83:443.
17. Marak GE, Font RL, Alepa FP. Experimental lens-induced granulomatous endophthalmitis. *Mod Probl Ophthalmol.* 1976;16:75.
18. Marak GE, Font RL, Alepa FP. Alepa: Arthus-type panophthalmitis in rats sensitized to heterologous lens protein. *Ophthalmol Res.* 1977;9:162.
19. Fauci AS, Haynes BF, Katz P. The spectrum of vasculitis: clinical, pathologic, immunologic, and therpeutic considerations. *Ann Intern Med.* 1978;89(pt 1):660.
20. Opremcak EM. Collagen disorders: retinal manifestations of collagen vascular diseases. In: Albert DM, Jakobiec FA, eds. *Principles and Practice of Ophthalmology* Philadelphia: WB Saunders; 1994;2:985.
21. Roitt IM, Brostoff J, Male DK. *Immunology.* 3 ed. St. Louis: CV Mosby; 1987.
22. Jakobiec FA, Marboe CC, Knowles DM, et al. Human smpathetic ophthalmia: an analysis of the inflammatory infiltrate by hybridoma-monoclonal antibodies, immunochemistry, and correlative electron microscopy. *Ophthalmology.* 1983;90:76.
23. Hirose S, Tanaka T, Nussenblatt RB, et al. Lymphocyte responses to retinal-specific antigens in uveitis patients and healthy subjects. *Curr Eye Res.* 1988;7:393.
24. Nussenblatt RB, Palestine AG, Magda ES, et al. Long-term antigen specific and non-specific T-cell lines and clones in uveitis. *Curr Eye Res.* 1984;3:299.
25. Nussenblatt RB, Gery I, Ballentine EJ, et al. Cellular immune reponsiveness of uveitis patients to retinal S-antigen. *Am J Ophthalmol.* 1980;89:173.

26. Smith RE, Nozik RA, eds. *Uveitis: A Clinical Approach to Diagnosis and Management*. 2 ed. Baltimore: Williams & Wilkins, 1989.

27. Nussenblatt RB, Palestine AG. *Uveitis: Fundamentals and Clinical Practice*. Chicago: Year Book Medical Publishers; 1989.

28. Perkins ES, Folk J. Uveitis in London and Iowa. *Ophthalmologica*. 1984;189:36.

29. Opremcak EM and Kocur I. Uveitis in middle and older aged populations. *Ophthalmology* 1994;35(Suppl):2093.

2
Symptoms and Signs of Uveitis

Symptoms

The eye has a limited repertoire of responses when confronted with inflammatory disease[1-6] (Table 2.1). Symptoms of acute forms of uveitis include ocular pain, photophobia, lacrimation, and redness. Patients with idiopathic iridocyclitis, herpes zoster, and human leukocyte antigen (HLA)-B27–associated iritis often present in this fashion. Their vision may be good, with only mild blurring or an occasional floater. In contrast, patients with chronic forms of uveitis often have minimal discomfort. They may complain of decreased vision and "floaters." In some forms of uveitis and particularly in children, patients may be completely asymptomatic, yet have multiple ocular findings. Juvenile rheumatoid arthritis (JRA)–associated iridocyclitis, cytomegalovirus (CMV) retinitis, ocular histoplasmosis, tuberculosis, toxocara, and toxoplasmosis can all be unrecognized by the patient.

Signs

Conjunctival and Scleral Signs

A red eye is the most commonly recognized sign of ocular inflammation. Conjunctival, limbal, or episcleral blood vessels may all become dilated, resulting in hyperemia. Although many ocular surface diseases can cause a red eye, it is important to distinguish these disorders from the hyperemia representing a potentially sight-threatening intraocular or systemic inflammatory disease.

Mild ocular surface diseases such as viral conjunctivitis often present with a diffuse pink or red color to the eye (Fig. 2.1). More serious inflammations of the episclera or sclera result in dilation of the episcleral vessels and often have a sectoral pattern of redness. In true scleritis, this pattern is accompanied by marked pain, tenderness, and scleral thickening. The most serious red eye presentation is a ring of redness around the cornea at the limbus. Limbal hyperemia or limbal flush indicates active intraocular inflammation. The overlying limbal blood vessels become dilated and tortuous as an outward sign of iris or ciliary body inflammation.

Other conjunctival findings, including conjunctivitis and conjunctival nodules, may be found in association with several conditions such as sarcoidosis, Wegener's granulomatosis, Reiter's syndrome, psoriasis, relapsing polychondritis, atopic keratoconjunctivitis (AKC), vernal keratoconjunctivitis (VKC), hay fever, and bacterial infections including tuberculosis (Fig. 2.2). Long-standing or severe inflammation of the conjunctiva may result in subepithelial fibrosis, scarring, and loss of goblet cells.

Table 2.1. Ocular symptoms and signs in common forms of ocular inflammation.

Anterior segment

Accommodative deficiency: Sympathetic ophthalmia

Band keratopathy: JRA, sarcoidosis, multiple myeloma, chronic uveitis

Conjunctival scarring: Ocular cicatricial pemphigoid, Stevens-Johnson syndrome, Sjögren's syndrome, sarcoidosis, chemical burns

Conjunctivitis/nodules: Sarcoidosis, Wegener's granulomatosis, Reiter's syndrome, psoriatic, atopy, vernal, hay fever, herpes simplex, *Chlamydia*, bacterial, tuberculosis, molluscum contagiosum, phlyctenulosis

Corneal infiltrate (peripheral): Inflammatory bowel syndrome, Reiter's syndrome, Wegener's granulomatosis, SLE, polyarteritis nodosa, psoriasis, rosacea

Corneal opacities (central): Herpes simplex, herpes zoster, psoriasis, inflammatory bowel syndrome

Corneal neovascularization: Syphilis, ocular cicatricial pemphigoid, atopy, trachoma, rosacea, phlyctenulosis, trauma

Glaucoma: Posner-Schlossman syndrome, herpes simplex, herpes zoster, Fuchs's heterochromia, reticulum cell sarcoma, JRA, sympathetic ophthalmia

Hypopyon: Behçet's disease, Reiter's syndrome, ankylosing spondylitis, gonorrhea, gram-positive keratitis, fungal keratitis, toxoplasmosis

Hyphema: Fuchs' heterochromia, reticulum cell sarcoma, herpes zoster

Iris nodules: Tuberculosis, lues, sarcoidosis, leprosy

Keratic precipitates (diffuse): Fuchs' heterochromia, herpes simplex

Keratitis (interstitial): Syphilis, herpes simplex, herpes zoster, leprosy, Cogan's, mumps, onchocerciasis, *Acanthamoeba*, psoriasis, inflammatory bowel syndrome

Parinaud's: Cat scratch agent, tuberculosis, tularemia, syphilis, sporotrichosis, chancroid

"Quiet eye": JRA, pars planitis, Fuchs' heterochromia, toxocara, CMV retinitis, masquerade

Scleritis: Vasculitis, rheumatoid arthritis, Wegener's granulomatosis, SLE, PAN, relapsing polychondritis, inflammatory bowel syndrome, lues, herpes simplex, herpes zoster, tuberculosis, sarcoidosis, leprosy, mumps

Scleritis (sectoral): Tuberculosis, syphilis, gout

Synechiae: JRA, syphilis, VKH syndrome, Behçet's disease, Reiter's syndrome, psoriatic, sarcoidosis, pars planitis, ankylosing spondylitis

Posterior segment

Cotton wool spots: SLE, AIDS/ARC, scleroderma, vasculitis

Granuloma (retinal): Tuberculosis, toxocara, sarcoidosis

Hemorrhage (vitreous): Pars planitis, VKH syndrome, ocular histoplasmosis

Neovascularization

  Retinal: SLE, Behçet's disease, Eales disease, sarcoidosis, VKH syndrome, pars planitis

  Subretinal: Ocular histoplasmosis, coccidiomycosis, toxoplasmosis, Behçet's disease, birdshot retinochoroidopathy, sarcoidosis, choroiditis, toxocara, VKH syndrome, rubella, serpiginous chorioretinitis

Optic nerve involvement: DUSN, ARN/BARN, temporal arteritis, VKH syndrome, sarcoidosis, toxoplasmosis, CMV, syphilis, sympathetic ophthalmia, Wegener's granulomatosis, toxocara, papillophlebitis, APMPPE, Leber's idiopathic stellate neuroretinitis, scleritis, Behçet's disease, SLE

Peripapillary choroiditis (Jensen's): Tuberculosis, toxoplasmosis, toxocara

Retinal detachment (exudative): Sympathetic ophthalmia, VKH syndrome, uveal effusion syndrome, scleritis, birdshot retinochoroidopathy, toxoplasmosis, toxocara, PAN, Crohn's disease

Retinal detachment (bilateral exudative): VKH syndrome

Retinal detachment (RPE): VKH syndrome, reticulum cell, sarcoma, sympathetic ophthalmia, leukemia

Retinal pigment changes:

  Increased: Syphilis, PIC, acute retinal pigment epitheliitis, VKH syndrome, APMPPE

  Decreased: Birdshot retinochoroidopathy, SFU, MEWDS, Acute retinal necrosis syndrome, Behçet's disease, PAN, DUSN

Retinitis: Toxoplasmosis, CMV, toxocara, herpes simplex, syphilis, tuberculosis, sarcoidosis

Vasculitis (arteriolitis):

  Infectious: ARN, syphilis, toxoplasmosis, CMV

  Immune: Idiopathic/Eales disease, Behçet's disease, Kawasaki's disease, PAN, Wegener's granulomatosis, sarcoidosis, scleroderma, MS associated, SLE

Vasculitis (periphlebitis): Tuberculosis, Eales disease, syphilis, sarcoidosis

Vessel attenuation: Behçet's disease, retinitis pigmentosa, ARN/BARN

JRA, juvenile rheumatoid arthritis; SLE, systemic lupus erythematosus; CMV, cytomegalovirus; VKH, Vogt-Koyanagi-Harada; PHPV, persistent hyperplastic primary vitreous; CRVO, central retinal vein occlusion; DUSN, diffuse unilateral subacute neuroretinitis; ARN, acute retinal necrosis; BARN, bilateral acute retinal necrosis; APMPPE, acute posterior multifocal placoid pigment epitheliopathy; RPE, retinal pigment epithelium; PIC, punctate inner choroiditis; SFU, subretinal fibrosis and uveitis syndrome; MEWD, multiple evanescent white dot syndrome; PAN, polyarteritis nodosa; MS, multiple sclerosis.

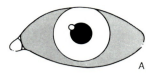

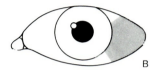

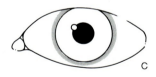

Figure 2.1. Patterns of ocular redness. Diffuse pink or red color to the eye may represent milder forms of ocular inflammation such as conjunctivitis or episcleritis (**A**). Sectoral redness often indicates scleritis (**B**). Limbal hyperemia is an indication of intraocular inflammation (**C**).

Ocular cicatricial pemphigoid (OCP), Stevens-Johnson syndrome (S-J syndrome), and Sjögren's syndrome may all develop such scarring. A directed conjunctival bi-

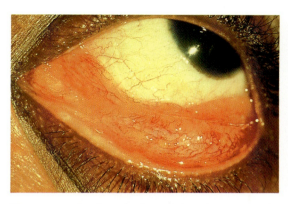

Figure 2.2. Conjunctival nodules. Conjunctival nodules in a patient with systemic sarcoidosis and a bilateral, diffuse granulomatous uveitis. Conjunctival nodules can be biopsied and may provide tissue confirmation in patients with suspected sarcoid-associated uveitis.

opsy is exceedingly safe and often helpful in establishing a specific diagnosis in these diseases.

Corneal Signs

Keratic precipitates (KP) are pathognomonic for intraocular inflammation. The type, location, number, and color of KPs provide useful clinical information.

The type of KP refers to whether the precipitates are granulomatous or nongranulomatous. Granulomatous KPs are larger than nongranulomatous KPs and are often yellow and "greasy" in appearance (Fig. 2.3).

Most KPs are distributed in a triangular pattern on the lower half of the cornea as a result of the normal convection currents within the anterior chamber (Fig. 2.4). A unique pattern of KPs also can be observed in Fuchs' heterochromic iridocyclitis: KPs are disseminated diffusely over the endothelium rather inferiorly. In corneal infections [herpes simplex virus (HSV), keratouveitis], discrete areas of KPs often underlie the involved area.

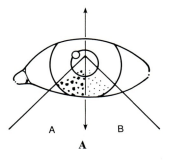

A

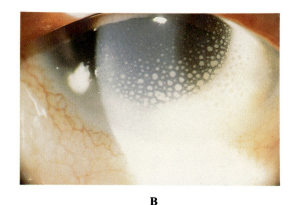

B

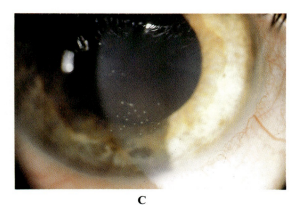

C

Figure 2.3. Keratic precipitates—appearance. Inflammatory precipitates may be granulomatous or nongranulomatous (**A**). Granulomatous KPs appear yellowish white "greasy" and are larger (**B**) than nongranulomatous KP (**C**).

The clinician should assess the number and color of KPs at each visit to help evaluate disease remission or activity and response to therapy. Active KPs are solid, round, and whitish yellow. Effective therapy should reduce the number and size of the KPs (Fig. 2.5). Old KPs often appear crenated and, with time, become pigmented (Fig. 2.6); they do not require treatment. With resolution, imprints of the KPs or "ghost KPs" often remain on the corneal endothelium.

Band keratopathy is the deposition of calcium in Bowman's layer and can occur in any form of chronic uveitis. It is frequently observed in patients with JRA and sarcoidosis (Fig. 2.7). The holes noted in the band are openings in Bowman's layer where the corneal nerves traverse to the corneal epithelium.

True keratitis can be associated with uveitis in several disorders. Herpes simplex virus and varicella-zoster virus (VZV) may cause a keratouveitis with marked corneal anesthesia. Interstitial keratitis can be accompanied by uveitis in syphilis, leprosy, Cogan's syndrome, mumps, onchocerciasis, acanthamoeba, psoriasis, and inflammatory bowel–associated diseases. Peripheral ulcerative keratitis, with or

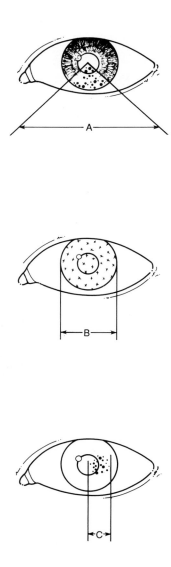

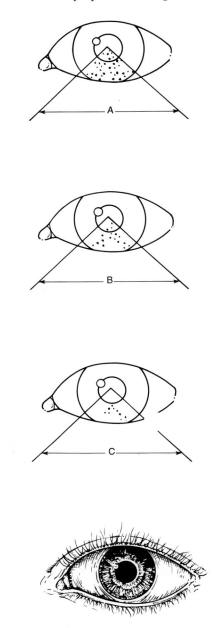

Figure 2.4. Keratic precipitates—distribution. Keratic precipitates are typically located on the inferior corneal endothelium (**A**). Stellate KPs distributed diffusely may be noted in Fuch's heterochromic iridocyclitis (**B**). Focal areas of KPs may be found underlying areas of keratitis (**C**).

Figure 2.5. Keratic precipitates—response to therapy. The number and size of KPs are useful clinical signs in determining activity of the uveitis and response to treatment. Keratic precipitates diminish in size and number with effective therapy.

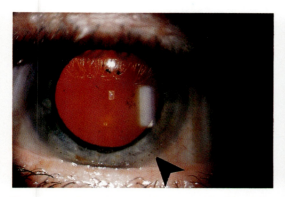

Figure 2.6. Keratic precipitates—old. The KPs in this patient with inactive Reiter's syndrome have become pigmented over time. The eye had no active cell or flare in the anterior chamber. The pigment seen in the red reflex is on the anterior lens capsule; remnants are from previous posterior synechiae. Old, crenated, pigmented KPs, may be slow to disappear and, in the absence of other signs, do not indicate active disease.

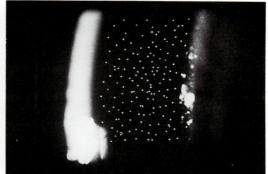

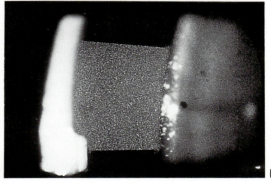

Figure 2.8. Aqueous cell and flare. Inflammatory cell (A) and flare (B) can be seen via biomicroscopy in the anterior and posterior chambers in patients with iridocyclitis. The presence of inflammatory cell within the eye is an indication of active disease. Flare may persist in these eyes and, in the absence of cell, is not an indication of active uveitis.

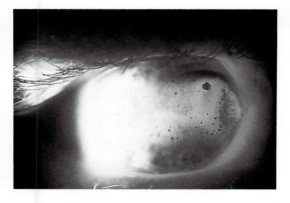

Figure 2.7. Band keratopathy. Band keratopathy in a patient with JRA and chronic, nongranulomatous anterior uveitis.

without uveitis, may be noted in several disorders. Infectious causes include HSV, chlamydia, staphylococci, actinomycosis, gonorrhea, and brucella. Systemic vasculitis and other collagen vascular diseases may also present with a peripheral corneal ulceration.

Anterior Chamber Signs

The hallmark of iritis is the presence of inflammatory cells and flare in the anterior and posterior chambers; in iridocyclitis, some cells may "spill over" into the anterior vitreous cavity (Fig. 2.8). The inflammatory cells characteristically circulate in the anterior chamber because of the normal thermal currents in the aqueous humor (Fig. 2.9). When the inflammation is severe, these cells may collect in the anterior chamber to form a hypopyon (Fig. 2.10).

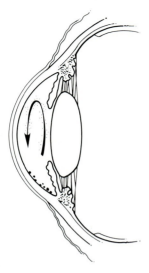

Table 2.2. Grading system for anterior chamber flare and cell.

Aqueous flare: (0–4 + flare/fibrin)	
0	Optically empty
1+	Faint
2+	Moderate—clear iris and lens
3+	Marked—hazy iris and lens
4+	Intense—fibrin with no motion of cells in aqueous
Aqueous cell: (1 × 3 mm beam at 5–10°)	
0	0
Rare	Rare
Occasional	1–2 cells
Trace	2–4 cells
1+	5–15
2+	16–25
3+	26–60
4+	>60 cells

Figure 2.9. Aqueous convection currents. Convection currents develop in the anterior chamber when the aqueous humor interfaces with the cooler corneal endothelium. Inflammatory cells can be seen circulating in the thermal currents.

The amount of cell and flare in an eye is an important clinical measure of activity and can be used to assess response to treatment. A representative grading system is listed in Table 2.2.

Iris and Ciliary Body Signs

The inflamed iris is typically miotic (Fig. 2.11). Normal iris vessels may become more tortuous and dilated and may be difficult to distinguish from iris neovascularization. Granulomatous forms of uveitis can

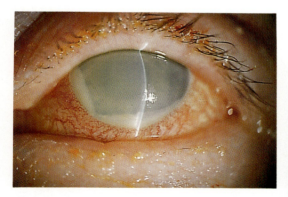

Figure 2.10. Hypopyon. A double hypopyon in a patient with lens-induced uveitis. The patient sleeps on the right side and inflammatory cell accumulates in both the inferior and nasal parts of the anterior chamber angle. Note the corneal edema from elevated intraocular pressure and the limbal hyperemia.

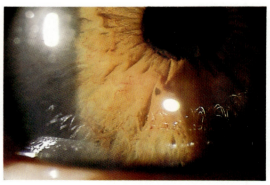

Figure 2.11. Miotic pupil. A miotic pupil in a patient with anterior, nongranulomatous uveitis secondary to syphilis. Note the mild limbal hyperemia and iris vessel dilation.

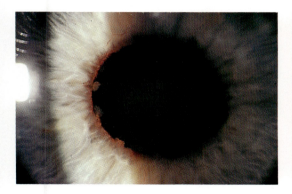

Figure 2.12. Iris Koeppe nodules. Granulomatous IPs in a patient with systemic sarcoidosis and a chronic, granulomatous anterior uveitis. Koeppe nodules can be seen at the pupillary margin. Busacca nodules occur in the iris stroma.

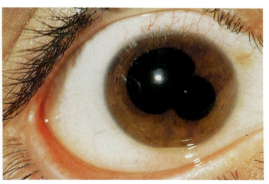

Figure 2.14. Posterior synechiae. Posterior synechiae in a patient with Behçet's disease and a nongranulomatous, diffuse uveitis. Note the small hypopyon and mild limbal hyperemia.

produce iris precipitates (IP) called Koeppe and Busacca nodules (Fig. 2.12). Koeppe nodules appear at the pupillary margin and Busacca nodules are found on the iris stroma. If the inflammation is chronic or severe, the iris may adhere to the peripheral cornea or the anterior lens capsule, resulting in anterior and posterior synechiae, respectively (Figs. 2.13 and 2.14). Seclusion

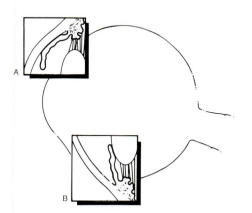

Figure 2.13. Anterior and posterior synechiae. The inflamed iris may adhere to the corneal endothelium, forming anterior synechiae (**A**). Posterior synechiae are inflammatory adhesions between the iris and anterior lens capsule (**B**).

of the pupil posteriorly may occur if the scarring is extensive.

Iris stromal atrophy and secondary iris heterochromia may occur with long-standing inflammation and is characteristic of Fuchs' heterochromic iridocyclitis (Fig. 2.15). Severe iris ischemia and infarction can occur in varicella zoster–mediated iritis, which is often characterized by a pathognomonic sector iris atrophy (Fig. 2.16). True iris neovascularization can occur in certain forms of posterior uveitis and indicates widespread ocular ischemia.

In pure iritis, cells are confined mainly to the anterior and posterior chambers. Cyclitis may result in inflammatory cells within the posterior chamber and the anterior vitreous. Some spillover cell may be found in the anterior chamber. Iridocyclitis is characterized by an equal cellular reaction in the anterior and posterior chambers, as well as in the anterior vitreous.

Inflammation of the ciliary body may result in impaired aqueous humor secretion and lower intraocular pressure. Cyclitic membrane formation and chronic traction on the ciliary body can also result in ciliary body dysfunction. Prolonged ocular hypotony results in phthisis and loss of the eye. A

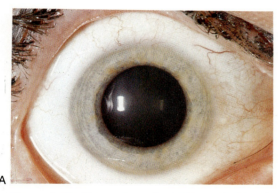 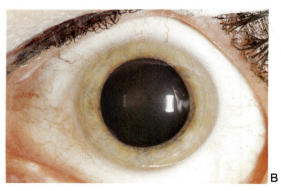

Figure 2.15. Heterochromia iridium. Subtle iris heterochromia in a patient with Fuchs's heterochromic iridocyclitis. The right eye (**A**) had a chronic, nongranulomatous anterior uveitis with a lighter colored iris and fine, stellate KPs. The left eye (**B**) was normal.

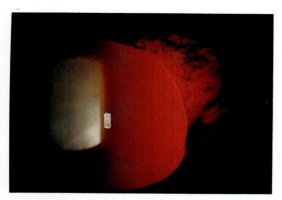

Figure 2.16. Sector iris atrophy. Sector iris atrophy in a patient with herpes zoster and a chronic, nongranulomatous anterior uveitis. Transillumination will often demonstrate the extent of iris atrophy.

major goal of medical and surgical therapy is to prevent these complications.

Angle and Trabecular Meshwork Signs

Damage to the filtration angle and trabecular meshwork (TM) is common in uveitis. The TM may be impaired as a result of direct inflammatory injury (trabeculitis), blockage by inflammatory debris, anterior synechiae, angle neovascularization, or cor-

ticosteroid therapy. Certain infectious diseases such as herpes simplex and herpes zoster appear to cause direct injury to the TM cells and, in contrast to most forms of uveitis, result in elevated pressure during active disease.

Inflammatory debris and trabecular meshwork precipitates (TP) may be observed in uveitis. This material can impair filtration capacity of the TM and result in elevated pressure. More often, however, this potential is balanced by the relative hyposecretion found during active uveitis and an increased alternative uveoscleral outflow. With resolution of the cyclitis, elevated intraocular pressure resulting from damage to the TM is not uncommon.

Inflammation of the iris may result in anterior synechiae, which can also block aqueous outflow. Posterior synechiae, if extensive, may cause iris bombé and produce angle-closure glaucoma (Fig. 2.17). One goal of therapy is to prevent the formation of synechiae by moving the pupil with dilating agents. Inadequate or excessive dilation of the iris may immobilize the pupil, allowing permanent adhesions to form.

Corticosteroid-induced glaucoma may be a result of topical, regional, or systemic therapy with these medications. Thirty-three percent of normal subjects experience

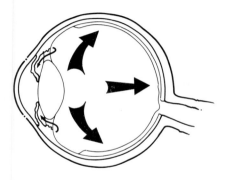

Figure 2.17. Secondary glaucoma. Seclusion of the pupil can block aqueous flow and result in iris bombé and secondary angle-closure glaucoma in uveitis.

an elevation in intraocular pressure in response to topical steroid therapy within 2 to 3 weeks of therapy.[7,8] Optic nerve damage can occur quickly in these patients because of the dynamic changes in intraocular pressure.

Lenticular Signs

Inflammatory debris can collect on the lens epithelium, forming lens precipitates (LP) (Fig. 2.18). Fibrin and scar tissue membranes can form across the pupil, causing

occlusion of the pupil. Pigment may be left behind on the lens capsule after the release of posterior synechiae (see Fig. 2.6).

One of the most common complications of uveitis and its therapy is the development of cataract. The avascular lens is nourished via the circulation of aqueous humor. With inflammation, the ciliary body produces less aqueous humor. In addition, the metabolically active inflammatory cells within the aqueous deplete many of these nutrients. Both these events result in a relative hypoxemia and nutritional deprivation of the lens. Inflammatory cells secrete a variety of enzymes, cytokines, and free radicals, which can be toxic to the lens epithelium. Posterior subcapsular cataract formation is a common sequela of all forms of ocular inflammation (Fig. 2.19).

Corticosteroid therapy can itself promote posterior subcapsular cataracts.[9–11] Corticosteroids inhibit Na^+–K^+ ATPase pump mechanism of the lens epithelium,[12] resulting in increased hydration of the lens and dispersion of light. These drugs also appear to promote cataracts via a mechanism

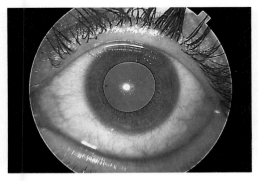

Figure 2.18. Lens precipitate. An inflammatory LP can be seen on the posterior lens capsule in this patient with idiopathic intermediate uveitis—pars planitis.

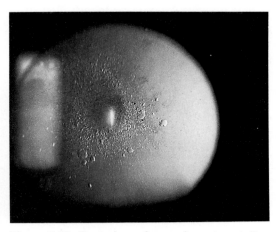

Figure 2.19. Posterior subcapsular cataract. Posterior subcapsular cataract formation in a patient with inflammatory bowel syndrome and recurrent nongranulomatous, anterior uveitis. The red reflex demonstrates the extent of cataract formation.

similar to that which causes glucose and galactose cataracts.[13] By reacting with the amino group on lysine in lens crystallins, corticosteroids result in a conformational change in the protein and secondary disulfide bond formation. These bonds change the refractive capacity of the lens. Interestingly, aspirin may inhibit the formation of corticosteroid-induced cataracts by preventing the binding of corticosteroids to the lens proteins.[13] Treatment regimens should prescribe the least amount of steroids needed to control the inflammation. By this approach both excessive inflammation and unnecessary steroid delivery can be minimized.

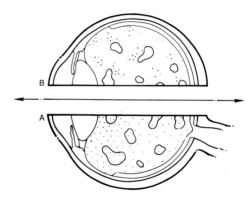

Figure 2.20. **Vitreous inflammatory cells—distribution.** Active inflammatory cells in the vitreous are often distributed evenly throughout the formed and liquid vitreous (**A**). The cells are white, "plump," and uniformly spaced. Inactive, old cells are often crenated, pigmented, clumped, and "trapped" within the formed vitreous (**B**). The liquid vitreous and syneresis cavities are often devoid of cells in inactive disease.

Vitreous Signs

Cell and flare in the vitreous cavity can be found in anterior, intermediate, posterior, and diffuse forms of uveitis. The severity of inflammation can be graded in a fashion similar to aqueous cell and flare (Table 2.3). Vitreous opacification has been standardized by a set of photographs developed by Nussenblatt et al.[14] Their system represents a composite of cells, flare, and debris and can be used to follow response to therapy.

Active inflammatory cells in the vitreous appear white, round, and "plump," with regular distribution throughout both formed and liquid vitreous (Fig. 2.20).

Table 2.3. Grading system for vitreous cell and opacification.

Flare (vitreous opacification)	
0	Good view of NFL
1+	Clear ON and vessels but hazy NFL
2+	ON and vessels hazy
3+	ON only
4+	No ON
Cell (1 × 3 mm beam in anterior vitreous)	
Trace	0–10 cells
1+	10–20
2+	20–30
3+	30–100
4+	>100

NFL, nerve fiber layer; ON, optic nerve.

When located close to the retina, they cast shadows that the patient perceives as floaters. Old vitreous inflammatory cells often remain "trapped" within the vitreous gel after an episode of uveitis and may be difficult to distinguish from active cells. Old cells are often small, irregular, and "crenated" with a pigmented appearance. They are often noted within the formed vitreous and not distributed evenly throughout the liquid vitreous and syneresis cavities. Resolving, old vitreous cells and inflammatory debris do not require treatment.

Collections of inflammatory cells can occur in the vitreous, forming vitreous precipitates, "strings of pearls" and vitreous "snowballs" (Figs. 2.21 and 2.22). Snowbanking at the vitreous base also may occur in chronic forms of intermediate uveitis (Fig. 2.23). It may evolve into firm "collagen bands" and often contains neovascular tissue. Progressive damage to the vitreous gel may result in vitreous membranes, vitreoretinal traction, and retinal detachment.

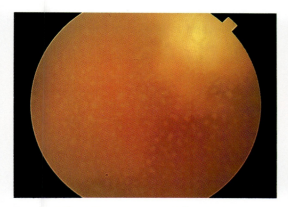

Figure 2.21. Vitreous precipitates. Vitreous precipitates (VP) in a patient with active retinal toxoplasmosis. The granulomatous VPs have formed on the posterior vitreous face overlying the area of active retinal infection.

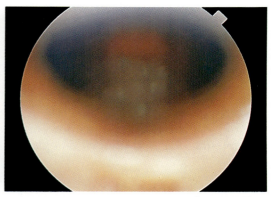

Figure 2.23. Vitreous inflammatory cells—pars plana and vitreous base. Inflammatory "snowball" and "snowbank" formation in the inferior vitreous base at the pars plana in a patient with multiple sclerosis and bilateral, chronic, intermediate uveitis. Scleral depression is required to obtain a clear view of the pars plana region in these eyes.

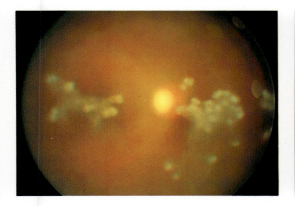

Figure 2.22. Vitreous inflammatory cells— "snowballs." Inflammatory cells may collect within the vitreous gel to form intravitreal "strings of pearls" or "snowballs," as in this patient with pars planitis.

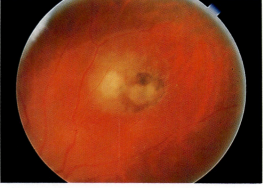

Figure 2.24. Retinitis and retinal vasculitis. Focal retinitis and secondary retinal vasculitis in a patient with active toxoplasmosis. The active area of infection is adjacent to an old, inactive, pigmented scar from a prior episode of toxoplasmosis. With active retinitis, the retina appears thickened, opacified, and yellowish white.

Sensory Retina and Retinal Pigment Epithelial Signs

Retinitis implies an inflammation process occurring predominantly within the sensory retina. Cellular infiltration and edema cause the retina to appear thickened and yellowish white with "soft," nondiscrete margins (Fig. 2.24). Adjacent retinal vessels are often inflamed in various forms of retinitis. Secondary retinal hemorrhage, focal ischemia, and retinal infarction may occur as a result of retinal vascular injury and occlusion. If the retinitis is severe, the contiguous vitreous, retinal pigment epithelium (RPE), and adjacent choroid become inflamed. Individual white cells can be seen with biomicroscopy and contact lens examination of the overlying posterior cortical vitreous (see Fig. 1.4). Retinal and subreti-

nal neovascular membranes may develop if the ischemia is prolonged or severe (Fig. 2.25).

Inflammation of the retinal arterioles, venules, and capillaries may be a primary disorder or may represent a secondary response to a more generalized breakdown in the blood–eye barrier. Primary retinal vasculitis implies direct damage to the vessel wall via several mechanisms, including

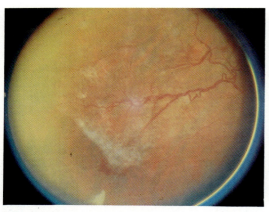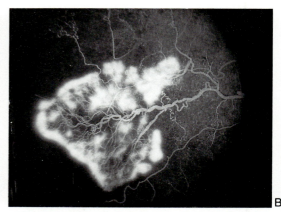

A   B

Figure 2.25. Peripheral RNV. Color photograph (**A**) and fluorescein angiogram (**B**) of an area of peripheral RNV in a patient with sarcoidosis and chronic, granulomatous, diffuse uveitis. Note the capillary nonperfusion distal to the area of neovascularization.

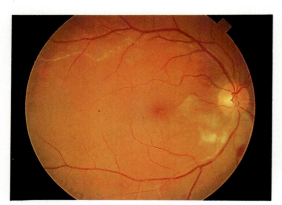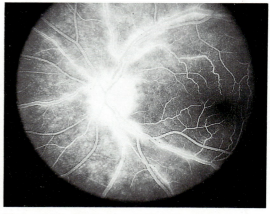

Figure 2.26. Retinal arteriolitis. Primary retinal vasculitis, intraretinal hemorrhage, and retinal infarction (cotton-wool spots) in a patient with PAN and posterior uveitis.

Figure 2.27. Retinal periphlebitis. Secondary retinal "vasculitis" involving the retinal venules in a patient with birdshot chorioretinitis. The fluorescein angiogram demonstrates a generalized breakdown of the blood–eye barrier and widespread fluorescein staining of the venules.

immune complex deposition. Fibrinoid necrosis of the vessel wall with vascular occlusion may result in retinal infarction (Fig. 2.26). Primary retinal vasculitis will often be focal and associated with cotton-wool spots and retinal hemorrhage. Polyarteritis nodosa, SLE, and Wegener's granulomatosis can present with a true retinal vasculitis.

Secondary retinal vessel inflammation can occur as a result of inflammatory cells exiting the eye via diapedesis through the postcapillary, high-endothelial venules. The resultant periphlebitis is typically generalized and not associated with focal retinal ischemia or hemorrhage (Fig. 2.27). Intermediate uveitis and birdshot chorioretinitis may be associated with such a secondary vascular inflammation.

It is important to distinguish between retinal arteriolitis and venulitis. Certain diseases such as PAN and acute retinal necrosis syndrome (ARN/BARN) affect the arterioles, whereas other diseases often affect the retinal venules (syphilis and sarcoidosis). Arteriolar attenuation may occur after widespread retinal destruction (CMV retinitis) or as a result of continual small vessel or capillary closure, as seen in Behçet's disease (Fig. 2.28).

Retinal edema, cystoid macular edema (CME), and retinal precipitates are other common sensory retinal findings in uveitis. Cystoid macular edema results from a breakdown of the perifoveal capillary tight junctions (Fig. 2.29). The characteristic "petaloid" appearance is due to fluid accumulating within the Henle's fiber layer in

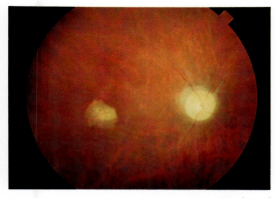

Figure 2.28. Arteriolar attenuation. Profound arteriolar attenuation from progressive small vessel occlusion in a patient with long-standing Behçet's disease and recurrent retinal arteriolitis.

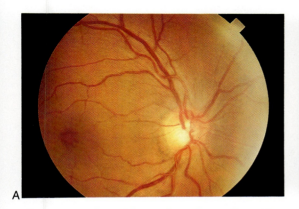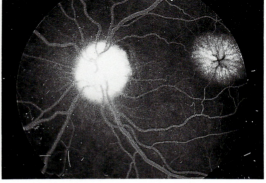

Figure 2.29. Cystoid macular edema. Cystoid macular and disc edema noted in a patient with idiopathic, intermediate uveitis—pars planitis. A: Characteristic petaloid, cystic edema in the macula. B: Fluorescein angiography is often dramatic and will define the extent and severity of the edema.

the macula. Cystoid macular edema may cause architectural damage in the retina and permanent "fixed cysts," with loss of central vision if not aggressively treated.

The retina may become ischemic or necrotic as a result of various infectious and autoimmune mechanisms. Retinal necrosis from ARN/BARN syndrome and CMV retinitis often results in destruction of the retina and secondary combined traction/rhegmatogenous retinal detachments (Fig. 2.30). Periretinal fibrosis and epiretinal membrane formation may occur as a result of intraocular inflammation and may also compromise visual acuity.

Several conditions appear to cause direct inflammation of the RPE. The RPE may be primarily involved in diseases such as acute posterior multifocal pigment epitheliopathy (APMPPE), acute retinal pigment epitheliitis (ARPE), syphilis, multiple evanescent white dot syndrome (MEWDS), and serpiginous chorioretinitis (Fig. 2.31). On fluorescein angiography, the swollen and inflamed RPE blocks the underlying choroidal fluorescence early in the study and becomes more hyperfluorescent in the later frames. The blood–eye barrier function of the RPE may be compromised in Vogt-Koyanagi-Harada (VKH) syndrome, syphilis, posterior scleritis, and sympathetic ophthalmia. The tight junctions between the RPE monolayer can be disrupted, thereby permitting the accumulation of exuda-

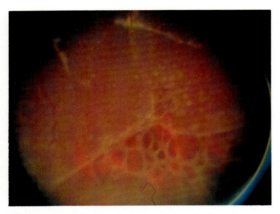

Figure 2.30. Retinal necrosis and detachment. Retinal necrosis with multiple, atrophic, posterior retinal tears and a combined traction, rhegmatogenous retinal detachment in a patient 6 months after BARN syndrome from HZV infection.

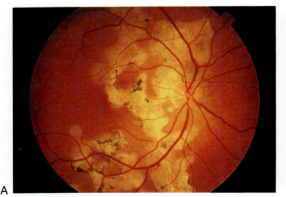

A

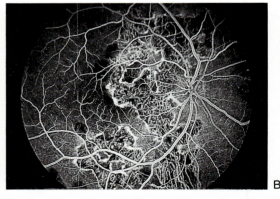

B

Figure 2.31. Inflammation of the retinal pigment epithelium. Retinal pigment epithelial damage after recurrent episodes of serpiginous chorioretinopathy. **A:** Areas of active RPE inflammation appear yellowish white and deep to the sensory retina. **B:** Fluorescein angiography demonstrates blocked fluorescence early in the study and staining late in the corresponding areas.

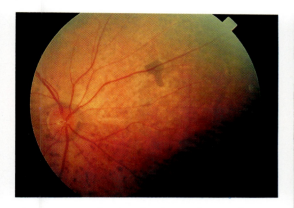

Figure 2.32. Chorioretinal scarring and atrophy. Widespread retinal pigment epithelial hypertrophy and atrophy after resolution of an exudative retinal detachment in VKH syndrome.

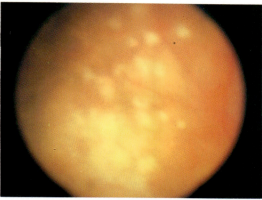

Figure 2.33. Choroiditis. Multiple areas of choroidal inflammation in a patient with idiopathic, multifocal choroiditis and panuveitis syndrome. In active choroiditis, the choroid appears thickened and yellow. The overlying cortical vitreous may have inflammatory cells.

tive fluid beneath the sensory retina. With healing, the RPE often reestablishes its barrier function and may develop hyperpigmentation or atrophy (Fig. 2.32).

Choroidal Signs

Inflammation of the choroid denotes a true form of uveitis. On biomicroscopic examination, areas of inflamed choroid appear thickened and yellow (Fig. 2.33). With severe or long-standing choroidal inflammation, significant vitritis also may develop. In many forms of choroiditis, however, the vitreous may be remarkably free of inflammatory cells [ocular histoplasmosis, punctate inner choroiditis syndrome (PIC), and exudative retinal detachments in VKH]. In these diseases, the RPE and sensory retina provide a physical barrier to cellular infiltration of the vitreous.

As mentioned previously, widespread inflammation in the choroid may effect a secondary breakdown of the RPE blood–eye barrier. This breakdown can produce localized or total exudative, sensory retinal de-

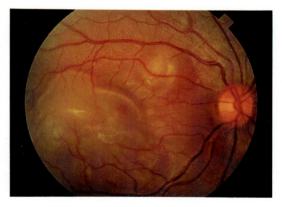

Figure 2.34. Exudative retinal detachment. Severe inflammation of the choroid can produce a breakdown of the blood–eye barrier and result in exudative retinal detachments, as observed in this patient with VKH syndrome. These detachments are not associated with retinal tears and are typically "shifting" in nature.

tachments (Fig. 2.34). Because of the inflammatory nature of this exudative fluid and a higher specific gravity, these detachments shift with positioning of the patient.

References

1. Hogan MJ, Kimura SJ, Thygeson P. Signs and sumptoms of uveitis. I. Anterior uveitis. *Am J Ophthalmol.* 1959;46:155.
2. Kimura SJ, Thygeson P, Hogan MJ. Signs and symptoms of uveitis. II. Classification of the posterior manifestations of uveitis. *Am J Ophthalmol.* 1959;47:171.
3. Tessler HH. Classification and sumptoms and signs of uveitis. In: Duane TD, Jaeger EA, eds. *Clinical Ophthalmology.* New York: Harper & Row, 1987.
4. Smith RE, Nozik RA. *Uveitis: A Clinical Approach to Diagnosis and Management.* 2nd ed. Baltimore: Williams & Wilkins, 1989.
5. Nussenblatt RB, Palestine AG. *Uveitis: Fundamentals and Clinical Practice.* Chicago: Year Book Medical Publishers; 1989.
6. Bloch-Michel E, Nussenblatt RB. International Uveitis Study Group recommendations for the evaluation of intraocular inflammatory disease. *Am J Ophthalmol.* 1987; 103:234.
7. Armaly MF. Statistical attributes of steroid hypertensive response in the clinically normal eye. *Invest Ophthalmol.* 1965;4:187.
8. Becker B. Intraocular pressure response to topical corticosteroids. *Invest Ophthalmol.* 1965;4:198.
9. Black RL, Oglesby RB, von Sallmann L, et al. Posterior subcapsular cataracts induced by corticosteroids in aptients with rheumatoid arthritis. *JAMA.* 1960;174:166.
10. Valerio M. Les dangers de la cortisonothérapie locale prolongée. *Bull Mem Soc Fr Ophthalmol.* 1963;76:572.
11. Urban RC, Cotlier E. Corticosteroid-induced cataracts. *Surv Ophthalmol.* 1986;31:102.
12. Mayman CI, Miller D, Tijerina ML. In vitro production of steroid cataract in bovine lens. II. Measurement of sodium-potassium adenosine triphosphatase activity. *Acta Ophthalmol.* 1979;57:1107.
13. Bucala R, Manabe S, Urban RC Jr, et al. Nonenzymatic modification of lens crystallins by prednisolone induces sulfhydryl oxidation and aggregate formation: in vitro and in vivo studies. *Exp Eye Res.* 1985;41:353.
14. Nussenblatt RB, Palestine AG, Chan C-C, Roberge F. Standardization of vitreal inflammatory activity in intermediate and posterior uveitis. *Ophthalmology.* 1985;92:467.

3
Clinical Approach to the Patient with Ocular Inflammation

Methods of Diagnosis in Uveitis

Successful treatment of uveitis depends on establishing a diagnosis and understanding the predominant pathophysiologic mechanism responsible for the intraocular inflammation. Thus, it is essential to obtain a specific syndrome diagnosis. Because of the often elusive nature of uveitis, however, efforts to establish a diagnosis may be prolonged and difficult. It is not uncommon to establish a syndrome diagnosis months or even years after the onset of uveitis. Several authors have proposed systems of diagnosis that emphasize one or more of the clinical features of uveitis.[1-8] For example, one method of diagnosis identifies patient age as the focal point for diagnosis. Other strategies have focused on the granulomatous or nongranulomatous nature of the disease, or whether the disease is acute or chronic.

Although each method has its own merits, the most useful systems incorporate as much clinical information as possible. The "name-meshing" system of diagnosis in uveitis emphasizes the need to consider all facets of the clinical presentation to form as clear a clinical picture as possible.[5] This system begins with a specific disease syndrome and describes its major clinical features to allow a match or "meshing" with an individual patient's clinical picture. In the clinical setting, however, the practitioner is often unsure of the ultimate diag-

nosis, so it is difficult to use a system that begins with a specific disease syndrome rather than with actual clinical features.

This chapter describes a differential-based diagnostic system (DBDS) for uveitis, which begins with a pattern of clinical findings and generates a list of plausible disease syndromes. This system evolved from the need to consider all diseases capable of presenting with a similar clinical picture. From this inclusive list of diseases, a diagnosis can often be made by additional clinical examination or laboratory testing (see Chapter 4).

Differential-Based Diagnostic System

The act of searching for a specific patient's disease is commonly referred to as *diagnosis* or *making the diagnosis*.[9] The process of making a diagnosis requires four basic steps: the acquisition of facts, the evaluation of facts, the listing of hypotheses, and the selection among the hypotheses. The *acquisition of clinical facts* is accomplished through the medical history and physical examination. In the *evaluation of facts*, the clinician determines which of the findings are pertinent and most consequential. The *listing of hypotheses*, the most difficult and exacting aspect of diagnosis, involves the diagnostic acumen and experience of the physician. Both knowledge of diseases and considerable experience with patients are required. During this step, a list of diseases is generated that fits the patient's clinical picture. The final diagnostic step is *selecting among the hypotheses* or differential diagnosis. The goal of this step is to choose a single disease that most likely explains all the patient's manifestations. This chapter presents such a diagnostic approach tailored for the patient with uveitis.

Acquisition of Facts

The tools of data collection in the uveitis patient are well known to physicians: (1) general biographic information, (2) description of chief complaint, (3) history of present illness, (4) past ocular history, (5) past medical history, (6) review of systemic complaints, (7) general physical examination, and (8) ocular examination (Table 3.1).

Biographical Information

Biographical information provides the age, sex, race, and geographic location of the patient. This information is often helpful in diagnosis, as certain diseases are more prevalent at particular age groups, in males or females, and in different races or geo-

Table 3.1. Practical information obtained from history and physical examination in uveitis.

Biographic information: Age, sex, race and geographic region
Chief complaint: Pain, photophobia, floaters, decreased acuity
HOPI: Acute/recurrent/chronic inflammation; response to therapy
Past ocular history: Trauma—surgical or nonsurgical; other ocular diseases
Past medical history: Known systemic diseases
Review of systems/immunologic survey: Symptoms of systemic involvement
Physical exam: Evidence for systemic disease
Ocular exam: Location of inflammation—anterior, intermediate, posterior, diffuse; type of inflammation—granulomatous or nongranulomatous; severity of inflammation

---

HOPI, history of present illness.

graphic locales. For example, juvenile rheumatoid arthritis (JRA) is most common in young girls, sarcoidosis is more common in blacks than in whites, and Behçet's disease is more prevalent in the Mideast and Japan.

Chief Complaint

The chief complaint (CC) establishes the patient's main concern. In uveitis the CC is often ocular pain, photophobia, redness, floaters, or reduced visual acuity (see Chapter 2). Typically, acute forms of uveitis, such as ankylosing spondylitis–associated iridocyclitis, are accompanied by pain, photophobia, and redness, whereas chronic forms, such as pars planitis, are characterized by floaters and reduced acuity. The CC must be acknowledged and addressed to establish a successful doctor–patient relationship.

History of Present Illness

The history of present illness (HOPI) confirms the nature of the disease and provides a chronology of events. The rate of disease progression also is established during this portion of the medical history. Profound pain or rapid vision loss can occur in diseases such as herpes zoster keratouveitis or herpetic retinitis. Modest complaints are typical in JRA-associated iridocyclitis. The acute, recurrent, or chronic nature of the disease is also established. Behçet's disease often presents with a history of recurrent exacerbations, whereas sarcoidosis is often associated with longstanding disease. Prior treatment successes or failures can also be helpful diagnostically. Infectious and neoplastic diseases such as syphilis and ocular lymphoma will be ultimately unresponsive to corticosteroid therapy alone.

Past Ocular History

The past ocular history (POH) documents prior surgeries, ocular trauma, or the presence of other eye diseases. Patients with lens-induced uveitis, chronic anaerobic endophthalmitis, uveitis-glaucoma-hyphema (UGH) syndrome, and sympathetic ophthalmia all have a history of surgical intervention or nonsurgical trauma. Other eye diseases such as preexisting glaucoma may influence the design of corticosteroid therapy.

Past Medical History

The past medical history (PMH) documents known, existing diseases. For example, it is helpful to establish that a patient who presents with necrotizing scleritis has longstanding rheumatoid arthritis. The presence of other diseases such as diabetes, hypertension, or peptic ulcer disease is important to consider when planning medical therapy involving nonsteroidal anti-inflammatory drugs (NSAIDs) or corticosteroids.

Review of Systemic Complaints

In uveitis, review of systemic complaints (ROS) is often the most rewarding component in diagnosis. It can provide evidence for the presence of associated disease elsewhere in the body. As such, ocular inflammation will be part of a more generalized, systemic disease or represent a local and primarily ocular disorder. Fuchs's heterochromia and pars planitis occur in otherwise healthy individuals, whereas patients with syphilis and relapsing polychondritis may have many systemic complaints.

To direct patient responses, the history and review of systems can be initiated by a uveitis questionnaire. This survey can be given to the patient before the office appointment. Questions are designed to elicit symptoms and signs that may indicate systemic infectious, autoimmune, or neoplastic diseases. Any positive response should be pursued to determine its clinical relevance. For example, painful oral ulcers, genital ulcers, and uveitis suggest Behçet's syn-

drome. Weight loss, night sweats, a productive cough, and exposure to tuberculosis should raise the possibility of tuberculosis-associated inflammation. Intermittent numbness, tingling, and weakness may suggest underlying neurologic disorders such as multiple sclerosis. Hearing loss, vitiligo, alopecia, and headaches with uveitis suggest Vogt-Koyanagi-Haradas (VKH) syndrome. Urethritis, large joint arthralgia, and iridocyclitis in a young male is the clinical triad of Reiter's syndrome. The uveitis survey, therefore, is time-saving and indispensable.

The Uveitis Service at the Ohio State University College of Medicine uses the questionnaire illustrated in Figure 3.1. The questionnaire is continually modified and updated as our understanding of inflammatory diseases expands. Organized into a family history section, social history, PMH, and a ROS, the questionnaire is constructed so that the practitioner may scan the YES column for positive responses. The medical history section is divided into general medical problems (e.g., anemia, cancer), infectious diseases (e.g., viral, bacterial, protozoal, helminthic), and autoimmune disorders (types I–IV hypersensitivities). This organization prompts the patient to consider thoroughly issues pertinent to diagnosis in uveitis.

General Physical Examination

Guided by the patient's responses, the physician may then examine pertinent areas of the body to confirm the patient's complaints. For example, the physician may inspect a palmar rash often found in active syphilis. Patients complaining of white patches of skin and hair loss should be examined for vitiligo and alopecia, which may be evidence for VKH syndrome. Examination of mucous membranes, skin, joints, ears, and the respiratory tract is particularly fruitful when searching for signs of a more generalized disease in uveitis (Table 3.2).

Figure 3.1. Uveitis questionnaire.

Ohio State University Immunology and Uveitis Service

Diagnostic Survey
This is a *confidential* survey. Please respond to all questions (front and back page) by circling the proper answer.

Family History
These questions refer to your grandparents, parents, aunts, uncles, brothers, sisters, children, or grandchildren.

Has anyone in your *family* had:

Tuberculosis_____	Yes	No
Syphilis_____	Yes	No
Arthritis or rheumatism_____	Yes	No
Diabetes_____	Yes	No
Allergies_____	Yes	No
Gout_____	Yes	No

Has anyone in your *family* had medical problems of the:

Eyes_____	Yes	No
Skin_____	Yes	No
Kidneys_____	Yes	No
Lungs_____	Yes	No
Intestines_____	Yes	No
Brain_____	Yes	No

Social History

Have you lived outside of the USA?_____	Yes	No
Where?_____		
Have you lived in states other than Ohio?_____	Yes	No
Where?_____		
Is your job harmful to your eyes?_____	Yes	No
How?_____		
Have you ever owned a puppy?_____	Yes	No
Have you ever owned a cat?_____	Yes	No
Have you ever eaten raw meat or hamburger?_____	Yes	No
Do you drink untreated stream or well water?_____	Yes	No
Have you ever been exposed to sick animals?_____	Yes	No
Do you smoke cigarettes?_____	Yes	No
Have you ever used IV drugs?_____	Yes	No
Have you ever had bisexual or homosexual relationships?_____	Yes	No
Have you been exposed to the AIDS virus (HIV)?_____	Yes	No
Have you ever taken birth control pills?_____	Yes	No

Personal Medical History
Have you ever had the following *diseases*?

Anemia_____	Yes	No
Cancer_____	Yes	No
Diabetes_____	Yes	No
Hepatitis_____	Yes	No

High blood pressure	Yes	No
Pleurisy	Yes	No
Pneumonia	Yes	No
Ulcers	Yes	No
Herpes	Yes	No
Chicken pox	Yes	No
Shingles or zoster	Yes	No
German measles or rubella	Yes	No
Measles or rubeola	Yes	No
Mumps	Yes	No
Chlamydia or trachoma	Yes	No
Syphilis	Yes	No
Gonorrhea	Yes	No
Tuberculosis or TB	Yes	No
Leprosy	Yes	No
Leptospirosis	Yes	No
Lyme disease	Yes	No
Ocular histoplasmosis	Yes	No
Candida or moniliasis	Yes	No
Coccidiomycosis	Yes	No
Sporotrichosis	Yes	No
Cryptococcal infection	Yes	No
Toxoplasmosis	Yes	No
Amoeba infection	Yes	No
Giardiasis	Yes	No
Toxocariasis	Yes	No
Cysticercosis	Yes	No
Trichinosis	Yes	No
Whipple's disease	Yes	No
Hay fever	Yes	No
Allergies	Yes	No
Pemphigoid	Yes	No
Vasculitis	Yes	No
Rheumatoid arthritis	Yes	No
Arthritis	Yes	No
Lupus or systemic lupus erythematosus	Yes	No
Scleroderma	Yes	No
Reiter's syndrome	Yes	No
Colitis	Yes	No
Psoriasis	Yes	No
Behçet's disease	Yes	No
Temporal arteritis	Yes	No
Erythema nodosa	Yes	No
Multiple sclerosis	Yes	No
Sarcoid	Yes	No

Personal Medical History
Have you ever had any of the following *symptoms*?

General Health

Chills	Yes	No
Fevers (persistent or recurrent)	Yes	No

Night sweats_____Yes   No
Fatigue or tire easily_____Yes   No
Poor appetite_____Yes   No
Recent weight loss_____Yes   No
Do you consider yourself healthy_____Yes   No

Head

Frequent or severe headaches_____Yes   No
Frequent or severe dizziness_____Yes   No
Fainting_____Yes   No
Numbness or tingling in your body_____Yes   No
Paralysis in parts of your body_____Yes   No
Seizures or convulsions_____Yes   No

Ears

Hard of hearing or deafness_____Yes   No
Ringing or noises in your ears_____Yes   No
Frequent or severe ear infections_____Yes   No
Painful or swollen ears_____Yes   No

Nose and Throat

Sores in your nose or mouth_____Yes   No
Severe or recurrent nosebleeds_____Yes   No
Frequent sneezing_____Yes   No
Stuffed up nose_____Yes   No
Sinus trouble_____Yes   No
Persistent hoarseness_____Yes   No
Tooth or gum infections_____Yes   No
Sore throat_____Yes   No
Dry Mouth_____Yes   No

Skin

Rashes_____Yes   No
Skin sores_____Yes   No
Sunburn easily (photosensitivity)_____Yes   No
White patches of skin or hair_____Yes   No
Loss of hair_____Yes   No
Tick or insect bites_____Yes   No
Painfully cold fingers_____Yes   No
Severe itching_____Yes   No

Respiratory

Severe or frequent colds_____Yes   No
Constant coughing_____Yes   No
Coughing up of blood_____Yes   No
Pneumonia_____Yes   No
Recent flu or viral infection_____Yes   No
Wheezing or asthma attacks_____Yes   No

Blood

Frequent or easy bruising_____	Yes	No
Frequent or easy bleeding_____	Yes	No
Shortness of breath_____	Yes	No
Blood transfusion_____	Yes	No

Gastrointestinal

Swallowing trouble_____	Yes	No
Diarrhea_____	Yes	No
Bloody stools_____	Yes	No
Severe heartburn or ulcers_____	Yes	No
Jaundice or yellow skin_____	Yes	No

Bones and Joints

Stiff joints_____	Yes	No
Painful joints_____	Yes	No
Swollen joints_____	Yes	No
Red and Hot joints_____	Yes	No
Stiff lower back_____	Yes	No
Back pain while sleeping_____	Yes	No
Neuralgia_____	Yes	No
Muscle aches_____	Yes	No

Genitourinary

Kidney problems_____	Yes	No
Bladder trouble_____	Yes	No
Blood in your urine_____	Yes	No
Urinary discharge_____	Yes	No
Genital sores or ulcers_____	Yes	No
Prostatitis_____	Yes	No
Testicular pain_____	Yes	No
Are you pregnant or plan to be?_____	Yes	No

What is your present weight?_____

What is your present height?_____

_____

Signature

Table 3.2. Symptoms and signs of systemic disease in uveitis.

Oral ulcers: Behçet's disease, mucocutaneous lymph node syndrome, ocular cicatricial phemphigoid, Stevens-Johnson syndrome, SLE, herpes, Reiter's syndrome, ulcerative colitis

Arthralgia/arthritis: Syphilis, brucella, Lyme disease, sporotrichosis, Whipple's disease, ankylosing spondylitis, Behçet's disease, SLE, relapsing polychondritis, ulcerative colitis, psoriatic arthritis, sarcoidosis, JRA, Reiter's syndrome

Asthma/wheeze: Systemic toxocara, ascariasis, aspergillosis, Churg-Strauss syndrome, sarcoidosis, tuberculosis

Bell's palsy: Lyme disease, sarcoidosis

Coughing: Tuberculosis, coccidiomycosis, Wegener's granulomatosis, sarcoidosis

Cystitis: Whipple's disease, Reiter's syndrome, chemotherapy

Diarrhea: Amoeba, Crohn's disease, *Giardia*, ascariasis, schistosomiasis, ARC/AIDS, ulcerative colitis, Cogan's syndrome, Whipple's disease

Ear/auditory/vestibular: Relapsing polychondritis, Wegener's granulomatosis, Cogan's syndrome, VKH syndrome, sarcoidosis, syphilis, temporal arteritis, Eales disease

Epididymitis: Polyarteritis nodosa, Behçet's disease

Flulike symptoms: Leptospirosis, APMPPE, acute retinal pigment epitheliitis, MEWDS, ascariasis

Fever: Reiter's syndrome, Behçet's disease, polyarteritis nodosa, temporal arteritis, colitis, ARC/AIDS, infectious uveitis, Whipple's disease, tuberculosis, brucella, leptospirosis, Lyme disease, *Candida*, coccidiomycosis, amoeba, mucormycosis, Cogan's syndrome, Stevens-Johnson syndrome, serum sickness, trypanosomiasis

Genital sores/ulcers: Ocular cicatricial pemphigoid, syphilis, Reiter's syndrome, Behçet's disease

Headache/meningitis: Behçet's disease, *Cryptococcus*, leptospirosis, VKH syndrome, tuberculosis, Lyme disease, herpes zoster, brucella, reticulum cell sarcoma, uveal effusion, Whipple's disease, Churg-Strauss syndrome, polyarteritis nodosa, sarcoidosis, giardiasis

"Healthy": DUSN, pars planitis, herpes simplex, ocular histoplasmosis, toxoplasmosis, toxocara, traumatic, Fuchs' heterochromia, birdshot retinochoroidopathy, sympathetic ophthalmia, serpiginous chorioretinitis

Hematuria: Polyarteritis nodosa, SLE, Wegener's granulomatosis

Hepatosplenomegaly: Leptospirosis, AIDS, brucella, sarcoidosis

Jaundice: Brucella, schistisomiasis, leptospirosis

Nephritis: Cogan's syndrome, polyarteritis nodosa, Wegener's granulomatosis, cryoglobulinemia

Neuritis:
   Cranial: Lyme disease, sarcoidosis, syphilis, subacute sclerosing panenchephalitis, Churg-Strauss syndrome
   Peripheral: Lyme disease, leprosy, herpes zoster, sarcoidosis

Night Sweats: Tuberculosis, coccidiomycosis, sarcoidosis

Pharyngitis/tonsillitis: Sarcoidosis, ARC/AIDS, Whipple's disease

Pneumonia/pneumonitis: CMV, ARC/AIDS, Whipple's disease, coccidiomycosis, aspergillosis, sporotrichosis, SLE, sarcoidosis, Wegener's granulomatosis

Prostatitis: Whipple's disease, Reiter's syndrome

Saddle nose: Syphilis, Wegener's granulomatosis, relapsing polychondritis

"Sick animal exposure": Brucella, trichinosis

Sinusitis: Sarcoidosis, Wegener's granulomatosis, Whipple's disease, Churg-Strauss syndrome, relapsing polychondritis

Skin nodules: Behçet's disease, ulcerative colitis, sarcoidosis, Crohn's disease, APMPPE, leprosy

Skin rash: Syphilis, Lyme disease, Reiter's syndrome, leprosy, toxoplasmosis, giardiasis, loaiasis, schistosomiasis, SLE, ulcerative colitis, sarcoidosis, Stevens-Johnson syndrome, psoriasis

Urethral discharge: Reiter's syndrome, *Chlamydia*, syphilis

Vasculitis (cerebral): APMPPE, Behçet's, syphilis, Lyme disease

---

SLE, systemic lupus erythematosus; JRA, juvenile rheumatoid arthritis; ARC, AIDS-related complex; AIDS, acquired immunodeficiency syndrome; VKH, Vogt-Koyanagi-Harada; APMPPE, acute posterior multifocal placoid pigment epitheliopathy; MEWDS, multiple evanescent white dot syndrome; DUSN, diffuse unilateral subacute neuroretinitis; CMV, cytomegalovirus.

Ocular Examination

Visual acuity, intraocular pressure, external and neurologic examination, slit-lamp biomicroscopy, and fundus examination are the components of a complete eye examination. Ocular symptoms and signs identified with uveitis are presented in greater detail in Chapter 2. In general, the ocular examination provides several pieces of information essential for diagnosis in uveitis: the location, type, and severity of inflammation. Inflammation may occur in the cornea/sclera or anterior, intermediate, posterior, or diffuse regions of the eye. The type or nature of the inflammation refers to whether the inflammation is granulomatous or nongranulomatous. "Mutton fat" precipitates are often noted in sarcoidosis, whereas fine nongranulomatous keratic precipitates (KP) are typical in Fuchs's heterochromia. Finally, the severity of inflammation can be graded, as reviewed in Chapter 2. Severe and acute forms of uveitis such as Reiter's syndrome or Behçet's disease often have a 4+ cellular reaction and hypopyon formation, whereas JRA-associated iridocyclitis may have only low-grade inflammation.

Evaluation of Facts

In this step of diagnosis, the ophthalmologist must decide which of the symptoms and signs collected are reliable, accurate, and pertinent. Patients may embellish the course of their illness or connect unrelated incidents with the disease. Alternatively, patients may downplay their experience. Past episodes of uveitis may be forgotten. The PMH and ROS initially may be unremarkable, but with questioning and persistence, important symptoms may be elicited. For example, it is not uncommon for young adults to minimize or deny lower back pain in ankylosing spondylitis. Only with directed questioning guided by the overall clinical picture are the suspected symptoms confirmed. Likewise, personal or emotional issues may not be readily disclosed; sexually transmitted diseases and genital lesions often go unreported.

Although it is essential to set aside unrelated systemic complaints, during this phase of the diagnosis it is often better to be inclusive. As the process evolves irrelevant concerns can then be discarded.

In evaluating the clinical findings, the ocular signs should also be critically appraised. The location of inflammation may be easy to determine in conditions such as in toxoplasmosis chorioretinitis. It may be more difficult to designate an anterior, intermediate, or diffuse location when there is cell present in both the anterior chamber and vitreous as in pars planitis. Priority should be asssigned to that tissue, layer, or region with the greatest amount of inflammation. Granulomatous disease also may be difficult to distinguish with certainty in individual patients. Medium-sized inflammatory precipitates may be particularly ambiguous; the clinician must judge whether they are to be considered granulomatous or nongranulomatous in different settings.

Listing of Hypotheses

Perhaps the most challenging aspect of diagnosis in uveitis is the creation of the list of possible entities that can present with the unique set of findings. This step requires knowledge of each syndrome and experience with patients and their presentations.

This section identifies diseases that present with certain characteristic patterns of ocular inflammation. As with general physical diagnosis, primary importance is placed on the location of the disease. For example, in internal medicine, conditions that cause chest pain are generally distinct from those associated with chronic diarrhea. Similarly, the location of inflammation within the eye is of foremost importance in diagnosis. A second pivotal piece of information is whether the inflammation is granulomatous or nongranulomatous. Unlike other areas of medicine, ophthalmologists can make this distinction via ocular examination and with the aid of direct tissue biomicroscopy. The final diagnostic feature of most consequence is whether the ocular inflammation is associated with a systemic disease.

In summary, the pattern of inflammation to be identified in this system of diagnosis includes three primary clinical features: (1) location of inflammation, (2) type of inflam-

Table 3.3. Primary and secondary diagnostic features of the uveitis and source of information.

Primary features
Location/region/layer of the eye primarily inflamed—
ocular exam
    Cornea/sclera
    Anterior
    Intermediate
    Posterior
    Diffuse
Type of inflammation–ocular exam
    Granulomatous forms
    Nongranulomatous forms
Extent of disease—ROS, physical Eexamination, labo-
ratory tests
    Local ocular disease
    Systemic disease

Secondary features
Biographic information
    Age
    Sex
    Race
    Geographic region
Clinical course—HOPI
    Acute
    Recurrent
    Chronic uveitis
Response to therapy—HOPI
Unilateral vs. bilateral disease—ocular exam
Severity of inflammation—ocular exam

ROS, review of systemic complaints; HOPI, history of present illness.

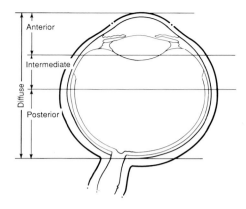

Figure 3.2. Location of the ocular inflammation. Biomicrosopic and fundus examination will determine the location of the inflllammation as either anterior, intermediate, posterior, or diffuse.

mation, and (3) extent of systemic disease (Table 3.3). Other facts, including biographic information, clinical course, response to therapy, laterality, and severity of inflammation, are ultimately useful but used as secondary underlying features.

These fundamental clinical features can be easily collected during the initial and subsequent office examinations. The location of the primary inflammation is determined by the ocular examination. External examination, slit-lamp biomicroscopy, and direct and indirect ophthalmoscopy usually reveal the region or layer of the eye that is inflamed (Fig. 3.2). The type of inflammation, whether granulomatous or nongranulomatous, can also be ascertained by slit-lamp biomicroscopy and fundus exami-

nation (Fig. 2.3). Granulomatous inflammation presents as large, yellow-white, "greasy" precipitates on the cornea, iris, lens, vitreous, retina, or vessels. Nongranulomatous disorders are characterized by small, fine, white precipitates. The presence of associated systemic disease is established by the PMH, ROS, general physical examination, and laboratory testing (Fig. 3.3).

Once the three primary features are determined, a list of possible diseases that are capable of presenting in such fashion can be considered. Table 3.4 provides a list of disorders known to present with these patterns of inflammation. Under each heading the diseases are divided into traumatic, infectious, autoimmune, and masquerade disorders.

Selection Among the Hypotheses

Each disease in the list is now considered with regard to the patient's overall clinical picture. In many cases, the differential diagnosis can be made on clinical grounds alone. For example, in a list that includes both Fuchs's heterochromic iridocyclitis and pars planitis, the diagnosis can be made via ocular examination. Fuchs's het-

Figure 3.3. Systemic disease vs. local ocular inflammation. The history of present illness, past medical history, review of systems, general physical examination, and ancillary laboratory testing will help determine whether the uveitis is a local ocular disease (**A**) or part of a more generalized systemic inflammatory disorder (**B**).

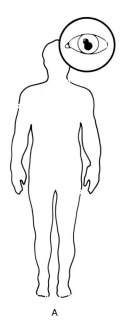

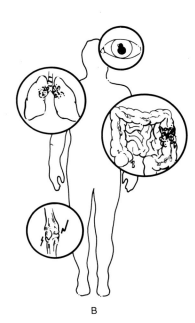

A   B

Table 3.4. Ocular inflammation and uveitis differential diagnosis.

Region/layer—conjunctiva/cornea/sclera
Nongranulomatous
  Systemic disease
    Infectious: Herpes zoster, *Chlamydia*, tuberculosis, syphilis
    Autoimmune: Rosacea, hay fever, atopy, ocular cicatricial pemphigoid, rheumatoid arthritis, Reiter's syndrome, Stevens-Johnson syndrome, SLE, polyarteritis nodosa, Wegener's granulomatosis, relapsing polychondritis, ulcerative colitis, ankylosing spondylitis, Cogan's syndrome, mucocutaneous lymph node syndrome
    Masquerade: Leukemia, lymphoma, amyloidosis
  Local ocular disease:
    Trauma: Surgical and nonsurgical trauma, suture reactions, graft rejection
    Infectious: *Staphylococcus*, herpes simplex, herpes zoster, *Chlamydia*, amoebiasis
    Autoimmune: Idiopathic episcleritis, contact dermatitis, vernal keratoconjunctivitis, giant papillary conjunctivitis, phlyctenulosis, Mooren's ulcer, primary autoimmune and acute idiopathic corneal endotheliitis
    Masquerade: Foreign bodies, amyloid
Granulomatous
  Systemic disease
    Trauma
    Infectious: Herpes zoster, Parinaud's syndrome, tuberculosis, syphilis, leprosy

Autoimmune: Sarcoidosis, Wegener's granulomatosis
    Masquerade
  Local ocular disease
    Trauma
    Infectious: Herpes simplex, herpes zoster, Parinaud's syndrome, amoebiasis, leprosy
    Autoimmune
    Masquerade: Ophthalmia nodosa (tarantula hair)

Region/layer—anterior uveitis
Nongranulomatous
  Systemic disease
    Infectious: Herpes zoster, syphilis, Lyme disease, leptospirosis, amoebiasis, *Giardia*
    Autoimmune: Joint—JRA, HLA-B27–associated, ankylosing spondylitis, psoriatic arthritis/uveitis, ulcerative colitis, Reiter's disease, Crohn's disease, Sjögren's syndrome
    Vasculitis—Behçet's disease, polyarteritis nodosa, relapsing polychondritis, Stevens-Johnson syndrome, serum sickness, rheumatoid arthritis (rare)
    Masquerade: Lymphoma (reticulum cell sarcoma), leukemia
  Local ocular disease
    Trauma: Surgical and nonsurgical trauma, uveitis-hyphema-glaucoma syndrome, graft vs. host disease, prolene reaction
    Infectious: Herpes simplex, herpes zoster, gonorrhea

Table 3.4. (*continued*)

Autoimmune: Idiopathic iridocyclitis, Fuchs'
heterochromic iridocyclitis, lens-induced
(phacogenic), glaucomatocyclitic crisis
Masquerade: Endophthalmitis
Granulomatous
Systemic disease
Infectious: Syphilis, tuberculosis, onchocerciasis,
toxoplasmosis, leprosy, brucella, helminthic
Autoimmune: sarcoid, VKH syndrome
Masquerade
Local ocular disease
Trauma
Infectious: Herpes simplex, herpes zoster, chronic
anaerobic endophthalmitis, schistosomiasis
Autoimmune: Sympathetic ophthalmia, lens-
induced (phacoanaphylaxis), Fuchs'
heterochromia (rare)
Masquerade

Region/layer—intermediate uveitis
Nongranulomatous
Systemic disease
Infectious: Syphilis, tuberculosis, Lyme disease
Autoimmune: MS
Masquerade: Reticulum cell sarcoma, amyloid
Local ocular disease
Trauma
Infectious
Autoimmune: Pars planitis, Fuchs' heterochromia,
idiopathic senile vitritis
Masquerade: Foreign body, endogenous
endophthalmitis, ophthalmia nodosa (tarantula
hair), familial exudative vitreoretinopathy
Granulomatous
Systemic disease
Infectious: Syphilis, tuberculosis, Lyme disease
Autoimmune: Sarcoidosis, MS
Masquerade: Endogenous endophthalmitis
Local ocular disease
Trauma
Infectious: Toxocara
Autoimmune: Pars planitis
Masquerade: Foreign body

Region/layer—posterior uveitis
Nongranulomatous
Systemic disease
Infectious: CMV retinitis, herpes zoster, syphilis,
tuberculosis, herpes simplex, Lyme disease,
trypanosomiasis, rubella, measles, Whipple's,
acanthamoeba, *Giardia*, rubella
Autoimmune: Behçet's disease, MS, SLE,
polyarteritis nodosa, relapsing polychondritis,
Crohn's disease, Wegener's granulomatosis,
antiphospholipid antibody syndrome,
scleroderma, dermatomyositis, cryoglobulinemia, Sjögren's syndrome, Eales disease,

uveal effusion syndrome
Masquerade: Endogenous endophthalmitis,
lymphoma (reticulum cell sarcoma), leukemia
Local ocular disease
Trauma: Radiation vasculitis
Infectious: Ocular histoplasmosis, CMV retinitis,
acute retinal necrosis syndrome (ARN),
varicella-zoster retinitis, diffuse unilateral
subacute neuroretinitis (DUSN),
ophthalmomyiasis
Autoimmune: APMPPE, MEWDS, birdshot
retinochoroidopathy, punctate inner
choroidopathy, serpiginous chorioretinitis,
subretinal fibrosis and uveitis syndrome (SFU),
acute retinal pigment epitheliitis, multifocal
choroiditis and panuveitis syndrome (MCP),
posterior scleritis
Masquerade: Retinitis pigmentosa, amyloid,
tumors, familial exudative vitreoretinopathy
syndrome
Granulomatous
Systemic disease
Infectious:
Viral
Bacterial—syphilis, tuberculosis, *Brucella*
Protozoal—toxoplasmosis
Fungal—coccidiomycosis
Helminthic—ascariasis, onchocerciasis,
microfilaria, cysticercosis, schistosomiasis
Autoimmune: Sarcoidosis, VKH syndrome
Masquerade: Fungal endophthalmitis, amyloid
Local ocular disease
Trauma
Infectious: Toxoplasmosis, ocular histoplasmosis,
ARN, toxocara
Autoimmune: Sympathetic ophthalmia
Masquerade: Foreign body

Region/layer—diffuse uveitis
Nongranulomatous
Systemic disease
Infectious: Syphilis, tuberculosis, Lyme disease,
brucella, *Giardia*
Autoimmune: Behçet's disease, polyarteritis
nodosa, Churg-Strauss syndrome
Masquerade: Lymphoma (reticulum cell sarcoma),
leukemia
Local ocular disease
Trauma
Infectious: ARN, toxoplasmosis
Autoimmune: Pars planitis, Fuchs' heterochromia,
birdshot retinochoroidopathy, MCP, SFU,
idiopathic senile vitritis, lens-induced uveitis
Masquerade: Endophthalmitis, reticulum cell
sarcoma
Granulomatous
Systemic disease

Table 3.4. (*continued*)

Infectious: Tuberculosis, helminthic,
  coccidiomycosis, sporotrichosis, brucella,
  cryptococcal
Autoimmune: Sarcoidosis, VKH syndrome,
  amyloid
Masquerade: *Candida*
Local ocular disease
Trauma
Infectious: Toxoplasmosis, toxocaraiasis, ARN
Autoimmune: Pars planitis, Fuchs' heterochromia,
  sympathetic ophthalmia, lens-induced uveitis
Masquerade: Foreign body, endophthalmitis

SLE, systemic lupus erythematosus; JRA, juvenile rheumatoid arthritis; VKH, Vogt-Koyanagi-Harada; MS, multiple sclerosis; CMV, cytomegalovirus; APMPPE, acute posterior multifocal placoid pigment epitheliopathy; MEWDS, multiple evanescent white dot syndrome; ARN, acute retinal necrosis.

erochromia is often unilateral with distinct ocular findings of heterochromia irides, iris transillumination defects, and stellate, diffuse KP. Secondary features often assist in narrowing the list. The age and sex of the patient help differentiate JRA and ankylosing spondylitis–associated iridocylitis, both being listed under anterior, nongranulomatous systemic disease. In other situations, additional clinical examinations and laboratory or ancillary testing may be required to narrow the differential diagnosis. Tests helpful in diagnosing uveitis are discussed further in Chapter 4.

Example #1: The differential diagnosis for an anterior, granulomatous uveitis associated with systemic disease includes the following: syphilis, tuberculosis, onchocerciasis, toxoplasmosis, leprosy, brucellosis, helminthic diseases, sarcoidosis, and VKH syndrome. The disorders under each subheading (i.e., infectious) are given in order of most to least commonly encountered.

Example #2: The differential diagnosis for a patient with an intermediate, nongranulomatous uveitis without systemic illness includes pars planitis, Fuchs' heterochromic iridocylitis, idiopathic senile vitritis, intraocular foreign body, endogenous endo-

phthalmitis, ophthalmia nodosa, and familial exudative vitreoretinopathy. The most common conditions are pars planitis and Fuchs's heterochromic iridocyclitis.

Example #3: Patients who present with posterior, nongranulomatous inflammation as a local ocular disease have a relatively large differential diagnosis. Radiation vasculitis, cytomegalovirus (CMV) retinitis, acute posterior multifocal placoid pigment epitheliopathy (APMPPE), serpiginous chorioretinitis, and retinitis pigmentosa are a few of the conditions included in the differential diagnosis. Most of the conditions can be ruled out on clinical grounds alone; for example, it is unlikely that CMV retinitis would be confused with serpiginous chorioretinitis. To narrow the differential diagnosis further, additional clinical examinations or ancillary testing may be required (see Chapter 4).

As with any diagnostic method, certain limitations should be acknowledged. Some diseases may begin in one region of the eye and progress to involve other tissues and layers. For example, sarcoidosis may begin as an anterior uveitis and evolve to a diffuse uveitis. Similarly, certain diseases may begin as a nongranulomatous inflammation but with time develop a granulomatous character (e.g., sarcoidosis, VKH syndrome, sympathetic ophthalmia). Finally, many systemic diseases present in the eye months or even years before the onset of more generalized symptoms. To account for these factors, certain diseases are cross-referenced under several headings (e.g., syphilis, sarcoidosis) to provide a more inclusive list for the differential diagnosis. The clinical approach to a patient with uveitis, therefore, is dynamic and often requires continual observation and vigilance.

References

1. Woods AC, Burgess AS. *Endogenous Uveitis.* Baltimore: Williams & Wilkins; 1956:1.
2. Duke-Elder WS, Perkins ES, eds. *Systems of*

Ophthalmology, vol. IX, Diseases of the Uveal Tract. St. Louis: CV Mosby; 1966.

3. Maumenee AE. Clinical entities in "uveitis": an approach to the study of intraocular inflammation. *Am J Ophthalmol.* 1970;69:1.

4. Schlaegel TF Jr. Differential diagnosis of uveitis. *Ophthalmol Digest.* 1973;72:34.

5. Smith RE, Nozik RA. *Uveitis: A Clinical Approach to Diagnosis and Management.* 2nd ed. Baltimore: Williams & Wilkins, 1989:2.

6. Nussenblatt RB, Palestine AG. *Uveitis: Fundamentals and Clinical Practice.* Chicago: Year Book Medical Publishers; 1989:80.

7. Bloch-Michel E, Nussenblatt RB: International Uveitis Study Group recommendations for the evaluation of intraocular inflammatory disease. *Am J Ophthalmol.* 1987;103:234.

8. Rosenbaum JT. An algorithm for the systemic evaluation of patients with uveitis: guidelines for the consultant. *Semin Arthritis Rheum.* 1990;19:248.

9. DeGowin EL, DeGowin RL. *Bedside Diagnostic Examination.* 3rd ed. New York: Macmillan Publishing Co; 1976.

4
Laboratory Testing

Laboratory testing and complementary examinations may not be indicated for all patients with uveitis. A specific diagnosis can be made on clinical grounds alone in certain circumstances. For example, patients with herpes simplex, varicella-zoster, cytomegalovirus (CMV) retinitis, ocular histoplasmosis, Behçet's disease, Reiter's syndrome, Vogt-Koyanagi-Harada (VKH) syndrome, and Fuchs' heterochromia often present with a distinct clinical picture and additional testing may be unnecessary. In addition, patients who are experiencing their first episode of a mild, nongranulomatous, anterior uveitis and whose history, review of systems, and physical examination are unremarkable may be treated empirically without undergoing an extensive work-up.

Laboratory testing is indicated if the inflammation is recurrent, chronic, or medically unresponsive or if it becomes granulomatous. Deeper forms of uveitis (intermediate, posterior, or diffuse) also should be evaluated. Perhaps the most important factor in determining whether laboratory testing is worthwhile is the history, review of systems, and physical examination. Any patient with uveitis who has symptoms or signs of an underlying systemic inflammatory process should undergo diagnostic testing.

There is no standard work-up for a patient with uveitis. Rather, a rational work-up must be directed by the patient's clinical presentation and differential diagnosis. Indiscriminate approaches to laboratory testing are rarely productive. Bayes' theorem would predict little success with such a "shotgun" approach.[1-3] This theorem addresses the statistical probability of a disease when the results of a test are known.[4] The predictive value of any test depends on the prevalence of the disease within the population being tested.[5]

The clinician should have a fundamental understanding of general medicine and a familiarity with infectious diseases and rheumatology to design a fruitful work-up. Laboratory evaluations should, at a minimum, help the physician determine whether the uveitis is systemic or local. It should also help establish whether it is autoimmune or infectious, as well as screen for masquerade syndromes. Successful work-ups may confirm a clinical impression and help establish a specific diagnosis. Laboratory testing may also be used to monitor side effects of drug therapy and to follow disease activity or remission.

Routine and Frequently Ordered Tests

Although the overall work-up is tailored to the differential diagnosis, most patients can benefit from a routine testing strategy

Table 4.1. Ancillary diagnostic tests in uveitis.

Routine screening tests
  CBC with differential (leukemia vs. infection)
  ESR/CRP (systemic vs. local ocular inflammation)
  VDRL/FTA-ABS (syphilis)
Frequently obtained tests
  Chest radiograph (tuberculosis and sarcoidosis)
  ACE/lysozyme (sarcoidosis and tuberculosis—
    "great imitators")
  ANA/RF/ANCA (autoimmune collagen vascular
    diseases)
  Skin testing (tuberculin and anergy panel)
Specific tests directed by the differential diagnosis
  Blood tests (autoantibodies, specific serologies,
    serum proteins)
  Radiologic studies (chest radiography, sacroiliac and
    lumbosacral spine, films, gallium scan, MRI, CT)
  Fluorescein angiography
  Ultrasound
  Tissue biopsy

CBC, complete blood count; ESR, erythrocyte sedimentation rate; CRP, C-reactive protein; VDRL, Venereal Disease Research Laboratory; FTA-ABS, fluorescent treponemal antibody absorption; ACE, angiotensin-converting enzyme; ANA, antinuclear antibody; RF, rheumatoid factor; ANCA, antineutrophilic cytoplasmic antibody; MRI, magnetic resonance imaging; CT, computed tomography.

designed to detect masquerade conditions, help ascertain whether there is an active, more generalized inflammatory condition, and screen for certain common and potentially curable conditions (Table 4.1). These routine tests include complete blood count (CBC) with differential, erythrocyte sedimentation rate (ESR), Venereal Disease Research Laboratory (VDRL), and fluorescent treponemal antibody absorption (FTA-ABS). Frequently ordered tests include chest radiography, angiotensin-converting enzyme (ACE), serum lysozyme, skin testing for tuberculosis and anergy (*Candida* and mumps antigens), and certain autoantibodies.

A CBC is obtained to rule out an underlying masquerade condition such as leukemia or systemic infection. An elevated white blood count may indicate a systemic infec-

tion or a neoplastic process. The white blood count and differential can help distinguish these two considerations.

The ESR is a nonspecific assay for active systemic inflammation. It is an indirect measure of acute-phase reactants in the serum. Acute-phase reactants are groups of serum proteins that are elevated in systemic inflammatory diseases. Local ocular forms of uveitis seldom affect these indirect measures of acute-phase reactants. An elevation of the ESR supports a more widespread systemic disorder. Other tests of acute-phase reactants, such as C-reactive protein (CRP) and a serum protein electrophoresis, can be used in a similar fashion.

Sarcoidosis, tuberculosis, and syphilis can present with any form of uveitis and should be considered in many different clinical settings. The VDRL and FTA-ABS are tests for syphilis. The VDRL is not specific for treponemal antigens, but is elevated during active infection. With appropriate therapy, the VDRL will return to normal. Both the FTA-ABS and microhemagglutination *Treponema pallidum* (MHA-TP) are specific tests for treponemal antigens and are indicators of prior exposure to syphilis. These two tests remain positive throughout life, even with appropriate treatment.

Other frequently obtained tests in uveitis include a chest radiograph, skin testing, serum lysozyme, ACE, and autoantibody screening. The incidence of tuberculosis has been increasing in the United States coincident with the acquired immunodeficiency syndrome (AIDS) epidemic. New, multidrug-resistant strains of tuberculosis have been identified, and extrapulmonary forms of infection including uveitis are not uncommon. As a result of this public health concern, more patients with uveitis are being routinely screened for tuberculosis via purified protein derivative (PPD) skin testing and chest radiograph. A 0.1-ml solution of 5 TU (tuberculin units) intermediate dose PPD is injected subcutaneously. A lower test dose (1 TU) can be given if a strong reaction is anticipated. Negative responses to the intermediate strength dose can be confirmed by using a 250-TU dose of PPD.

Sarcoidosis is a relatively common cause of uveitis in most published reviews. Serum lysozyme and ACE can be elevated in sarcoidosis as well as active tuberculosis. Chest radiography findings and skin testing for anergy to a panel of common antigens such as *Candida* and mumps can differentiate tuberculosis from sarcoidosis.

Autoantibodies including antinuclear antibody (ANA), rheumatoid factor (RF), anticardiolipin antibody, and antineutrophilic cytoplasmic antibody (ANCA) can be elevated in many collagen vascular and connective tissue diseases. The presence of these autoantibodies suggests an active systemic autoimmune disorder rather than an infectious process. These tests can be helpful when an underlying autoimmune, collagen vascular disease is suspected. Only rarely, however, do they establish a specific diagnosis.

Table 4.2. Ocular inflammation and uveitis: laboratory evaluation.

Region/layer—conjunctiva/cornea/sclera
Nongranulomatous
  Systemic disease
    Infectious: Tuberculosis skin test, CXR, VDRL, FTA-ABS, MHA, TP, immunofluorescence for *Chlamydia*
    Autoimmune: Conjunctival biopsy, RF, CH_{50}, ANA, U/A, ESR, CXR, CBC with Diff, CIC, C3, C4, SPE, CRP, EKG, cryoglobulins, hearing test
    Masquerade: CBC
  Local ocular disease
    Trauma
    Infectious: Scraping and smear and culture, corneal Bx, Rose Bengal staining, corneal sensitivity
    Autoimmune: CXR, ACE, lysozyme, scraping, smear and cultures
    Masquerade
Granulomatous
  Systemic disease
    Trauma
    Infectious: Tuberculosis skin test, VDRL, FTA-ABS
    Autoimmune: RF
    Masquerade
  Local ocular disease
    Trauma
    Infectious: Tuberculosis skin test, corneal sensation
    Autoimmune
    Masquerade

Region/layer—anterior uveitis
Nongranulomatous
  Systemic disease
    Infectious: Corneal sensitivity, VDRL, FTA-ABS, Lyme titer
    Autoimmune
      Joint: L/S spine film, S/I joint x-ray, ANA (JRA),

      RF, ESR, uric acid, VDRL, FTA-ABS, HLA-B27, barium enema, Schirmer's testing, salivary Bx
    Vasculitis: CRP, ESR, SPE, cryoglobulins, C3, C4, ear biopsy, CH50, CIC, skin Bx, CBC with Diff, ANA, RF, CXR, tuberculosis skin test, U/A, properdin factor B, serum lysozyme, alpha-1-acid glycoprotein
    Masquerade: Aqueous/vitreous Bx
  Local ocular disease
    Trauma: Aqueous Bx
    Infectious: Corneal sensitivity, sector iris atrophy, urethral culture
    Autoimmune: Iris transillumination defects, angle vessels, heterochromia, aqueous Bx
    Masquerade: Aqueous Bx
Granulomatous
  Systemic disease
    Infectious: Tuberculosis skin test, VDRL, FTA-ABS, CBC with Diff, toxoplasmosis titer
    Autoimmune: ACE, serum Ca^{2+}, anergy, CXR, conjunctival Bx, gallium, examination for poliosis, vitiligo, hearing loss
    Masquerade
  Local ocular disease
    Trauma
    Infectious: Corneal anesthesia, sector iris atrophy, aqueous culture
    Autoimmune: HLA-A11, retinal S-Ag testing vitreous Bx, fluorescein angiography
    Masquerade

Region/layer—intermediate uveitis
Nongranulomatous
  Systemic disease
    Trauma
    Infectious: VDRL, FTA-ABS, lyme titer,

Table 4.2. (*continued*)

tuberculosis skin test, CXR
  Autoimmune: MRI, LP, neurologic exam
  Masquerade: vitreous Bx
Local ocular disease
  Trauma
  Infectious
  Autoimmune: Examination for heterochromia, iris transillumination, angle vessels
  Masquerade: Vitreous biopsy
Granulomatous
  Systemic disease
    Trauma
    Infectious: VDRL, FTA-ABS, tuberculosis skin testing, CXR, Lyme titer
    Autoimmune: MRI, neurologic exam, ACE, lysozyme, CXR, skin tests for anergy
    Masquerade: Vitreous biopsy
  Local ocular disease
    Trauma
    Infectious: *Toxocara* titer
    Autoimmune: ESR
    Masquerade: Ultrasound

Region/layer—posterior uveitis
Nongranulomatous
  Systemic disease
    Trauma
    Infectious: CMV titers, HIV testing, VDRL, FTA-ABS, tuberculosis skin test, CXR, TORCH titers, jejunal Bx, toxoplasmosis titers, lyme titers, measles titer
    Autoimmune: ANA, ANCA, RF, cryoglobulins, ESR, CIC, tuberculosis skin testing, MRI, lumbar puncture, SIEP, HB-SAg, CXR, sinus x-ray, alpha-1-acid glycoprotein, properdin factor B, ear pinna Bx
    Masquerade: CBC with Diff, vitreous Bx
  Local ocular disease
    Trauma
    Infectious: CBC with Diff, SGOT, LDH, photos/FA, HIV testing
  Autoimmune: FA, ERG, EOG, S-Ag testing, HLA-A29, examination for vitiligo (birdshot), EBV-EA, IgM
  Masquerade
Granulomatous

Systemic disease
  Trauma
  Infectious: Tuberculosis skin test, VDRL, FTA-ABS, CXR, *Toxocara* titer, CBC with Diff, serologies
  Autoimmune: ACE, serum Ca^{2+}, CXR, gallium scan anergy, conjunctival Bx, examination for poliosis, vitiligo, hearing loss
  Masquerade: Vitreous Bx
Local ocular disease
  Trauma
  Infectious: Toxoplasmosis titer, *Toxocara* titer
  Autoimmune: FA, S-Ag testing
  Masquerade: Ultrasound

Region/layer—Diffuse uveitis
Nongranulomatous
  Systemic disease
    Infectious: VDRL, FTA-ABS, anergy, lyme titer, CXR, tuberculosis skin test, *Giardia* in stool
    Autoimmune: CBC with Diff, CIC, C3, C4, RF, ANA, ESR, serum lysozyme, alpha-1-acid glycoprotein, properdin factor-B
    Masquerade: CBC with Diff, vitreous Bx
  Local ocular disease
    Trauma
    Infectious: Toxoplasmosis titer
    Autoimmune: Iris heterochromia, angle vessels, EBV titers, vitreous Bx
    Masquerade: Vitreous Bx, CBC Diff, ultrasound, x-ray for foreign body
Granulomatous
  Systemic disease
    Infectious: Tuberculosis skin test, CXR, *Toxocara* titer, toxoplasmosis titer, CBC with Diff, *Brucella* agglutination titers, vitreous Bx
    Autoimmune: ACE, Ca^{2+}, CXR, gallium scan, anergy, conjunctival Bx, examination for poliosis, vitiligo, hearing loss
    Masquerade
  Local ocular disease
    Trauma
    Infectious: *Toxocara* ELISA, toxoplasmosis titer
    Autoimmune: History for ocular injury, examination for vitiligo, FA, ultrasound
    Masquerade: Vitreous Bx

CBC with Diff, complete blood count with differential; ESR, erythrocyte sedimentation rate; CRP, C-reactive protein; SPE, serum protein electrophoresis; SIEP, serum immunoelectrophoresis; CIC, circulating immune complexes; C3, complement 3; C4, complement 4; ACE, angiotensin converting enzyme; RF, rheumatoid factor; ANA, antinuclear antibody; HB-SAg, hepatitis B surface antigen; U/A, urinalysis; CXR, chest radiograph; MRI, magnetic resonance imaging; FA, fluorescein angiography; U/S, ultrasonography; EKG, electrocardiogram; Bx, biopsy; MHA, microhemagglutination; JRA, juvenile rheumatoid arthritis; SGOT, serum glutamic-oxaloacetic transaminase; LDH, lactate dehydrogenase; ERG, electroretinogram; ANCA, antineutrophilic cytoplasmic antibody; EOG, electrooculography; LP, lumbar puncture; VDRL, venereal disease research laboratory; FTA-ABS, fluorescent treponemal antibody absorption; CH$_{50}$, hemolytic complement; TP, *Treponema palldon*; HIV, human immunodeficiency virus; TORCH, toxoplasmosis, rubella, cytomegalovirus, herpes simplex; MRI, magnetic resonance imaging; EBV-EA, Epstein-Barr virus early antigen; LDH, locate dehydrogenase; HLA, human leukocyte antigen; IgM, immunoglobulin M; L/S, liver/spleen; S/I, Saozoillac; ELISA, enzyme-linked immunoabsorbent assay.

Tests Individualized for the Differential Diagnosis

Beyond this set of screening tests, each work-up is tailored to the patient's differential diagnosis. As discussed in Chapter 3 and as listed in Table 3.4, a differential diagnosis can be generated for most patients with ocular inflammation. Many of the possibilities within a patient's differential diagnosis can be ruled out on clinical grounds alone. As discussed, it would be unlikely that juvenile rheumatoid arthritis would be confused with Behçet's disease, yet both can present with an anterior, nongranulomatous uveitis in a patient with evidence of systemic disease. After the clinician eliminates the obvious diagnoses from the differential list, a directed laboratory evaluation can be designed to address the remaining diseases.

Table 4.2 lists ancillary tests that may be appropriate for the corresponding diseases listed in Table 3.4. For example, in the patient with an anterior, granulomatous uveitis and a history and physical examination suggesting possible systemic involvement, a tuberculosis skin test, VDRL, FTA-ABS, ACE, lysozyme, anergy panel, chest radiograph, gallium scan, and examination for hearing loss, vitiligo, and poliosis would be appropriate to rule out most of the considerations listed in the Table 3.4.

Similarly, laboratory testing may include a Lyme titer, additional neurologic testing, magnetic resonance imaging (MRI) scan, ACE, lysozyme, VDRL, and an FTA-ABS for the patient with a nongranulomatous, intermediate uveitis with systemic neurologic complaints (see Table 3.4 and Table 4.2 under Intermediate Uveitis). These tests differentiate sarcoidosis from multiple sclerosis–associated intermediate uveitis, syphilis, and Lyme disease.

Finally, in a patient with a posterior, nongranulomatous, local ocular disease, human immunodeficiency virus (HIV) testing, fluorescein angiography, electrophys-

iologic testing, HLA-A29, Ebstein-Barr virus (EBV) serologies, and liver function tests would help differentiate birdshot retinochoroidopathy from acute posterior multifocal placoid pigment epitheliopathy (APMPPE), multifocal choroiditis, and panuveitis (MCP) from rheumatoid arthritis–associated posterior scleritis, and multiple evanescent white dot syndrome (MEWDS) from diffuse unilateral subacute neuroretinitis (DUSN). It is likely, however, that CMV retinitis would present a distinct enough picture to distinguish it from ophthalmomyiasis (subretinal Bot-fly maggot). Depending on the overall acumen of the clinician, not all these tests need be performed.

Special Blood Tests

Antiphospholipid antibodies (APLA) include anticardiolipin antibodies and lupus anticoagulant. The autoantibodies are prevalent in patients with systemic lupus erythematosus (SLE) and other connective tissue diseases that may produce thrombosis and vascular occlusion.[6,7] Several visual symptoms and ocular conditions have been associated with anticardiolipin antibodies, including transient visual obscuration, ischemic optic neuropathy, diplopia, vertebrobasalar insufficiency, branch retinal vein occlusion, and branch retinal artery occlusion. These tests should be ordered in patients presenting with vaso-occlusive disease in whom an underlying autoimmune/collagen vascular disease is suspected.

ANCA are autoantibodies that are specific for intracellular components of the neutrophil.[8] There are two types of ANCA: C-ANCA, which identify lysosomal granules of neutrophils, and P-ANCA, which are specific for myeloperoxidase. Both types are found in the serum of patients with systemic necrotizing vasculitis, Wegener's granulomatosis, polyarteritis nodosa, Churg-Strauss syndrome, and "overlap" systemic vasculitis.[8] Patients with inflammatory bowel disease may also have P-ANCA.[9] The sensitivity of this test for necrotizing systemic vasculitis is between 85% and 96%.

The presence of ANCA often helps establish a diagnosis of underlying systemic vasculitis at an earlier stage of the disease.[10,11] Appropriate systemic immunosuppression can then be initiated and permanent injury prevented. ANCA can also be used to follow clinical disease activity and response to therapy. Patients who are well controlled or in disease remission exhibit falling ANCA titers; exacerbation of the underlying vasculitis is accompanied by elevation in these antibodies.

Other tests that help establish the presence of active systemic vasculitis include circulating immune complexes and complement levels. Behçet's disease has been reported to cause elevation of serum lysozyme, alpha-1-acid glycoprotein, and properdin factor B.[12]

Human leukocyte antigen (HLA) tissue typing is most helpful in diagnosing the HLA-B27–associated diseases. Patients with Reiter's syndrome, ankylosing spondylitis, inflammatory bowel disease, or psoriatic arthritis–associated iridocyclitis are often HLA-B27–positive.[13,14] This test can help support the clinical diagnosis, limit further laboratory evaluations, and direct appropriate systemic and ocular therapy.

Patients who present with a clinical picture compatible with birdshot retinochoroiditis may also benefit from HLA-A29 testing.[15,16] More than 95% of patients with this condition are HLA-A29–positive. These patients often require long-term, systemic immunosuppressive therapy, and an accurate diagnosis is essential.

As discussed previously, other laboratory tests including HIV testing, titers for *Toxocara*, toxoplasmosis, Lyme disease, and EBV uveitis can be ordered in the proper clinical setting. It is not common to obtain these tests routinely. These tests are dis-

cusssed further in each specific disease section.

Radiologic Testing

Chest radiographs can be helpful in the patient with suspected sarcoidosis, tuberculosis, Wegener's granulomatosis, and masquerade conditions (see Fig. 4.1). Characteristic pulmonary findings of apical scarring, Ghon complexes, and infiltration can be seen in mycobacterial disease. Sarcoidosis may cause hilar adenopathy and interstitial lung changes. Cavitary lesions may be seen in both Wegener's granulomatosis and tuberculosis. In patients with metastatic endophthalmitis, an occult pneumonia may be the primary source.

Radiography of the lumbosacral spine and sacroiliac joints should be obtained when ankylosing spondylitis is suspected. Patients may present with an anterior, nongranulomatous, acute uveitis and sig-

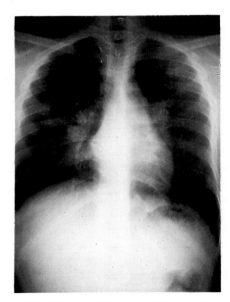

Figure 4.1. Chest radiograph. Chest radiograph from a patient with a chronic, bilateral granulomatous, diffuse uveitis. The study demonstrates hilar adenopathy supporting the working diagnosis of sarcoidosis.

nificant lower back pain and stiffness. Radiologic confirmation not only helps establish the diagnosis but promotes appropriate physical therapy for the vertebral complications of this disease. Bone scans are a more sensitive test for patients with early or mild disease.

MRI and computed tomography (CT) scanning can be helpful in several clinical settings. Patients who present with uveitis and neurologic complaints may have multiple sclerosis, primary central nervous system lymphoma, sarcoidosis, or Lyme disease. These studies often reveal central nervous system lesions, and thereby assist in the diagnosis. Patients with primary central nervous system lymphoma often have widespread paraventricular infiltration on MRI. Patients with intermediate uveitis due to multiple sclerosis have multifocal white matter lesions on MRI.

Gallium scans use low-level radioactive gallium to image inflammatory tissue in the body. Often patients with sarcoidosis

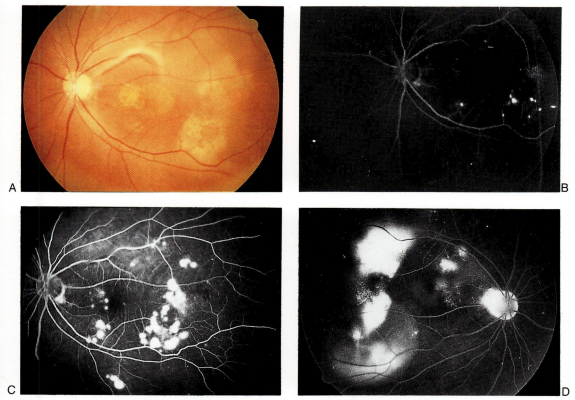

Figure 4.2. Fluorescein angiogram—exudative retinal detachment. Color photographs and fluorescein angiogram from a patient with VKH syndrome. **A:** Moderate vitreous opacification, multifocal areas of choroiditis, and areas of exudative retinal detachment. **B:** Fluorescein angiogram demonstrates blocked fluorescence early in the study. In the later stages of the angiogram, multifocal punctate areas of hyperfluorescence intensify (**C**) and leak into the subretinal space (**D**).

have increased lacrimal gland, liver, spleen, and pulmonary uptake. These findings can be used to support a working diagnosis of sarcoidosis in certain clinical settings.

Fluorescein Angiography

Fluorescein angiography can provide information not available on biomicroscopic and fundus examination. It can be particularly useful in the clinical setting of unexplained visual loss. For example, media opacities such as cataract or vitreous debris can complicate the diagnosis of cystoid macular edema (CME). Angiography can often show CME even through a clinically significant cataract and, therefore, is useful for documenting the presence and severity of the disease (see Fig. 2.30), as well as its response to therapy.

Fluorescein angiography can also be used to define the nature of retinal vaso-occlu-

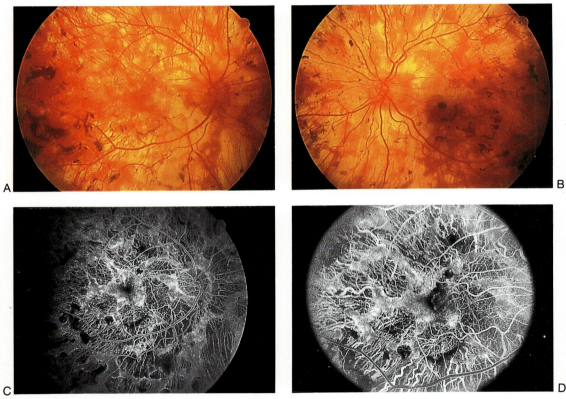

Figure 4.3. Fluorescein angiogram—subretinal neovascularization. Color photographs and fluorescein angiogram from a patient with serpiginous chorioretinitis. **A** and **B** show extensive bilateral chorioretinal scarring. Visual acuity was 20/20 OD and counting fingers OS due to a subfoveal disciform scar. **C:** Fluorescein angiogram shows a disease-free area in the fovea of the right eye. Nine months later the patient complained of decreased acuity in the right eye. Vision had fallen to 20/400 OD. **D:** Fluorescein angiography demonstrates the development of a subfoveal neovascular membrane.

sive disorders and vasculitis. It can help characterize retinal vasculitis as predominantly a phlebitis, capillaritis, or arteriolitis and can demonstrate the extent of capillary nonperfusion and retinal ischemia (see Fig. 2.28). In addition, angiography can better differentiate the presence of secondary retinal neovascularization from other microvascular changes.

Active choroiditis can be distinguished from old chorioretinal scarring: on angiography active choroidal inflammation will block early and stain late in the study. Several diseases such as VKH syndrome and sympathetic ophthalmia have characteristic findings of multifocal punctate hyperfluorescent areas at the level of the choroid and retinal pigment epithelium (RPE) that pool fluorescein dye later in the study (Fig. 4.2).

Subretinal neovascular membranes can occur in any choroidal inflammatory disease and can be well defined via angiography (Fig. 4.3). Determining the location and extent of these membranes is critical when evaluating the feasibility of laser surgical therapies.

Finally, several retinal white dot syndromes (see Chapter 19) and inflammatory diseases of the RPE can be diagnosed and characterized via angiography. APMPPE, serpiginous chorioretinitis, acute retinal pigment epitheliitis, birdshot retinochoroiditis, diffuse unilateral subacute neuroretinitis (DUSN), ocular histoplasmosis syndrome, and punctate inner choroiditis all have characteristic fluorescein angiographic findings that can aid in diagnosis.

Ultrasonography

Patients with uveitis often have media opacification that limits direct visualization of the eye. Corneal opacities, posterior synechiae, cataracts, and vitreous debris can impair examination. Posterior involvement or secondary complications cannot be determined without the use of ultrasonography. Intraocular tumors, foreign bodies,

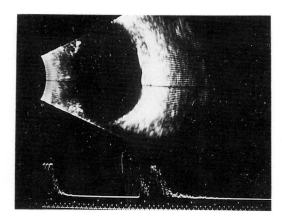

Figure 4.4. Ultrasonography. Ultrasound study of a patient with sympathetic ophthalmia and dense cataract formation. The right eye had been injured with a knife several years before the onset of uveitis and was phthisical. The left eye developed a granulomatous iridocyclitis and a dense cataract. B scan demonstrates thickening of the choroid and the diffuse nature of the contralateral uveitis.

retinal detachment, vitreous debris, choroidal thickening, scleritis, and Tenon's capsule fluid can be detected via ultrasonography (Fig. 4.4).

Tissue Biopsy

Tissue biopsy is frequently necessary to manage patients with uveitis. Biopsy information can be invaluable when clinical findings, blood tests, radiologic studies, and other noninvasive testing have failed to establish or confirm a diagnosis. Patients with a suspected masquerade process such as intraocular lymphoma also should be considered for tissue biopsy.

Conjunctival biopsies can be particularly helpful in the diagnosis of sarcoidosis and ocular cicatricial pemphigoid (OCP). Conjunctival nodules can form in sarcoidosis and can be sampled more easily and safely than lung biopsy. Noncaseating granulomas with giant cells and epithelioid cells confirm the diagnosis of sarcoidosis (Fig.

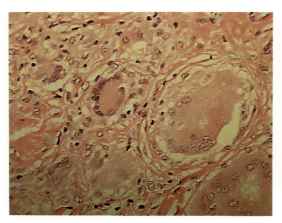

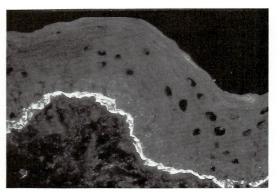

Figure 4.6. Conjunctival biopsy—immunohistology. Conjunctival biopsy from a patient with chronic conjunctivitis, subepithelial scarring, and symblepharon formation. Immunohistochemical studies demonstrated a linear deposition of IgG at the level of the basement membrane, supporting a diagnosis of cicatricial pemphigoid.

Figure 4.5. Conjunctival biopsy—histology. Conjunctival biopsy from a patient with a chronic, diffuse, granulomatous uveitis. A conjunctival nodule was biopsied and showed noncaseating granuloma with giant cell and epithelioid cell formation.

4.5). Conjunctival biopsies are also helpful in the diagnosis of OCP. This disorder routinely requires systemic immunosuppression and tissue confirmation can be quite supportive. Immunoprecipitates at the level of the conjunctival basement epithelium are diagnostic (Fig. 4.6).

Anterior chamber aspirates are most helpful in cases of masquerade conditions.[17,18] Patients who do not have an established diagnosis for their ocular inflammation or who do not respond to appropriate therapy can also benefit from aqueous biopsy. In this setting, neoplastic or infectious processes such as large cell lymphoma and chronic anaerobic endophthalmitis may be responsible for the uveitis. Anterior chamber aspirates, however, often contain too little material for accurate cytologic examination and comprehensive microbial analysis. Vitreous sampling is often necessary to complement aqueous humor aspirates. Witmer quotients have been used to compare the level of intraocular antibody production to serum levels.[19–21] A higher titer of antibody in the eye to varicella-zoster virus has been used

to support a mediating role for this virus in the acute retinal necrosis syndrome. Unfortunately, a high degree of clinical suspicion is required to decide which antibody to assay for using this technique.

Vitreous biopsy may be worthwhile in certain cases of diffuse, posterior, or intermediate forms of uveitis when other methods of establishing a diagnosis have failed.[22,23] It also may be helpful when masquerade conditions are suspected. Both vitreous needle aspirate and pars plana vitrectomy techniques can be performed to obtain a vitreous sample. Pars plana vitrectomy optimizes the amount of vitreous material for analysis, minimizes vitreoretinal trauma, and can help clear the media for ophthalmologic examination. Needle aspirates provide a much smaller sample for analysis and, without the cutting action of a vitrectomy handpiece, can potentially produce vitreoretinal traction and retinal detachment.

The vitrectomy specimen should be divided into aliquots and processed for viral, fungal, and aerobic and anaerobic bacterial cultures. Gram and special staining should

Figure 4.7. Laboratory evaluation of the immunology and uveitis service.

Laboratory Evaluation
Immunology and Uveitis Service

Name _____ Date _____

Blood	*Tissue/fluids*
CBC	Urinalysis _____
WBC _____	HLA _____
Hgb/Hct _____	Aqueous _____
Plates _____	Vitreous _____
Diff _____	Chorioretinal Bx _____
Chemistry	CSF _____
BUN/Cr _____	Conjunctiva Bx _____
LDH/SGOT _____	Ova and Parasite _____
SGPT/Bili _____	Other _____
Calcium _____	*Radiology*
Uric acid _____	CXR _____
Serum Proteins	CT/MRI
ESR _____	Brain _____
C-reactive protein _____	Ocular _____
SPE _____	Orbit _____
SIEP _____	Sinus _____
Cryoglobulins _____	SI joint _____
CIC-Raji _____	Knee _____
CIC-C1Q _____	Gallium scan _____
C3/C4 _____	BaE _____
CH 50 _____	Other _____
Properdin Factor B _____	*Skin tests*
Alpha-1-Acid glycoprotein _____	PPD _____
Lysozyme _____	Candida _____
ACE _____	Mumps _____
Other _____	Tetanus _____
Serology	Histoplasmin _____
VDRL _____	S Ag _____
FTA-ABS _____	Lens Ag _____
Toxocara _____	*Consults*
HB SAg _____	Rheumatology _____
Toxoplasma _____	Allergy _____
Viral titers _____	Hematology _____
HIV _____	Dermatology _____
Autoantibodies	ENT/Audio _____
RF _____	EOG/ERG _____
ANA/Hep2 _____	Ultrasound _____
ds DNA _____	Fluorescein angiogram _____
ss DNA _____	_____
ENA	
Sm _____	*Other*
RNP _____	_____
Anti-Ro (SSA) _____	_____
Anti-La (SSB) _____	_____
Anti-Microsomal _____	_____
APLA _____	_____
ANCA _____	_____

be performed as indicated by the clinical picture. Another portion of the vitreous sample should be sent to the pathology laboratory for standard cytologic examination. The specimen should be fixed in glutaraldehyde to allow for light and electron microscopic evaluation. The results of this investigation should provide supporting evidence for an infectious, autoimmune, neoplastic, or degenerative process and will often establish a more specific diagnosis.

Retinal and chorioretinal biopsies are much more invasive procedures. They should be limited to situations with severe, sight-threatening, medically unresponsive ocular inflammatory diseases.[24–27] Retinal biopsy should be considered when the disease is located posterior to the equator and primarily within the sensory retina. In contrast, chorioretinal biopsy techniques can only access tissues anterior to the equator. However, chorioretinal biopsy has the advantage of providing uveal tissue for analysis. As with vitreous biopsy, these biopsies provide information that help differentiate among infectious, autoimmune, neoplastic, and degenerative processes and thus direct subsequent therapy. Because hemorrhage, retinal detachment, and hypotony are serious complications of these procedures, however, they should be considered as an alternative to a diagnostic enucleation.

Figure 4.7 is a form used to assist in the design of a laboratory evaluation in the patient with uveitis. Test results can be summarized and followed as indicated by the clinical course. A more in-depth analysis of laboratory testing has been published and is valuable in many clinical settings.[28]

References

1. Sox HC. Probability theory in the use of diagnostic tests: an introduction to critical study of the literature. *Ann Intern Med.* 1986;104:60.
2. Schlaegel TF Jr. *Essentials of Uveitis.* Boston: Little, Brown; 1969.
3. Rosenbaum JT, Wernick R. Selection and interpretation of laboratory tests for patients with uveitis. *Int Ophthalmol Clin.* 1990;30:238.
4. Havener WH. *Ocular Pharmacology.* St. Louis: Mosby-Year Book; 1983.
5. Rosenbaum JT, Wernick R. The utility of routine screening of patients with uveitis for systemic lupus erythematosus or tuberculosis. *Arch Ophthalmol.* 1990;108:1291.
6. Love PE, Santoro SA. Antiphospholipid antibodies: anticardiolipin and the lupus anticoagulant in systemic lupus erythematosus (SLE) and in non-SLE disorders. *Ann Intern Med.* 1990;112:682.
7. Levine SR, Crofts JW, Lesser GR, et al. Visual symptoms associated with the presence of a lupus anticoagulant. *Ophthalmology.* 1988;95:686.
8. Goeken JA. Antineutrophil cytopalsmic antibody—a useful serological marker for vasculitis. *J Clin Immunol.* 1991;11:161.
9. Saxon A, Shanahan F, Landers C, et al. A distinct subset of antineutrophil cytoplasmic antibodies is associated with inflammatory bowel disease. *J Allergy Clin Immunol.* 1990;86:202.
10. de Keizer RJ, van der Woude FJ. cANCA test and the detection of Wegener's disease in sclerokeratitis and uveitis. *Curr Eye Res.* 1990;9(suppl):59.
11. Mills RA, Weeramanthri TS, Hollingsworth PN, Cooper RL. Antineutrophil cytoplasmic antibody in uveitis and scleritis. *Aust NZ J Ophthalmol.* 1991;19:71.
12. Lehner T, Adinolfi M. Acute phase proteins, C9, factor B, and lysozyme in recurrent oral ulceration and Behçet's syndrome. *J Clin Pathol.* 1980;33:269.
13. Calin A. Ankylosing spondylitis. In: Kelley WN, Harris ED Jr, Ruddy S, Sledge CB, eds. *Textbook of Rheumatology.* 2nd ed. Philadelphia: WB Saunders; 1985;2.
14. Brewerton DA, Caffrey M, Nicholls A, et al. Acute anterior uveitis and HLA-B27. *Lancet.* 1973;2:994.
15. Nussenblatt RB, Mittal KK, Ryan S. Birdshot retinochoroidopathy associated with HLA-A29 antigen and immune responsiveness to retinal S-antigen. *Am J Ophthalmol.* 1982;94:147.
16. Priem HA, Kijlstra A, Noens L, et al. HLA typing in birdshot chorioretinopathy. *Am J Ophthalmol.* 1988;105:182.
17. Green WR. Diagnostic cytopathology of ocu-

lar fluid specimens. *Ophthalmology.* 1984;91:
726.

18. Stulting RD, Leif RC, Clarkson JG, Bobbitt
D. Cenrifugal cytology of ocular fluids. *Arch
Ophthalmol.* 1982;100:822.

19. Witmer R. Clinical implications of aqueous
humor studies in uveitis. *Am J Ophthalmol.*
1978;86:39.

20. Baarsma GS, Luyendijk L, Kijlstra A, et al.
Analysis of local antibody production in the
vitreous humor of patients with severe uveitis. *Am J Ophthalmol.* 1991;112:147.

21. Kijlstra A, van den Horn GJ, Luyendijk L, et
al. Laboratory tests in uveitis. New develop-
ments in the analysis of local antibody production. *Doc Ophthalmol.* 1990;75:225.

22. Davis JL, Solomon D, Nussenblatt RB, et al.
mmunocytochemical staining of vitreous
cells. *Ophthalmology.*1992;99:250.

23. Nussenblatt RB, Palestine AG. Surgical treatment in uveitis. In: Nussenblatt RB, Palestine
AG, eds. *Uveitis: Fundamentals and Clinical
Practice.* Chicago: Year Book Medical Publishers; 1989.

24. Chan C-C, Palestine AG, Davis JL, et al. Role
of chorioretinal biopsy in inflammatory eye
disease. *Ophthalmology.* 1991;98:1281.

25. Freeman WR, Wiley CA, Gross JG, et al. En-
doretinal biopsy in immunosuppressed and
healthy patients with retinitis. *Ophthalmology.* 1989;96:1559.

26. Schneiderman TE, Faber DW, Gross JG, et al.
The agar-albumin sandwich technique for
processing retinal biopsy specimens. *Am J
Ophthalmol.* 1989;108:567.

27. Fujikawa LS, Haugen J-P. Immunopathology
of vitreous and retinochoroidal biopsy in
posterior uveitis. *Ophthalmology.* 1990;97:
1644.

28. Wallach J. *Interpretation of Diagnostic Tests: A
Synopsis of Laboratory Medicine.* 4th ed. Boston: Little, Brown; 1986.

5
Medical Therapy for Uveitis

General Principles

Optimal therapy for uveitis is predicated on an understanding of the predominant pathophysiologic mechanism(s) responsible for the specific disorder. To that end, antiviral, antibacterial, antiprotozoal, and antihelminthic agents, as well as specific anti-inflammatory and immunosuppressive medications, can be delivered via topical, regional, and systemic routes in specific circumstances. Whatever the form of therapy, the general goals are similar: to improve comfort, to reduce the severity and frequency of the inflammation, to prevent complications of the uveitis, to avoid treatment complications and drug side effects, and ultimately to preserve sight.

The practitioner can use several strategies to accomplish these goals (Table 5.1).[1] The first course of action is to eliminate the offending agent. The cause of the inflammation may be continual exposure to noxious material (intraocular foreign body), persistent trauma [e.g., uveitis-hyphema-glaucoma (UHG) syndrome], microorganisms (e.g., toxoplasmosis), or an ongoing immunologic reaction to an external or autoantigen (e.g., atopic diseases and lens-induced uveitis). If the agent(s) mediating the disease can be identified, treatment strategies can be designed to remove the source. For example, an intraocular foreign body can be removed via vitreoretinal surgical techniques. An ill-fitting intraocu-

lar lens can be explanted or exchanged in the UHG syndrome. Antiparasitic drugs can be used in ocular toxoplasmosis, and remaining lens proteins and antigens can be removed from the eye via cataract surgery in lens induced uveitis. The rationale for removing or avoiding contact with allergens that cause type I hypersensitivity responses or type IV–mediated contact dermatitis also falls within this principle of eliminating the causative agent.

Unfortunately, the inciting agent is not always apparent or cannot be completely removed, as in presumed autoimmune retinal diseases or idiopathic forms of inflammation. Even in situations where the offending microorganism is killed, a secondary inflammatory response is often driven by tissue injury, dead organisms, and possibly secondary autoreactivity. In these situations, the inflammatory response can be nonspecifically suppressed. Nonsteroidal anti-inflammatory drugs (NSAIDs), corticosteroids, cytotoxic agents, and cyclosporin can all be used in prescribed circumstances. Specific immunization strategies, tolerization schema, and promotion of T suppressor cell functions are promising therapeutic modalities under investigation that should expand the armamentarium in the future.

A third mode of therapy involves the inhibition of cellular actions. Several drugs can interfere with the inflammatory cell actions and function. Chemotaxis can be im-

Table 5.1. General treatment strategies.

Eliminate Agent
Toxic material: Remove noxious agents
Trauma: Minimize surgical and nonsurgical trauma
Infectious: Eliminate infectious organisms via specific
   antibiotics
Inflammatory/immune: Address the predominant
   hypersensitivity mechanism (i.e., remove the
   allergen)

Suppress inflammatory/immune response
Nonspecific: NSAIDs, corticosteroids, cytotoxic agents,
   cyclosporine A
Specific: Immunization, tolerization, T-cell suppression

Interfere with cell actions
Chemotaxis: Cobra venom C
Phagocytosis: Colchicine
Degranulation: Cromolyn, corticosteroids

Inactivate mediators
Hydrolytic: EDTA, collagenase
Arachidonic acid pathway: Corticosteroids
Prostaglandin: NSAID
Lipogenase: Lipoxygenase inhibitors
Coagulation: Antiplatelet NSAID, anticoagulants
   (heparin, Coumadin, streptokinase, tissue
   plasminogen activating factor)
Histamine: Antihistamines

Enhance immune response
Humoral: Gamma globulin
Cellular: IL-2, transfer factor, interferon, growth factors

Tissue reconstruction
Replace: Uveal prolapse
Remove devitalized or inciting tissue: Photoablation,
   vitrectomy, lensectomy, removal band keratopathy,
   synechiae, enucleation

EDTA, ethylenediamine-tetraacetic acids; NSAID, non-steroidal anti-inflammatory drug; IL-2, interleukon-2.

paired via cobra venom, phagocytosis can be disrupted by colchicine, and degranulation of mast cells can be impeded with cromolyn or lodoxamine.

The humoral mediators of inflammation also may be blocked via several mechanisms. Antihistamine agents can be used to counteract the effects of this vasoactive amine in type I hypersensitivity disorders such as atopic diseases. Many cyclooxygenase and lipoxygenase inhibitors are available that block the formation of prostaglandins and other arachidonic acid metab-olites. NSAIDs inhibit prostaglandin and thromboxane formation from arachidonic acid through the inhibition of the enzyme cyclooxygenase. Lipoxygenase products, including leukotrienes and 5-hydroperoxy-eicosatetraenoic acid (5-HPETE), can be blocked with newer lipoxygenase inhibitors. The metabolites from both these pathways have a wide range of action that promotes inflammation, which can be moderated by these agents.

In certain settings, it is helpful to enhance the immune response to assist in the elimination of an invading organism. Patients on high-dose chemotherapy and immunosuppressive regimens and patients with acquired immunodeficiency syndrome (AIDS) may benefit from drugs that stimulate the immune system. These drugs include gammaglobulin, various cytokine and interleukins, growth factors, and interferons.

Finally, inflammation may be modulated by surgical techniques discussed in the next chapter. Surgery can be designed to reconstruct tissue and remove inciting material and antigens, which may be driving an immunologic response. For example, the clinical course in sympathetic ophthalmia may be improved if the inciting eye is removed within 2 weeks of the onset of this autoimmune disease. Vitrectomy may improve the course of pars planitis by removing type II collagen found in the vitreous gel.

Nonspecific Therapy—General Considerations

Without a specific etiologic diagnosis or early in the evaluation of a patient, treatment often must be initiated before obtaining the results of laboratory testing to prevent complications from unbridled intraocular inflammation. In addition, certain disease syndromes are not characterized well enough to understand the predominant mechanism of injury and require less specific therapy. It is helpful to consider several tenets in these settings (Table 5.2).

Table 5.2. Nonspecific therapy strategies and considerations.

Route of administration
Topical: Cycloplegics, mydriatics, and topical
    corticosteroids
Regional: Subconjunctival, sub-Tenon's, transeptal,
    retrobulbar corticosteroid
Systemic: NSAID, corticosteroids, cytotoxic agents,
    cyclosporin A
Intraocular: Antibiotics, dexamethasone

Extent of systemic involvement
Systemic disorder: PO, intravenous routes of
    administration
Local ocular disease: Topical, regional, systemic routes
    of administration

Clinical course
Acute forms of uveitis: Avoid cytotoxic and systemic
    agents
Chronic forms of uveitis: Consider systemic and
    cytotoxic agents

Location
Anterior inflammation: Topical delivery
Intermediate, posterior, or diffuse inflammation:
    Regional, PO, intravenous delivery

Type of inflammation
Nongranulomatous: NSAID
Granulomatous: Avoid NSAID (theoretical)

NSAID, nonsteroidal anti-inflammatory drug; PO, by
mouth.

Medications can be delivered to the eye via topical, regional, systemic, and intraocular routes. Often the route of administration is determined by the character of inflammation. Anterior forms of uveitis lend themselves particularly well to topical medications. Deeper forms of uveitis (intermediate, posterior, and diffuse uveitis) cannot be treated adequately by topical medications alone. They usually require regional or oral routes of delivery. Similarly, local ocular forms of uveitis can be well managed by topical or regional therapies, but systemic diseases such as syphilis, Behçet's disease, and sarcoidosis respond better to oral medications. Not only does the eye respond favorably to this approach, but such treatment also addresses other areas of the body likely to be inflamed and injured by ongoing disease.

Other factors to consider in the design of nonspecific therapy are the clinical course of the uveitis and the type of inflammation. In acute forms of uveitis with a predictably short clinical course, long-acting, slow-acting, and potent systemic medications should be used with caution. Topical, periocular, and short pulses of oral corticosteroids should be considered as first-line therapy. The long-term, systemic, immunosuppressive regimens are more appropriate for chronic, recurrent, and severe forms of inflammation. Theoretically, NSAIDs could shunt arachidonic acid metabolites into the lipoxygenase pathway, thereby promoting a granulomatous uveitis. This problem has not been documented in clinical practice but may be considered when designing the overall medical strategy.

Specific Therapy—General Considerations

When a syndrome diagnosis has been made, the physician should explore the literature regarding any known or postulated disease mechanism. This knowledge facilitates the design of the most precise treatment strategies (Table 5.3). Antibiotics can be chosen that target the known sensitivities of the viral, bacterial, fungal, protozoal, helminthic, or insect organism. Similarly, the four major autoimmune hypersensitivity responses can be approached more specifically (see Fig. 1.3).

Ocular inflammation associated with a predominant type I hypersensitivity response can be treated by eliminating the responsible allergen, stabilizing mast cell degranulation with cromolyn, and impeding the action of vasoactive amines with antihistamine and corticosteroids. Type II diseases can be moderated by removing the tissue, cells, or proteins toward which the antibodies are directed. Lens-induced uveitis may have such a mechanism and can be cured via removal of lens antigens. Alternatively, type II diseases such as ocular cicatricial pemphigoid (OCP) can be

Table 5.3. Specific strategies for uveitis.

Infectious (antibiotics)
Antiviral agents
Antibacterial agents
Antifungal agents
Antiprotozoal agents
Anthelminthic agents

Inflammatory and immunologic (antiinflammatory)
Type I: Eliminate agents, cromolyn, antihistamine, corticosteroids
Type II: Dapsone, corticosteroids, cytotoxic agents, surgical removal
Type III: NSAIDs, corticosteroids, immunosuppressive and cytotoxic agents, plasmapheresis
Type IV: NSAIDs, corticosteroids, immunosuppressive and cytotoxic agents, cyclosporine

NSAID, nonsteroidal anti-inflammatory drug.

treated with dapsone and cytotoxic agents, targeting the B-cell side of the immune response. Type III hypersensitivity disorders are antibody driven as well. Immune complex deposition and complement activation result in vasculitis and Arthus reactions. Plasmapheresis can help remove circulation immune complexes and temporarily assist in controlling a crisis such as occurs in Behçet's disease. Collagen vascular diseases with a component of vasculitis often respond to corticosteroids and other immunosuppressive and cytotoxic drugs. Finally, diseases thought to have a predominant cell-mediated immune mechanism (type IV hypersensitivity) respond to strategies designed to down-regulate the autoreactive T lymphocyte. Corticosteroids, cytotoxic agents, and cyclosporin can be used in these cases. Cyclosporin specifically has the ability to block the interleukin-2 (IL-2) receptor T cells, thereby blocking T cell–mediated processes.

Topical Medical Therapy for Uveitis

Topical delivery of medication is often the safest and most effective mode of therapy in uveitis.[2] Inflammatory disease that in-

volves the anterior segment of the eye benefits from these drugs.

Mydriasis and Cycloplegia

The rationale behind the use of mydriatic agents in iritis is to prevent the formation of iris adhesions posteriorly to the lens and anteriorly to the cornea. This goal can be achieved by preventing prolonged iris-lens and iris–cornea contact through effective dilation. Only rarely do synechiae directly interfere with visual function. More commonly, extensive anterior and posterior synechiae result in secondary forms of glaucoma that can be difficult to manage. Although newly formed synechiae can often be "broken" through aggressive dilation, the goal of mydriasis in iritis is to prevent their formation by "moving the pupil."

Table 5.4 lists commonly used dilating agents. Errors can be made by using too strong a drug such as atropine, which allows prolonged iris–cornea, or iris-lens apposition, or too weak of a drug, which allows miosis and posterior synechiae formation. Homatropine and scopolamine offer an intermediate duration of effect, which explains their clinical utility in managing these patients. Cyclopentolate has been reported to be a chemoattractant for

Table 5.4. Mydriatic and cycloplegic agents.

Agent	Percent	Duration of mydriasis/ cycloplegia
Sympathomimetic (mydriatic)		
Phenylephrine·HCL	2.5 & 10	3 hr
Cocaine	2–10	2 hr
Hydroxyamphetamine	1	40 min
Parasympatholytic (mydriatic and cycloplegic)		
Atropine sulfate	0.5–3	1-2 weeks
Scopolamine	0.25	Days to 1 week
Homatropine	2–5	Several days
Cyclopentolate	0.5–2	1 day
Tropicamide	0.5–1	6 hr

leukocytes in vitro and, theoretically may aggravate intraocular inflammation.[3] This response has not been noted in clinical settings.

The parasympathomimetic agents cause both mydriasis and cycloplegia through blocking acetylcholine receptors on the pupillary sphincter and ciliary muscles. Cycloplegia is desirable in anterior uveitis to prevent photophobia from iris sphincter spasm and painful ciliary muscle action associated with iridocyclitis.

Mydriatic/cycloplegic agents should be used whenever inflammatory cells are noted in the anterior chamber or when the patient notes pain and photophobia. Homatropine, 5% twice a day, or scopolamine, 0.25% twice a day, is a typical starting dose, with a slow taper to one drop in the evening corresponding to improvement in the clinical course. Unpleasant side effects from the use of these drops, including transient burning and loss of accommodation, can be expected. The patient should be informed about these symptoms to encourage maximum compliance. In milder forms of iritis, the use of shorter acting drops (tropicamide 1%) before bedtime facilitates movement of the pupil and minimal cycloplegia during the day to allow some accommodative function.

Broad, or chronic, synechiae may be impossible to break with topical medications. Some patients, however, respond to an aggressive dilation "cocktail" consisting of a pledget of 10% phenylephrine, 5% homatropine, and 10% cocaine. Systemic absorption can occur and patients should be monitored for side effects including hypertension, tachycardia, diaphoresis, and anxiety.

Topical Corticosteroids

Topical corticosteroid preparations are the mainstay of therapy for anterior uveitis. The beneficial effect of steroids is a result of their rapid, broad, anti-inflammatory action and the ability of topical preparations to penetrate the eye.[4] Corticosteroid drugs work by entering cells, binding to intracellular receptors, and influencing the generation of messenger ribonucleic acid (mRNA) specific for corticosteroid-induced products. These mediators in turn result in (1) the inhibition of the arachidonic acid pathway, (2) stabilization of cell membranes and subsequent degranulation, (3) decreasing vascular permeability, (4) augmentation of intracellular cyclic adenosine monophosphate (cAMP), (5) reduction of leukocyte chemotaxis and the number of immune cells in tissues, (6) inhibition of macrophage function, and (7) down-regulation of interleukin production. Each of these actions reduces the degree of the inflammatory response.

There are many topical corticosteroid compounds with differing potencies and bioavailability. Table 5.5 lists the most common preparations. Corticosteroid suspensions in animal models have penetrated the cornea better than solutions. These preparations, in contrast to solutions, require vigorous shaking to attain maximum effect.[5] Clinically, all prednisolone and dexamethasone preparations, when applied frequently, provide therapeutic levels of the drug and have an equivalent beneficial effect on anterior uveitis.

When the decision is made to treat anterior uveitis with topical corticosteroids, therapy should be initiated with very high dosing schedules. A common reason for treatment failure is a timid initial dosing schedule. To optimize intraocular levels of steroid, one drop every hour should be administered, with a taper according to the clinical response. In severe cases one drop every minute for 5 minutes every hour can be prescribed. Ocular irritation and corneal toxicity can be expected with this regimen if continued for more than several days.

Whereas cataract and glaucoma are frequent complications of poorly controlled iridocyclitis, excessive use of corticosteroids can result in posterior subcapsular cataract, steroid-induced glaucoma,

Table 5.5. Ophthalmic corticosteroid preparations.

Agent	Trade Name	Concentration (%)
Hydrocortisone		
Acetate suspension	Hydrocortone	2.5%
Solution	Optef	0.2%
Prednisolone		
Acetate suspension	Pred Forte, Pred Mild, Econopred/Plus,	0.12–1
	Ak-Tate	0.125–1
Phosphate solution	Inflamase/Forte, Ak-Pred	0.12–1
	B-H Prednisolone	0.125–1
	Hydeltrasol, Metreton	0.5
Dexamethasone		
Phosphate solution	Ak-Dex, Decadron	0.1
Suspension	Maxidex	0.1
Progesterone-like		
Medrysone suspension	HMS	1.0
Fluorometholone	FML, Flarex	0.1

and increased susceptibility to ocular infections.[6–10] The risks are more prevalent when these drugs are used at relatively high doses and for long periods of time. There does not appear to be a difference in complication rates between the acetate suspensions and phosphate solutions when delivered at equivalent strengths and frequencies.[11,12] In most cases, the patient should be informed about the risks and should be assured that the benefits of controlling intraocular inflammation universally outweigh these potential complications.

Efforts should be made to achieve the lowest possible dose to minimize the side effects of topical corticosteroids. This is accomplished by prescribing a tapering course and by drug adjustment and titration guided by clinical response. It is often helpful for the physician not only to discuss the medication regimen with the patient, but also to provide written instructions. The patient often will not remember verbal instructions and will benefit from written information about the specific medication dose and tapering course.

If the patient returns for follow-up on one medication schedule and clinical improvement is noted, it is reasonable to advise a continued taper; however, if a patient demonstrates persistent or increased cellular reaction, the medication should be either maintained or increased. It is not uncommon to observe a flare-up while on a tapering course of medication. This response is useful, as it helps define the lowest maintenance dose of drug required to control the disease.

While the patient is on topical corticosteroid therapy, intraocular pressures should be carefully monitored. Steroid-induced glaucoma can progress at a much more rapid rate than primary forms of glaucoma. Topical beta-blocking agents or oral carbonic anhydrase inhibitors are effective in lowering the intraocular pressure in uveitis. Strong miotics and epinephrine promote inflammation and should be avoided in inflamed eyes.

Topical therapy with mydriatics, cycloplegics, and corticosteroid preparations should be continued for as long as the disease remains active with cells in the anterior chamber. It is important to note that many forms of uveitis produce a long-lasting breakdown of the blood–eye/blood–aqueous barrier. These eyes may have a prolonged or even permanent intraocular flare. The presence of flare is not an indication for therapy. Aggressive topical steroids seldom eliminate all aqueous protein, and "chasing the flare" results in steroid overdose and an increased risk of adverse drug reactions. Additionally, certain chronic forms of iritis/iridocyclitis, such as Fuchs' heterochromia and juvenile rheumatoid arthritis (JRA), can be quite resistant to attaining complete cellular quiescence. The practitioner may find that relatively high doses of steroids are required to eradicate all inflammatory cells. Steroid-sparing drugs should be considered in these refractory cases, as discussed later. In Fuchs's heterochromia, however, a mild amount of cell can be tolerated to minimize long-term complications of high-dose steroids.

The development of topical NSAIDs, cyclosporin, and other classes of immunosuppressive agents will add new treatments to our armamentarium[13] (Table 5.6). Flurbiprofen sodium 0.03% (Ocufen), ketorolac 1% (Acular), and diclofenac sodium (Voltaren) are currently approved for inhibition of prostaglandin-mediated miosis during intraocular surgery, but their role in treating anterior uveitis is not well established.[13–15]

Several investigators have demonstrated that topical NSAIDs reduce the disruption of the blood–eye barrier and lessen postoperative inflammation after cataract surgery.[16–20] In these studies, blood–eye barrier integrity was assessed by clinical evaluation of cell and flare and by fluorophotometry. After intracapsular or extracapsular cataract extractions with intraocular lens implantation, postoperative inflammation was reduced with the topical application of flurbiprofen (0.03%), indomethacin (1%), and ketorolac (0.5%).[20–24] The anti-inflammatory effect was equal

or superior to the use of topical corticosteroid.[21,22] Topical NSAIDs did not have significant adverse side effects and did not elevate intraocular pressure. Both topical flurbiprofen (0.03%) and dexamethasone phosphate (0.1%) were ineffective in preventing postoperative inflammation after more aggressive and destructive surgical procedures such as cyclocryoablation.[25] Topical NSAIDs appear to be safe and effective in controlling postoperative inflammation after routine cataract surgery.

Cystoid macular edema (CME) is a common complication of uveitis and intraocular surgery.[26–28] Postoperative inflammation and prostaglandin release have been postulated to play a role in this condition.[29,30] Several studies have demonstrated that topical indomethacin in combination with corticosteroids can prevent the development of angiographic proven CME after both intracapsular and extracapsular cataract surgery.[31-33] These studies evaluated 948 eyes and demonstrated an overall 50% reduction in incidence of postoperative CME with the use of topical NSAIDs.

In another study of 98 eyes, a 70% reduction in fluorescein angiographic CME was noted with the use of topical flurbiprofen (0.03%) alone. This study concluded that flurbiprofen may be more effective than indomethacin and that corticosteroids may have an antagonistic action when used with NSAIDs. Topical indomethacin also has been used to prevent CME after retinal detachment surgery.[34] Postoperative CME was reduced from 33% (placebo-treated group) to 13% (indomethacin-treated group) in 63 eyes after scleral buckle procedure.

The treatment of clinically significant postoperative CME has been more challenging. Burnett et al.[35] treated 14 patients with aphakic CME with topical fenoprofen (11%) and found no significant effect when compared to placebo alone. Another randomized study found no significant visual improvement using oral indomethacin compared with placebo in patients with se-

Table 5.6. Nonsteroidal antiinflammatory drugs: topical ocular preparations.

Diclofenac (Voltaren 0.1%)
Indomethacin (Indocin 1.0%)
Suprofen (Profenal 1%)
Flurbiprofen (Ocufen 0.03%)
Ketorolac (Acular 0.5%, Toradol 0.5%)

vere CME.[30] More recently, Yannuzzi[30] reported two trials using topical indomethacin alone or in combination with topical corticosteroids. Treatment with topical indomethacin (1%) alone neared significance with respect to benefit in this small pilot study. When topical indomethacin was combined with corticosteroid drops in 40 consecutive patients with chronic CME, 80% achieved improved visual acuity by 6 weeks. More recently, a larger randomized trial was performed comparing topical ketorolac (0.5%) four times a day to placebo therapy in 120 patients with chronic pseudophakic CME.[36] A statistically significant improvement in visual acuity was noted in the ketorolac-treated group after 30, 60, and 90 days of therapy. The role of topical NSAIDs in uveitis remains unclear. While topical NSAIDs are not strong enough to treat acute anterior uveitis alone, they can be used as steroid sparing agents in chronic disorders.

Topical cyclosporin has been used recently to reduce corneal graft rejection and assist in the control of autoimmune forms of ocular sicca. Poor intraocular penetration and lack of an adequate vehicle cur-

rently limit the application of this drug for use in iritis.[37]

Regional Medical Therapy for Uveitis

Severe forms of anterior uveitis such as HLA-B27–associated diseases (e.g., ankylosing spondylitis, Reiter's syndrome) often require more intense therapy than is afforded by topical medications. Regional injection of medication also is an effective route for treating deeper intermediate, posterior, and diffuse forms of uveitis.[38] Subconjunctival, transeptal, sub-Tenon's, and retrobulbar spaces can be accessed for placement of injectable corticosteroid preparations (Fig. 5.1). The most commonly used medications are triamcinolone (40 mg/ml), methylprednisolone (80 mg/ml), and betamethasone (4 mg/ml). One milliliter of each preparation is injected into the potential periocular space. The clinical effect of these drugs can be as short as several days (betamethasone) or as long as 6 weeks or more (triamcinolone) after the injection. Frequently, remission of the uveitis

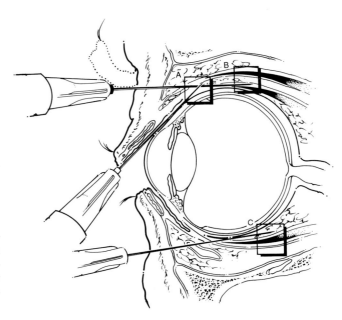

Figure 5.1. Periocular spaces. The potential space beneath the conjunctiva (**A**), Tenon's capsule (**B**), and retrobulbar area (**C**) can be accessed by injection for regional delivery of medications.

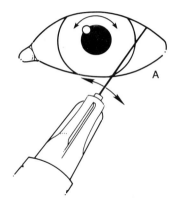
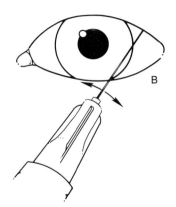
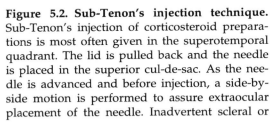

Figure 5.2. Sub-Tenon's injection technique. Sub-Tenon's injection of corticosteroid preparations is most often given in the superotemporal quadrant. The lid is pulled back and the needle is placed in the superior cul-de-sac. As the needle is advanced and before injection, a side-by-side motion is performed to assure extraocular placement of the needle. Inadvertent scleral or globe penetration will produce a cyclorotary motion to the eye (**A**). The injection should not proceed if such motion is observed. Correct placement in the sub-Tenon's space will not produce this movement, and injection will result in drug deposition behind the insertion of the Tenon's capsule (**B**).

continues well beyond the duration of action as a result of the powerful effect this route of delivery has on local inflammation.

Many uveitis specialists prefer the sub-Tenon's route (Fig. 5.2). The superotemporal conjunctiva is anesthetized via topical proparacaine and a pledget of 10% cocaine. Insulin syringes are preferable to tuberculin syringes, as the needle is fixed on the former. Incidents of needle plugging have occurred, and the tip of a removable needle has been propelled off the syringe with the extra effort required for injection. Depending on the agent used periocular injection can be repeated as frequently as every 1–8 weeks as necessary. Because the vehicle found in methylprednisolone can remain in the orbit for a long time, repeated use of this drug is not always possible.

Inadvertent intraocular injection is the most feared complication of periocular injection. Smith and Nozik[39] emphasize the importance of using a side-by-side motion of the needle to determine that it is not within the globe. Inadvertent penetration results in a cyclorotation of the eye and should warn the physician to withdraw the needle.

Another risk of periocular steroid use is a prolonged elevation of intraocular pressure. Posterior drug placement is thought to provide a certain degree of protection from steroid-induced glaucoma. In a review of 80 consecutive patients treated for CME over 2 years at the Department of Ophthalmology, Ohio State University College of Medicine, only one patient had an elevated intraocular pressure as measured 4 to 6 weeks postinjection. Nevertheless, intraocular pressure needs to be monitored carefully in all patients with uveitis and, in particular, those receiving any form of steroid. Prolonged or severe elevation of intraocular pressure may require the surgical removal of the deposited steroid.

Regional immunosuppression can be quite profound after a sub-Tenon's injection of triamcinolone. Patients with active infectious disease should be treated only rarely with this form of therapy and should receive concomitant specific antibiotic drug therapy. A focal area of retinal toxoplasmosis can rapidly expand into widespread acute retinal necrosis if the patient is not on concurrent antiprotozoal therapy.

Rare cases of scleral melting after the use of sub-Tenon's methylprednisolone have been reported.[40] It is possible that the vehicle in methylprednisolone may cause this response. Triamcinolone may have a therapeutic advantage in this disease. Direct placement of the medication against the inflamed sclera also may play a role in scleral melting; therefore, a retrobulbar location may be preferable in these patients.

Systemic Medical Therapy for Uveitis

Systemic medications are often used when patients have not responded to local therapies. It is not uncommon for patients with severe, bilateral posterior or diffuse forms of uveitis to fail to respond to topical and regional therapies. The addition of oral medications can help gain control in this setting. Patients who are unable to tolerate the side effects of local treatments are also candidates for oral therapy. For example, in patients who develop high intraocular pressure on topical or periocular steroids, oral agents can be used to minimize this side effect. Patients with toxoplasmosis retinochoroiditis and other infectious forms of uveitis often require control of their intraocular inflammation through the use of oral prednisone. Oral medications can avoid the risks of long-acting, intense immunosuppression produced by periocular delivery.

The most important reason to consider oral medications is the presence of an underlying systemic disease. Patients with disorders such as sarcoidosis, JRA, Behçet's disease, syphilis, tuberculosis, and Reiter's syndrome can benefit from proper oral therapy. Although local treatments can be adjunctive in these diseases, one can seldom achieve a successful outcome using this approach. The response of the eye to proper systemic therapy is often dramatic. Syphilic uveitis can resolve within days of antibiotic therapy. Often these patients have had "medically unresponsive" ocular inflammation for several months. The role of specific antibiotics for infectious forms of uveitis is discussed under each disease. Patients with collagen vascular diseases such as polyarteritis nodosa, rheumatoid arthritis, and relapsing polychondritis can achieve similar dramatic remission through the prudent use of systemic immunosuppressive agents.

It is often necessary to consult with an internist, family practitioner, rheumatologist, or hematologist when a patient with uveitis requires oral medications, especially when recommending oral corticosteroids or immunosuppressive agents. The potential drug interactions, side effects, and toxicities are often complex. The impact of these drugs on any other underlying disease such as diabetes mellitus, hypertension, and peptic ulcer disease is also important to consider. Although often manageable, these concerns are best handled by a team approach.

Oral Nonsteroidal Anti-Inflammatory Drugs

NSAIDs have been used widely in general medicine as a result of their analgesic, antipyretic, antiplatelet, and anti-inflammatory actions.[13] Approximately 14% of Americans are currently taking an oral NSAID, and more than 100 million prescriptions are dispensed each year.[41–43] Historically, the role for NSAIDs in ophthalmology has been less well defined. Recently, this class of drugs has been used in several clinical trials, and indications for the use of NSAIDs in ocular disease are expanding.

NSAIDs inhibit prostaglandin (PG) and thromboxane formation from arachidonic acid through the inhibition of the enzyme cyclooxygenase.[44] Another newer class of

NSAIDs blocks the enzyme lipoxygenase. Lipoxygenase products are also generated from arachidonic acid and include leukotrienes and 5-HPETE.[45]

The metabolites from both enzymatic pathways have a wide range of biologic activities. PGs are a large group of 20 carbon, unsaturated fatty-acid derivatives that promote a nonspecific inflammatory response.[46] They are synthesized de novo after tissue injury. In the eye, PGs increase vascular permeability, produce miosis, and result in breakdown of the blood–eye barrier.[16,47,48] Inhibition of cyclooxygenase in platelets blocks thromboxane formation and the ability of platelets to induce clotting. Lipoxygenase products and leukotrienes also have a potent effect on the immune response and, similar to PGs, promote inflammation after tissue injury.[42] The widespread use and clinical effectiveness of NSAIDs are due largely to their inhibitory action on these two enzymes.

Several classes of NSAIDs differ in their chemical structure, serum half-lives, and pharmacokinetics[43] (Tables 5.6 and 5.7). NSAIDs are absorbed rapidly from the gastrointestinal (GI) tract and have high protein-binding to albumin in the bloodstream.[49] Drug distribution depends in part on the lipid solubility of the individual drug. Agents such as naproxen and ketoprofen, with higher lipid solubility, exhibit greater ocular and central nervous system penetration, action, and side effects.[50,51] Certain NSAIDs have longer half-lives and thus are more conducive to patient compliance (Table 5.7). These agents, however, including naproxen, diflunisal, phenylbutazone, and sulindac require a loading dose to achieve an earlier therapeutic blood level.

Clinical trials comparing the various NSAIDs have demonstrated little difference in anti-inflammatory efficacy.[52–54] Individual patient preferences, however, vary significantly. It is not uncommon for a patient to respond poorly to one agent or

Table 5.7. Nonsteroidal anti-inflammatory drugs: classification and serum half-lives of common agents.

Carboxylic acids
Acetylated: aspirin (0.25 hr)
Nonacetylated: diflunisal (Dolobid) (13 hr)

Acetic acids
Tolmectin (Tolectin) (1 hr)
Diclofenac (Voltaren) (1 hr)
Etodolac (Lodine) (3 hr)
Indomethacin (Indocin) (5 hr)
Sulindac (Clinoril) (14 hr)

Propionic acids
Ketoprofen (Orudis) (2 hr)
Ibuprofen (Advil, Motrin, Nuprin) (2 hr)
Suprofen (Profenal) (2 hr)
Fenoprofen (Nalfon) (3 hr)
Flurbiprofen (Ansaid, Ocufen) (4 hr)
Naproxen (Anaprox, Naprosyn) (14 hr)

Fenamic acids
Meclofenamic acid (Meclomen) (2 hr)
Metafenamic acid (Ponstel) (2 hr)

Fenolic acids
Phenylbutazone (Butazolidin) (77 hr)
Piroxicam (Feldene) (57 hr)

Pyrrole-pyrrole
Ketorolac (Toradol) (5 hr)

group of NSAIDs but benefit from a trial with a second drug or class of NSAIDs. In certain disorders, one drug may appear to have a better anti-inflammatory effect than other NSAIDs. For example, rheumatoid scleritis and HLA-B27–associated diseases (e.g., ankylosing spondylitis, Reiter's syndrome) appear to respond to indomethacin better than other drugs.[55,56]

As a group, oral NSAIDs are associated with several potentially serious side effects. The most commonly reported adverse symptoms are gastrointestinal. PG increases gastric blood flow and mucin production and decreases acid production. PGE_2 has 2000 times more potency than cimetidine as an inhibitor of gastric acid secretion. NSAIDs block these protective actions of PG through inhibition of cyclooxygenase in the mucosal cell lining of the stomach. Gastric erosion, dyspepsia, ulceration, perforation, and hemorrhage are all associated with the use of NSAIDs.[42,57,58] Relative risk for peptic ulcer disease is estimated to be between two and four times greater in patients taking NSAIDs than case-controlled subjects not receiving these drugs.[59,60] Elderly patients or those with a history of peptic ulcer disease have a higher risk for these systemic side effects. Additionally, patients receiving anticoagulants should avoid NSAIDs because of potentially serious GI hemorrhage. Patients at higher risk for GI complications may benefit from the use of histamine H_2 antagonists and prostaglandin analogs. Misoprostol, cimetidine, and ranitidine are agents that can reduce endoscopically diagnosed gastric and duodenal ulceration.[61,62]

Long-term use of NSAIDs have other potentially serious side effects. Renal failure, hyperkalemia, and interstitial renal necrosis have been reported with oral NSAID administration.[41,63,64] All classes of NSAID have these potential side effects and renal function should be monitored accordingly. Potentially serious drug–drug interactions may also be noted with the use of NSAIDs. These interactions, which include reduced clearance of digoxin, methotrexate, lithium, and aminoglycosides, can result in elevated blood levels of these medications.[43]

Oral NSAIDs have been used to treat scleritis and patients with uveitis.[40,65] The scleral coat of the eye can be inflamed as an idiopathic condition or as a result of several infectious or autoimmune systemic diseases. In several series, rheumatoid arthritis is the most common etiology for this disorder. Topical corticosteroid therapy is often ineffective in controlling disease progression. Several clinical studies have suggested that oral indomethacin (75–150 mg/day) is the drug of choice for the treatment of scleritis.[40] Adjunctive oral corticosteroids may be needed for recalcitrant cases. Patients with necrotizing rheumatoid scleritis may even require second-generation immunosuppressive agents such as cyclophosphamide to control both ocular and systemic manifestations of the disease.[66]

Surprisingly, few studies have investigated the role of oral NSAIDs in uveitis.[13] Granulomatous inflammation was better controlled in a rat model of lens-induced uveitis with lipoxygenase inhibitors than cyclooxygenase inhibitors.[67] The authors postulated that lipoxygenase inhibitors interfere better with macrophage functions that play an important role in this model of granulomatous uveitis. In a rabbit model of an endotoxin-induced iridocyclitis, both parenteral indomethacin and aspirin were effective in reducing uveitis.[68] Only one clinical trial has used oral NSAIDs in patients with uveitis. Olson et al.[69] reported a beneficial effect from adjunctive use of oral NSAIDs in chronic childhood iridocyclitis. In a cross-over study of 14 patients, intraocular inflammation was significantly improved in all eyes on oral agents. A corticosteroid-sparing effect was noted in patients receiving NSAIDs.

Oral Corticosteroids

Oral corticosteroids are the first-line therapy for most sight-threatening bilateral forms of ocular inflammation because of their rapid onset of action and their widespread effect on inflammation and the immune system. The action of corticosteroid preparations is immediate. Because so few other medications provide this response, steroids are typically used in the initial phases of therapy.

Corticosteroids have many potential serious side effects and adverse reactions. Whereas some patients tolerate relatively high-dose, long-term steroid therapy remarkably well, most patients develop significant adverse side effects. A partial list of these side effects is summarized in Table 5.8.

Table 5.8. Complications and side effects of corticosteroid therapy.

Skin: Ecchymosis, telangiectasia, acne, hirsutism, delayed wound healing
Neurologic: Depression, sleep disturbance, psychosis, cerebral pseudotumor, convulsions
Gastrointestinal: Peptic ulcer, increased appetite, pancreatitis
Metabolic: Glucose intolerance, sodium retention, potassium loss, weight gain, Cushing's syndrome, growth stunting in children, adrenal suppression, fluid retention, hyperosmotic coma
Immune: Susceptible to infections, may complicate neoplasia
Vascular: Hypertension, thromboembolism
Musculoskeletal: Osteoporosis, steroid myopathy, weakness, bilateral hip necrosis, stunted growth in children

Table 5.9. Relative potencies of corticosteroids.[39]

Preparation	Systemic equivalent (mg)	Anti-inflammatory potency
Cortisone	25	0.8
Hydrocortisone	20	1.0
Prednisone	5	4.0
Prednisolone	5	4.0
Methylprednisolone	4	5
Triamcinolone	4	5
Betamethasone	0.6	33
Dexamethasone	0.75	26

Rheumatologists and ophthalmologists who treat many patients with uveitis have intimate knowledge of these troublesome and potentially fatal complications, which limit their use. The risks of these agents need to be weighed against their potential benefits and the natural history of the ocular inflammation. In most settings, their sight-saving benefits in severe forms of uveitis warrant their use.

Side effects are more common at higher doses of steroid. Many can be moderated by using lower doses or controlled by other medical means. Insulin therapy can be adjusted in patients with diabetes mellitus. Blood pressure can be monitored and peptic ulcers can be treated more aggressively during treatment. Comanagement with the patient's internist or general practitioner is often necessary. Once the disease is under control, efforts to find the lowest effective dose should be made.

The practitioner should initiate corticosteroid therapy in earnest and with resolve. Table 5.9 lists the various steroid preparations and their relative potencies.[39,70] Typically, oral prednisone is the drug of choice, but any agent may be used. Once the decision has been made to commit

a patient to prednisone, a 1 to 1.5 mg/kg/day dosage schedule should be started. Maximum anti-inflammatory effect can be achieved through divided doses, but this strategy is also associated with more side effects. Typically, the prednisone is given as a single dose in the morning. The peak steroid blood level will then coincide with the normal diurnal peak of cortisol, that is, highest in the morning. The most frequent error is prescribing too low an initial dose. It is more efficacious to start out with a high dose, gain rapid control, and begin a judicious taper than to begin "safe" and try to "catch up" with the inflammation. Firefighters understand this principle in their endeavors to extinguish their own kind of fire.

Alternate-day therapy can minimize systemic side effects of oral corticosteroids. Unfortunately, many forms of uveitis (e.g., sarcoid uveitis) do not respond well to such a dosing schedule. Daily dosing is frequently required because of the short-term effects of steroids on the immune system.

Duration of treatment is determined by the nature of the disease and the clinical response. Chronic disease such as sarcoidosis and Wegener's granulomatosis may require long-term therapy. Acute diseases such as ankylosing spondylitis–associated uveitis may require only a short "pulse" of corticosteroid to achieve control of the severe inflammation. Thus tapering the corticosteroid therapy requires knowledge of the underlying disorder and the "art" of medicine. A typical adult schedule is 80 mg/day for 2 days followed by a taper such as 60 mg/day for 2 days, 40 mg/day for 2 days, and 20 mg/day thereafter as dictated by treatment effect and side effects.

Corticosteroids can be used alone or in combination with other antibiotic and immunosuppressive drugs. It is not uncommon in ophthalmology to use both an antibiotic to eradicate an infectious process while paradoxically using an agent that hinders the body's ability to fight the infection. This is a consequence of the eye's low tolerance to severe intraocular inflammation. Rapid and permanent destruction of the delicate ocular tissues can develop without simultaneous attention to the host's inflammatory response. Prednisone can also be used as a component of various immunosuppressive regimens. By using corticosteroids in conjunction with dapsone, methotrexate, cyclophosphamide, or cyclosporin, lower doses of each agent can be administered, thus minimizing adverse reactions.

The clinician must also determine the safe dose for prednisone. This amount cannot be determined easily and is quite variable among patients. Some may tolerate relatively high doses (40–100 mg/day) without experiencing significant side effects, but these patients are rare. Most patients cannot tolerate maintenance doses greater than 20 mg/day. Typically, if a patient can be controlled with 20 mg or less of prednisone, long-term therapy can be attempted. Side effects are monitored every 4 to 6 weeks. Effort should be made to reduce the dose continually as dictated by the level of intraocular inflammation. In general, patients who require doses greater than 20 mg/day or who develop too many side effects with a regimen of 20 mg/day or less are considered steroid resistant or intolerant. Other immunosuppression strategies should be considered for these patients.

Cytotoxic and Immunosuppressive Agents

Cytotoxic immunosuppressive agents interfere with the synthesis of nucleic acids and proteins[39,70–79] (Table 5.10). Thus, they affect tissues such as lymphoid or bone marrow cells, which proliferate rapidly. Although an in-depth discussion of cytotoxic drug therapy is outside the scope of this chapter, ophthalmologists should be aware of the principles regarding their use and their ocular indications.

Patients who require cytotoxic and immunosuppressive therapy typically have severe, sight-threatening inflammations that are unresponsive to appropriate corticosteroid therapy (Table 5.10). Patients with severe idiopathic forms of uveitis who are intolerant to corticosteroid side effects are also candidates for second-generation immunosuppressive agents. Certain diseases mandate the use of these drugs. For example, without systemic immunosuppression, patients with Beçhet's disease will uniformly lose useful vision and patients with polyarteritis nodosa face a 50% to 90% mortality rate.

Cytotoxic drugs (Table 5.11) are often combined with other agents such as predni-

Table 5.10. Common ophthalmic indications for cytotoxic immunosuppression.

Type I
Autoimmune diseases: few indications
Type II
Autoimmune diseases: ocular cicatricial pemphigoid, severe lens-induced uveitis
Type III
Autoimmune/collagen vascular associated diseases: Beçhet's disease, PAN, Wegener's granulomatosis, SLE, rheumatoid arthritis
Type IV
Autoimmune diseases: sympathetic ophthalmia, VKH syndrome, birdshot retinochoroidopathy, pars planitis

PAN, polyarteritis nodosa; SLE, systemic lupus erythematosus; VKH, Vogt-Koyanagi-Harada.

Table 5.11. Cytotoxic immunosuppressive agents: application in severe uveitis.

Class	Agent
Alkylating drugs	Cyclophosphamide (Cytoxan)
	Chlorambucil (Leukeran)
Purine analogs	Azathioprine (Imuran)
Pyridine analogs	Fluorouracil
Folic acid analogs	Methotrexate
Antibiotics	Mitomycin C
	Doxorubicin (Adriamycin)
	Cyclosporin A
Miscellaneous	Colchicine
	Vincristine

sone to induce and maintain disease remission.[39,70-72] They are usually used for an extended time (5–72 months), with an average of 18 months, to "cure" the disease. Most of these agents have a slow onset of action ranging between 2 and 12 weeks, with a maximum effect later in the course of treatment.

Patients must have salvageable vision to assume the potential risks of these medications. They must also be able to provide informed consent before beginning therapy. Although cytotoxic drugs have markedly fewer side effects compared with prednisone, several are serious and even potentially fatal without careful and skilled monitoring. Patients should be tested for complications as frequently as every week when beginning therapy. Once they are on a stable dose, they require monthly observation for serious side effects.

Each drug has its own side effect profile. For example, methotrexate can cause liver damage and mucosal lesions, whereas cyclophosphamide may affect the bone marrow, bladder, and lung. Typically, the chemotherapist works with a limited number of these drugs to gain familiarity with their beneficial actions as well as anticipated complications. Contraindications include pregnancy, infectious diseases, and preexisting liver, renal, pulmonary, and hematologic disorders. Patients who plan to

have children need to be aware of potential fertility problems with the use of these agents.

The indications and choice of which drug to use is discussed further in subsequent chapters under the individual diseases. The side effect profile greatly affects this decision. Preexisting renal or hepatic disease often dictates the use of one agent over another. The choice of drug also is influenced by its proven efficacy for a particular disorder. For instance, methotrexate works well for Reiter's syndrome and severe rheumatoid arthritis. Cytoxan, however, is often the drug of choice for polyarteritis nodosa, relapsing polychondritis, and Wegener's granulomatosis.

Specific Immunosuppressive Agents

Alkylating Drugs

Cyclophosphamide (Cytoxan) and chlorambucil (Leukeran) are both alkylating agents.[72] These drugs interfere with cell division by permanently cross-linking the 7-nitrogen of guanine of DNA.[72] Cyclophosphamide has enjoyed wider use in the United States. As a prodrug, it must be converted by the liver to its active form. Thus it cannot be used as a topical drug and should not be used in the presence of severe liver disease. Both B cells and T cells are affected by these agents.

As cytoxic agents, these drugs are capable of killing clones of actively proliferating, autoreactive immune cells. Clinically, the drugs are the most potent of the immunosuppressive drugs and can induce a true immune tolerance. Cyclophosphamide has been used in severe, corticosteroid-unresponsive forms of ocular inflammation including cicatricial pemphigoid, Behçet's disease, relapsing polychondritis, polyarteritis nodosa, Wegener's granulomatosis, pars planitis, Vogt-Koyanagi-Harada (VKH) syndrome, serpiginous chorioretinopathy, and sympathetic ophthalmia (see relevant chapters).[39,70,71,75-77]

Cyclophosphamide is initiated at a dose of 1 to 2 mg/kg/day.[39,70,71,75–77] Medication should be taken in the mornings and used with 2 to 3 liters of fluid daily to reduce the incidence of cystitis. Blood counts should be obtained weekly until a stable dose is achieved. White blood counts should not be lower than 3000 to 3500 cells/mm, with neutrophil counts of 1500 to 2000 cells/mm. With a positive clinical response, the dose may be lowered.[72] Urine samples should be obtained every 4 weeks, and liver function tests should be performed every 3 months.[72]

Anemia, leukopenia, thrombocytopenia, azoospermia, hemorrhagic cystitis, and pulmonary fibrosis are possible complications of this drug. The long-term side effects of alkylating agents, including the potential for secondary malignancies, must be considered when prescribing these drugs. Secondary neoplasms are not as problematic in patients with autoimmune disorders as in patients with cancer and the propensity for neoplasia who use these agents. Secondary infections may occur while on any immunosuppressive medication.

Purine Analogs

Azathioprine (Imuran) inhibits the formation of purine bases in DNA synthesis.[72] Azathioprine is converted in the liver to its active forms. Because this agent appears to have a greater impact on T cells, it plays a greater role in presumed T cell–mediated diseases such as sympathetic ophthalmia, VKH syndrome, and possibly pars planitis.[39,70–72,78,79] T cell–independent, antibody-associated, or immune complex diseases do not respond as well to this agent. It has been used however to treat systemic lupus erythematosus (SLE), Wegener's granulomatosis, OCP, and JRA.

Azathioprine is typically initiated at a dose of 1 to 3 mg/kg/day.[39,70–72,78,79] The clinical response and potential side effects are monitored weekly during treatment induction. Anemia, leukopenia, thrombocyto-

penia, nausea, and vomiting are potential complications of this drug.

Folic Acid Analogs

Methotrexate is an antimetabolite that works by blocking the formation of tetrahydrofolic acid.[72] Thymidine and subsequent deoxyribonucleic acid (DNA) synthesis are inhibited. Methotrexate is variably absorbed by oral routes. It is bound to plasma proteins (50%) and can displace salicylates, tetracycline, and sulfa antibiotics.[39,70,71] Both proliferating T and B cells are affected by this drug, but the humoral response is affected to a greater extent. Methotrexate is typically administered weekly. Low doses (5–25 mg) in three divided doses, 12 hours apart, is often the range for immune disorders.[70,71,73,74] Rheumatoid scleritis, ankylosing spondylitis, Reiter's syndrome, SLE, and JRA-associated iridocyclitis respond well to this agent (see relevant chapters). Side effects include mucosal ulceration, GI disturbances, hepatotoxicity, meylotoxicity, and increased susceptibility to infection. Liver function tests and complete blood count need to be performed when this drug is prescribed.

Cyclosporin

Cyclosporin is a third-generation immunosuppressive medication that works via the reversible inhibition IL-2 release and IL-2 receptors on T cells.[80–85] Consequently, it has been used extensively in organ transplantation to inhibit the cell-mediated immune responses toward the heterologous donor tissue antigens. It has also been used to control presumed cell-mediated and other autoimmune disorders. In ophthalmology cyclosporin should be considered in patients with bilateral, sight-threatening, posterior or diffuse forms of uveitis. Birdshot retinochoroidopathy, sympathetic ophthalmia, VKH syndrome, Behçet's disease, serpiginous chorioretinitis, and severe idiopathic forms of uveitis have responded favorably to this drug.[82,86–88]

In most instances, cyclosporin is considered as a second-line therapy after corticosteroid therapy. Patients who are intolerant to the side effects of corticosteroids or are unresponsive at safe doses should be considered candidates for cyclosporin therapy.

The action of cyclosporin is not as rapid as prednisone, and it is often used in combination with other medications to achieve control of inflammation. As with other immunosuppressive medications, the patient should be compliant and be able to give informed consent regarding the risks and benefits of immunosuppressive therapy. In addition to the general risks of immunosuppression, kidney injury was noted frequently when high-dose cyclosporin was used at 10 mg/kg/day.[89,90] When used at initial doses below 5 mg/kg/day, it has been shown to be less nephrotoxic.[91] Patients typically start at 300 to 400 mg/day and can be gradually tapered to 200 to 300 mg/day, depending on their clinical response. Monthly blood urea nitrogen and creatinine testing and careful monitoring of blood pressure are essential. Serum creatinine should not rise more than 30% above baseline. Other complications and side effects include paresthesias, fatigue, hirsutism, and gingivitis.

FK506 is an oral immunosuppressive agent that has been used somewhat successfully to treat uveitis refractory to corticosteroids and other second-generation agents.[91,92] Renal toxicity and neurologic and GI side effects have limited its use.

References

1. Aronson SB. Potential pathways for anti-inflammatory therapy. *Trans Am Acad Ophthalmol Otolaryngol.* 1975;79:62
2. Opremcak EM. Topical therapy for iritis. *Focal Points.* 1991;9:1.
3. Tsai I, Till GO, Marak GE Jr. Effects of mydriatic agents on neutrophil migration, *Ophthalmic Res,* in press.
4. Clamen HN. Anti-inflammatory effects of corticosteroids. *Clin Immunol Allergy.* 1984;4: 317.
5. Leibowitz HM, Kupferman A. Bioavailability and therapeutic effectiveness of topically administered corticosteroids. *Trans Am Acad Ophthalmol Otolaryngol.* 1975;79:78.
6. Urban RC Jr, Cotlier E. Corticosteroid-induced cataracts. *Surv Ophthalmol.* 1986;31: 102.
7. Black RL, Oglesby RB, von Sallmann L, et al. Posterior subcapsular cataracts induced by corticosteroids in patients with rheumatoid arthritis. *JAMA.* 1960;174:166.
8. Hodapp EA, Kass MA. Corticosteroid-induced glaucoma. In: Ritch R, Shields MB, eds. *The Secondary Glaucomas.* St. Louis: CV Mosby; 1982.
9. Armaly MF. Statistical attributes of steroid hypertensive response in the clinically normal eye. *Invest Ophthalmol.* 1965;4:187.
10. Becker B. Intraocular pressure response to topical corticosteroids. *Invest Ophthalmol.* 1965;4:198.
11. Mindel J, Goldberg J, Tavitian H. Similarity of the intraocular pressure response to different corticosteroid esters when compliance is controlled. *Ophthalmology.* 1979;86:98.
12. Cantrill HL, Palmberg PF, Zink HA, et al. Comparison of in vitro potency of corticosteroids with ability to raise intraocular pressure. *Am J Ophthalmol.* 1975;79:1012.
13. Opremcak EM. Nonsteroidal anti-inflammatory drugs. In: Haverner WH, ed. *Havener's Ocular Pharmacology.* St. Louis: Mosby-Year Book; 1994.
14. Keates RH, McGowan KA. Clinical trial of flurbiprofen to maintain pupillary dilation during cataract surgery. *Ann Ophthalmol.* 1984;16:919.
15. Flurbiprofen—an ophthalmic NSAID. *Med Lett Ther.* 1987;29:58.
16. Araie M, Sawa M, Takase M. Topical flurbiprofen and diclofenac suppress blood-aqueous barrier breakdown in cataract surgery: a fluorometric study. *Jpn J Ophthalmol.* 1983; 27:535.
17. Araie M, Sawa M, Takase M. Effect of topical indomethacin on the blood-aqueous barrier after intracapsular extraction of a senile cataract—a fluorophotometric study. *Jpn J Ophthalmol.* 1981;25:237.
18. Eguchi K, Ohara K, Tobari I, et al. Effects of topical indomethacin on suppression of in-

flammation after ocular surgeries—double
mask study of anti-inflammatory effects on
the intracapsular lens extraction. *Acta Soc
Ophthalmol Jpn.* 1982;86:2198.

19. Mochizuki M, Sawa M, Masuda K. Topical
indomethacin in intracapsular extraction of
a senile cataract. *Jpn J Ophthalmol.* 1977;21:
215.

20. Sanders DR, Kraff MC, Leiberman HL, et al.
Breakdown and re-establishment of blood-
aqueous barrier with implant surgery. *Arch
Ophthalmol.* 1982;100:588.

21. Flach AJ, Kraff MC, Sanders DR, Tanenbaum
L. The quantitative effect of 0.5% ketorolac
tromethamine solution and 0.1% dexamethasone sodium phosphate solution on postsurgical blood-aqueous barrier. *Arch Ophthalmol.* 1988;106:480.

22. Flach AJ, Jaffe NS, Akers WA. The effect of
ketorolac tromethamine in reducing postoperative inflammation: double mask parallel
comparison with dexamethasone. *Ann Ophthalmol.* 1989;21:407.

23. Sabiiston D, Tessler H, Sumers K, et al. Reduction of inflammation following cataract
surgery by the nonsteroidal anti-inflammatory drug flurbiprofen. *Ophthalmic Surg.*
1987;18:873.

24. Flach AJ, Lavelle CJ, Olander KW, et al. The
effect of ketorolac tromethamine solution
0.5% in reducing postoperative inflammation after cataract extraction and intraocular
lens implantation. *Ophthalmology.* 1988;95:
1279.

25. Hurvitz LM, Spaeth GL, Zakhour I, et al. A
comparison of the effect of flurbiprofen dexamethasone and placebo on cyclocryother-
apy-induced inflammation. *Ophthal Surg.*
1984;15:394.

26. Stark WJ, Worthen DM, Halladay JT. The
FDA report on intraocular lenses. *Ophthalmology.* 1983;90:311.

27. Irvine AR. Cystoid macular edema. *Surv
Ophthalmol.* 1976;21:1.

28. The Miami Study Group. Cystoid macular
edema in aphakic and pseudophakic eyes.
Am J Ophthalmol. 1979;88:45.

29. Jampol LM. Pharmacologic therapy of
aphakic and pseudophakic cystoid maculae
edema. *Ophthalmology.* 1985;92:807.

30. Yannuzzi LA. A perspective on the treatment of aphakic cystoid macular edema.
Surv Ophthalmol. 1984;28:540.

31. Miyake K, Sakamura S, Miura H. Long-term
follow-up study on prevention of aphakic
cystoid macular edema by topical indomethacin. *Br J Ophthalmol.* 1980;64:324.

32. Yannuzzi LA, Landau AN, Turtz AI. Incidence of aphakic cystoid macular edema
with the use of topical indomethacin. *Ophthalmology.* 1981;88:947.

33. Kraff MC, Sanders DR, Jampol LM, et al.
Prophylaxis of psuedophakic cystoid macular edema with topical indomethacin. *Ophthalmology.* 1982;89:885.

34. Miyake K. Indomethacin in the treatment of
postoperative cystoid macular edema. *Surv
Ophthalmol.* 1984;28:554.

35. Burnett J, Tessler H, Isenberg S, Tso MOM.
Double-masked trial of fenoprofen sodium:
treatment of chronic aphakic cystoid macular edema. *Ophthal Surg.* 1983;14:150.

36. Flach AJ, Jampol LM, Weinberg D, et al. Improvement in visual acuity in chronic
aphakic and psuedophakic cystoid macular
edema after treatment with topical 0.5%
ketorolac tromethamine. *Am J Ophthalmol.*
1991;112:514.

37. BenEzra D, Maftzir G, de Courten C, Timo-
nen P. Ocular penetration of cyclosporin A.
III. The human eye. *Br J Ophthalmol.* 1990;
74:350.

38. Schlaegel TF Jr. *Essentials of Uveitis.* Boston:
Little Brown; 1969:41.

39. Smith RE, Nozik RA. The nonspecific treat-
ment of uveitis. In: Carol-lynn Brown, ed.
*Uveitis. A Clinical Approach to Diagnosis and
Management.* 2nd ed. Baltimore: Williams &
Wilkins; 1989:51.

40. Watson PG. The diagnosis and management
of scleritis. *Ophthalmology.* 1980;87:716.

41. Clive DM, Stoff JS. Renal syndromes associated with nonsteroidal anti-inflammatory
drugs. *N Engl J Med.* 1984;310:563.

42. Langman MJS. Ulcer complications and
nonsteroidal anti-inflammatory drugs. *Am J
Med.* 1988;84(suppl 2A):15.

43. Brooks PM, Day RO. Nonsteroidal anti-
inflammatory drugs—differences and similarities. *N Engl J Med.* 1991;324:1716.

44. Hamberg M, Svenson J, Samuelsson B.
Thromboxanes: new group of biologically
active compounds derived from prostaglandin endoperoxides. *Proc Natl Acad Sci* 1975;
72:2994.

45. Samuelsson B, Borgeat P, Hammarstrom S,

et al. Leukotrienes: a new group of biologically active compounds. In: Samuelsson B, Ramwell PW, Paoletti R, eds. *Leukotrienes and Other Lipoxygenase Products.* New York: Raven Press; 1980:1.

46. Kass MA, Holmberg NJ. Prostaglandin and thromboxane synthesis by microsomes of rabbit ocular tissues. *Invest Ophthalmol Vis Sci.* 1979;18:166.

47. Bhattacherjee P, Eakins KE. A comparison of the inhibitory activity of compounds on ocular prostaglandin biosynthesis. *Invest Ophthalmol Vis Sci.* 1974;13:967.

48. van Haeringen NJ, Oosterhuis JA, van Delft JL, et al. A comparison of the effects on nonsteroidal compounds on the disruption of the blood-aqueous barrier. *Exp Eye Res.* 1982;35:271.

49. Van den Ouweland FA, Gribnau FWJ, van Ginneken CAM, et al. Naproxen kinetics and disease activity in rheumatoid arthritis: a within patient study. *Clin Pharmacol Ther.* 1988;43:79.

50. Goodwin JS, Regan M. Cognitive dysfunction associated with naproxen and ibuprofen in the elderly. *Arthritis Rheum.* 1982;25:1013.

51. Netter P, Lapicque F, Bannwarth B, et al. Diffusion of intramuscular ketoprofen into the cerebrospinal fluid. *Eur J Clin Pharmacol.* 1985;29:319.

52. Orme M, Baber N, Keenan J, et al. Pharmacokinetics and biochemical effects in responders and non-responders to nonsteroidal anti-inflammatory drugs. *Scand J Rheum.* 1981;9(suppl):19.

53. Huskisson EC, Woolf DL, Balme HW, et al. Four new anti-inflammatory drugs: responses and variations. *Br Med J.* 1976;1:1048.

54. Gall EP, Caperton JF, McComb JE, et al. Clinical comparison of ibuprofen, fenoprofen calcium, naproxen, tolmectin sodium in rheumatoid arthritis. *J Rheumatol.* 1982;9:402.

55. Heller CA, Ingelfinger JA, Goldman P. Nonsteroidal anti-inflammatory drugs and aspirin—analyzing the scores. *Pharmacotherapy.* 1985;5:30.

56. Watson PG, Hayreh SS. Scleritis and episcleritis. *Br J Ophthalmol.* 1976;60:163.

57. Bjarnason I, Zanelli G, Prowse P, et al. Blood and protein loss via small intestinal inflammation induced by nonsteroidal anti-inflammatory drugs. *Lancet.* 1987;2:711.

58. Henry DA. Side effects of nonsteroidal anti-inflammatory drugs. *Baillieres Clin Rheumatol.* 1988;2:425.

59. Beard K, Walker AM, Perera DR, Jick H. Nonsteroidal anti-inflammatory drugs and hospitalization for gastroesophageal bleeding in the elderly. *Arch Intern Med.* 1987;147:1621.

60. Sommerville K, Faulkner G, Langman M. Non-steroidal anti-inflammatory drugs and bleeding peptic ulcer. *Lancet.* 1986;1:462.

61. Hawkey CJ. Non-steroidal anti-inflammatory drugs and peptic ulcers. *Br Med J.* 1990;300:278.

62. Soll AH. Pathogenesis of peptic ulcer and implication for therapy. *N Engl J Med.* 1990;322:909.

63. Garella S, Matarese RA. Renal effects of prostaglandins and clinical adverse effects of nonsteroidal anti-inflammatory agents. *Medicine.* 1984;64:165.

64. Lifschitz MD. Prostaglandins and renal blood flow: in vivo studies. *Kidney Int.* 1981;19:802.

65. Mondino BJ, Phinney RB. Treatment of scleritis with combined oral prednisone and indomethacin therapy. *Am J Ophthalmol.* 1988;106:473.

66. Foster CS. Immunosuppressive therapy for external ocular inflammatory disease. *Ophthalmology.* 1980;87:140.

67. Rao NA, Patchett R, Fernandez MA, et al. Treatment of experimental granulomatous uveitis by lipoxygenase and cyclo-oxygenase inhibitors. *Arch Ophthalmol.* 1987;105:413.

68. Howes EL, McKay DG. The effect of aspirin and indomethacin on the ocular response to circulating bacterial endotoxin in the rabbit. *Invest Ophthalmol.* 1976;15:648.

69. Olson NY, Lindsley CB, Godfrey WA. Nonsteroidal anti-inflammatory drug therapy in chronic childhood iridocyclitis. *Am J Dis Child.* 1988;142:1289.

70. Nussenblatt RB, Palestine AG. Philosophy, goals, and approaches to medical therapy. In: David K. Marshall, ed. *Uveitis. Fundamentals and Clinical Practice.* Chicago: Year Book Medical Publishers; 1989:104.

71. Dinning WJ. Therapy—selected topics. In:

Kraus-Mackiw E, O'Connor GR, eds. Uveitis. Pathology and Therapy. 2nd rev. ed. New York: Thieme Medical Publishers; 1986:204.

72. Fauci AS. Clinical aspects of immunosuppression: use of cytotoxic agents and corticosteroids. In: Bellanti JA, ed. Immunology II. Philadelphia: WB Saunders; 1978.

73. Wong VG. Methotrexate treatment of uveal disease. Am J Med Sci. 1966;251:239.

74. Wong VG. Immunosuppressive therapy of ocular inflammatory diseases. Arch Ophthalmol. 1969;81:628.

75. Foster CS. Immunosuppressive therapy for external ocular inflammatory disease. Ophthalmology (Rochester). 1980;87:140.

76. Buckley CE III, Gills JP Jr. Cyclophosphamide therapy of Behçet's disease. J Allergy. 1969;43:273.

77. Buckley CE III, Gills JP Jr. Cyclophosphamide therapy of peripheral uveitis. Arch Intern Med. 1969;124:29.

78. Andrasch RH, Pirofsky B, Burns RP. Immunosuppressive therapy for severe chronic uveitis. Arch Ophthalmol. 1978;96:247.

79. Newell FW, Krill AE. Treatment of uveitis with azathioprine (Imuran). Trans Ophthalmol Soc UK. 1967;87:499.

80. Palacios R, Moller G. Cyclosporin A blocks receptors for HLA-DR antigens on T cells. Nature. 1981;290:792.

81. Beveridge T. Pharmacokinetics and metabolism of cyclosporin A. In: White DJG, ed. Cyclosporin A. New York: Elsevier Biomedical Press; 1982:35.

82. Nussenblatt RB, Palestine AG. Cyclosporine: immunology, pharmacology, and therapeutic uses. Surv Ophthalmol. 1986;31:159.

83. Bunjes D, Hardt C, Rollinghoff M, et al. Cyclosporin A mediates immunosuppression of primary cytotoxic T cell respones by impairing the release of interleukin 1 and interleukin 2. Eur J Immunol. 1981;11:657.

84. Kaufman Y, Chang AE, Robb RJ, et al. Mechanism of action of cyclosporin A: inhibition of lymphokine secretion studied with antigen-stimulated T-cell hybridomas. J Immunol. 1984;133:3107.

85. Bendtzen K, Dinarello CA. Mechanism of action of cyclosporine A. Scand J Immunol. 1984;20:43.

86. Nussenblatt RB, Palestine AG, Chan CC. Cyclosporin A therapy in the treatment of intraocular inflammatory disease resistant to systemic corticosteroids and cytotoxic agents. Am J Ophthalmol. 1983;96:275.

87. Nussenblatt RB, Palestine AG, Rook AH, et al. Treatment of intraocular inflammatory disease with cyclosporin A. Lancet. 1983;2:235.

88. Nussenblatt RB, Palestine AG, Chan CC. Cyclosporine therapy for uveitis: long-term follow-up. J Ocular Pharmacol. 1985;1:369.

89. Feutren G, Mihaatsch MJ. Risk factors for cyclosporine-induced nephropathy in patients with autoimmune diseases. International Kidney Biopsy Registry of Cyclosporine in Autoimmune Diseases. N Engl J Med. 1992;326:1654.

90. Austin HA III, Palestine AG, Sabnis SG, et al. Evolution of cyclosporin nephrotoxicity in patients treated for autoimmune uveitis. Am J Nephrol. 1989;9:392.

91. Mochizuki M, Ikeda E, Shirao M, et al. Preclinical and clinical study of FK506 in uveitis. Curr Eye Res. 1992;11(suppl):87.

92. Mochizuki M, Masuda K, Sakane T, et al. A clinical trial of FK506 in refractory uveitis. Am J Ophthalmol. 1993;115:763.

6
Surgical Treatments in Uveitis

General Information

Uncontrolled, chronic, or severe forms of uveitis often result in structural damage to the various intraocular tissues. Sequelae common to all forms of uveitis include glaucoma, synechiae, cataract, pupillary membranes, vitreous opacification, epiretinal membranes, subretinal neovascular membranes, macular edema and retinal detachment (Table 6.1). Many of these complications can be treated surgically.

In most situations, establishing a diagnosis, instituting proper medical therapy, and gaining control of the inflammation should precede elective surgery. The literature contains many accounts of failure and postoperative complications that developed after surgery performed on an eye with active uveitis. More urgent situations of uncontrolled glaucoma and retinal detachment are exceptions to this rule. Medically unresponsive forms of uveitis and patients with lens-induced uveitis may also require surgery without first gaining complete control of the inflammation.

Surgery in uveitis can be either diagnostic or therapeutic (Table 6.2). Diagnostic surgery is indicated when a patient presents with sight-threatening, medically unresponsive disease and the information gained will help direct therapy (Table 6.3). Often an infectious disease is suspected such as in endogenous endophthalmitis, chronic anaerobic endophthalmitis, or viral retinitis. In addition, patients suspected of having intraocular neoplasm, such as large cell lymphoma, benefit from diagnostic surgery. Paracentesis, vitrectomy, retinal biopsy, and chorioretinal biopsy are viable alternatives to diagnostic enucleation in these situations.

The goals of therapeutic surgery include visual rehabilitation, prevention of further loss of vision, and control of the inflammatory process. To achieve these goals, removal of band keratopathy, corneal transplantation, glaucoma surgery, cataract removal, vitrectomy, epiretinal membrane removal, pars plana cryopexy, repair of retinal detachment, and laser photocoagulation are commonly used procedures in patients with uveitis.

Surgical Challenges in the Patient with Uveitis

Although many of the sequelae of uveitis can be corrected by surgery, the procedures can be challenging and the outcomes are more uncertain in these patients. Surgeons are confronted with numerous intraoperative and postoperative concerns when caring for the patient with uveitis (Table 6.4).

Many eyes will have media opacities such as band keratopathy, corneal edema, synechiae, miotic pupils, cataract, and vitreous debris that compromise the surgeon's

Table 6.1. Complications of uveitis.

Corneal opacification
Glaucoma/hypotony
Iris neovascularization and synechiae
Cataract
Cyclitic and pupillary membranes
Vitreous opacification and membranes
Maculopathy—CME, epiretinal membranes, subretinal
  neovascular membranes
Retinal detachment

CME, cystoid macular edema.

Table 6.2. Indications for surgery in uveitis.

Diagnostic procedures—indications
Severe, sight-threatening disease
Medically unresponsive inflammation
When information can aid in diagnosis and alter
  therapy

Therapeutic procedures—indications
Media opacification with decreased vision
Medically unresponsive inflammation, CME, or
  glaucoma
Retinal detachment and epiretinal membrane
  formation

CME, cystoid macular edema.

Table 6.3. Surgical treatments.

Diagnostic surgical techniques
Paracentesis
Vitrectomy
Retinal or chorioretinal biopsy
Enucleation

Therapeutic surgical techniques
Cornea: Removal band keratopathy, penetrating
  keratoplasty, epikeratophakia
Angle/glaucoma: Synechialysis, iridotomy/
  iridectomy, filtration surgery, seton's,
  cyclodestructive procedures
Lens: ICCE, ECCE, ECCE-IOL, lensectomy, combined
  lensectomy-vitrectomy
Vitreous: Vitrectomy for vitreous opacification,
  traction, cyclitic membrane, hypotony, medically
  unresponsive disease, diagnosis, persistent CME,
  removal of epiretinal membranes
Retina: Retinal detachment repair, ablation or removal
  of subretinal neovascular membranes
Cryoretinopexy/laser photocoagulation: pars planitis,
  retinal neovascularization

ICCE, intracapsular cataract extraction; ECCE, extracapsular cataract extraction; IOL, intraocular lens;
CME, cystoid macular edema.

Table 6.4. Surgical challenges in uveitis.

Intraoperative
Band keratopathy
Miosis/synechiae/neovascularization
Glaucoma/hypotony/cyclitic membrane
Vitreous opacities
Retinal detachment, epiretinal membranes

Postoperative
IOL complications
Hemorrhage
Glaucoma
Activation of the uveitis or excessive surgical
  inflammation
Preexisting macular/retinal disease

IOL, intraocular lens.

view and access to tissues. Band keratopathy can be removed before intraocular procedures via chelation with sodium ethylenediamine-tetraacetic acid (EDTA) and gentle debridement. Corneal edema should be addressed preoperatively by lowering intraocular pressure and controlling inflammation as much as possible. Removal of the corneal epithelium, and in extreme cases penetrating keratoplasty or temporary keratoprosthesis, may be required prior to other procedures such as cataract extraction or retinal detachment repair. Cataract surgery and/or vitrectomy can be performed when opacification of the lens or vitreous limits the surgeon's view in the repair of posterior segment disorders. Patients with retinal detachment due to bilateral acute retinal necrosis (BARN) often require cataract removal and vitrectomy to permit repair of a necrotic and detached retina.

Posterior synechiae and miotic pupils often need to be addressed intraoperatively. In some cases, synechialysis can be performed directly using the cyclodialysis spatula. A gentle sweeping motion through an open area under the iris often can break these adhesions and allow iris dilation. In more chronic cases, the lysis of adhesions alone does not allow for adequate iris dilation. Bimanual techniques using a hand-held iris hook can open segments of the pupil during cataract extraction. In other situations, translimbal, Silastic iris hooks can be used to retract the iris mechanically. Often pupiloplasty, sphincterotomy, marginal iridectomy, or even sector iridectomy can be performed to provide an improved surgical field. Iris bleeding, which is common in uveitis, usually can be stopped by temporarily increasing the intraocular pressure. Intraocular diathermy may be needed in patients with severe anterior segment neovascularization.

The postoperative course can be equally demanding. Patients with inflamed and congested eyes will experience more hemorrhage postoperatively. Elevation of the intraocular pressure is common as a result of marked synechiae, fibrin formation, and bleeding.

The most common postoperative problem is excessive inflammation. Instituting measures to control perioperative inflammation is critical (Table 6.5). First, all cellular activity should be eliminated before surgery. Once the appropriate medical regimen has been established, the level of therapy should be increased the week before surgery. This often requires doubling the topical drops or pulsing the patient with increased oral prednisone. In certain conditions, periocular steroids also can be given preoperatively.

The surgical procedure should be as

Table 6.5. Perioperative management considerations.

Preoperative diagnosis and control of inflammation
   NSAID
   Steroids—topical, regional, oral
   Second-generation immunosuppressives
Intraoperative control of inflammation
   Intraocular dexamethasone (300–400 μg/0.1 ml)
   Sub-Tenon's triamcinolone (40 mg/1 ml)
Postoperative control of inflammation

NSAID, nonsteroidal anti-inflammatory drug.

atraumatic as possible to minimize surgical injury. In most cases, periocular corticosteroid (40 mg triamcinolone) and intraocular dexamethasone (400 μg/0.1 ml) are given at the end of the procedure. Regional corticosteroids should be used with caution in infectious forms of uveitis. Topical and oral medications are continued postoperatively, often at an increased dose, and tapered according to the clinical course.

Postoperative visual acuity is often limited by preexisting optic nerve damage or macular disease. Cystoid macular edema (CME), epiretinal membranes, fixed macular cysts, macular hole formation, and scarring in the posterior pole are common findings in patients with uveitis.

Surgical Procedures and Considerations in Uveitis

Apprenticeship during medical school, internship, residency and fellowship, and surgical textbooks provide the basic information, skills, and experience necessary to perform ocular surgery. This section addresses only the unique aspects of surgery in the uveitis patient.

Corneal Surgery

Band keratopathy may occur in any form of chronic uveitis such as juvenile rheumatoid arthritis (JRA) and sarcoidosis. It can be removed via debridement of the epithelium and either mechanical scraping or Na-EDTA chelation of the calcium from Bowman's layer with 0.37% solution of Na-EDTA.[1,2] The goal of surgery is to remove the opacity and restore a smooth corneal surface. Superficial keratotomy and diamond burr removal can also be considered in difficult cases.[3,4] Care should be taken to avoid vigorous scraping and subsequent subepithelial scar formation.

Corneal edema may occur rarely as a result of active intraocular inflammation. It can often be treated medically by controlling the uveitis. Persistent edema and corneal scarring from herpetic keratouveitis often require penetrating keratoplasty.[5] Patients who undergo these high-risk transplantations require frequent treatment with antiviral drugs and topical corticosteroids for recurrent disease.[6] It is often difficult to distinguish a rejection episode from a flareup of the underlying uveitis. Aggressive anti-inflammatory therapy is required in both situations to prevent graft failure.

Glaucoma Surgery

Secondary forms of glaucoma are common in uveitis and can occur in 20% to 50% of patients. Fuchs' heterochromic iridocyclitis, JRA-associated iridocyclitis, herpetic keratouveitis, lens-induced uveitis, and toxoplasmosis are often associated with elevated intraocular pressure.[7,8] The filtration angle can be compromised by inflammatory cells, fibrin, granuloma, synechiae, scarring, and steroid-induced mechanisms. Pressure elevation may occur as a result of effective anti-inflammatory therapy and the resulting increased aqueous humor production.

In the patient with glaucoma and active uveitis, therapy should begin with measures aimed at controlling the inflammation. Topical, regional, and oral corticosteroids may be used. The intraocular pressure often may respond to this therapy alone. Aggressive anti-inflammatory therapy will also improve the chances of filtration bleb survival if the patient requires glaucoma surgery.

Much of the armamentarium used to treat glaucoma is ineffective or cannot be used effectively in the patient with uveitis. Pilocarpine and epinephrine agents compromise the blood–eye barrier and promote further intraocular inflammation. Laser iridotomy sites used to correct angle closure from pupillary block and seclusion from extensive posterior synechiae, frequently close because of marked fibrin formation, bleeding, and postsurgical inflam-

mation. Laser trabeculoplasty has not been effective in patients with uveitis and open-angle glaucoma.[9,10] Laser trabeculoplasty can aggravate the uveitis and promote further anterior synechiae and may be associated with a dramatic rise in postoperative pressure. When laser surgery is performed, aggressive perioperative topical corticosteroids should be used to minimize these complications.

Patients who fail medical therapy with beta blockers and oral carbonic anhydrase inhibitors often require filtration surgery, seton procedures, or cycloablation. Perioperative control of inflammation is critical in these high-risk patients. Topical corticosteroids, periocular triamcinolone, oral prednisone, and intraocular dexamethasone (400 μg/0.1 ml) should be used aggressively. Antimitotic agents such as mitomycin C and 5-fluorouracil should be considered to reduce bleb failure in these high-risk patients.[11] Intraocular tissue plasminogen-activator factor (tPA) has been used to clear excessive fibrin formation after glaucoma surgery to ensure continued bleb function.

Seton procedures are associated with a higher failure rate in this group of patients because of increased bleeding and excessive fibrin and inflammatory membrane formation.[12] Cyclodestructive procedures via cyclocryopexy or endolaser ablation can be performed but are associated with significant postoperative inflammation. These eyes require aggressive attention to inflammation and should receive periocular corticosteroids and intraocular dexamethasone during surgery. Postoperative topical and oral corticosteroids also are necessary in these patients.

Cataract Surgery

Cataracts, a common complication of uveitis, can occur in up to 50% of patients.[13] Free radical formation, nutritional deprivation, hypoxia, inflammatory medications, and corticosteroid-induced mechanisms can all play a role in their formation. Cataracts can be removed by several techniques. Pars plana lensectomy, pars plana endocapsular extraction, phacoemulsification, and extracapsular (ECCE) and intracapsular (ICCE) techniques have specific advantages and disadvantages in the patient with uveitis. Often, cataract surgery is combined with other surgical procedures such as glaucoma surgery, therapeutic vitrectomy, or other vitreoretinal operations.

Indications for cataract removal are more exacting in patients with uveitis.[14-16] Because of the higher surgical risks, visual acuity is often worse than 20/40 at the time of cataract removal. The ideal patient should have inactive disease or complete control of the uveitis before elective cataract surgery. The longer this period of inactivity, the better the chances for success. At a minimum, the patient should have no cellular activity for 6 to 8 weeks before elective surgery.

More controversial is the use of intraocular lenses (IOLs). Few large, well-controlled studies have been performed. It is difficult to control the numerous variables in uveitis, including specific etiology (JRA vs. Fuchs' heterochromia), stage of disease (acute vs. burned out), medical therapy (topical vs. chemotherapy), and surgical philosophies and techniques. The long-term placement of a prosthesis in an eye with chronic or recurrent inflammation has been considered a contraindication. Only recently have IOLs been implanted in selected patients with varying degrees of success. Better surgical techniques, implant design, and meticulous attention to control of the uveitis have reduced IOL-associated complications in the patient with uveitis. The short-term benefit of IOL implantation must be weighed against the increased risk during surgery and the long-term complications that arise in relatively young patients with recurrent or chronic ocular inflammation. Over time, the complication

rate will likely increase in patients with intraocular prostheses and chronic uveitis.

Anterior chamber, iris fixated, and ciliary sulcus–placed lenses should be avoided in patients with a history of uveitis. Direct, mechanical irritation of the iris and ciliary body will result in medically unresponsive inflammation, hyphema, and persistent CME; therefore, surgical aphakia and contact lens or spectacle correction should be used in these situations.

In well-selected patients, IOLs should be placed in the posterior chamber within the capsular bag (Table 6.6).[13,17] All polymethylmethacrylate (PMMA) lenses have a theoretical advantage of activating the complement system less than prolene-looped implants.

High-risk patients appear to be those without complete control of the uveitis or patients with expected recurrent or chronic disease.[13] Patients with systemic diseases such as JRA and sarcoidosis are at much higher risk for IOL complications than those with local ocular diseases such as Fuchs' heterochromic iridocyclitis and idiopathic iridocyclitis.[15,18] Posterior forms of uveitis such as histoplasmosis, acute posterior multifocal placoid pigment epitheliopathy (APMPPE), and acute retinal pigment epitheliitis (ARPE) would obviously have a better prognosis than those with anterior inflammation involving the iris and ciliary body. Forms of uveitis such as Fuchs' heterochromia, which are not associated with marked synechiae formation, respond better than "sticky" forms of uveitis.

Table 6.6. Indications for cataract extraction and IOL in patients with history of uveitis.

Inactive or controlled disease
Local ocular diseases: Fuchs' heterochromia, pars planitis
Minimal synechiae: Fuchs' heterochromia
Minor anterior inflammation: histoplasmosis, APMPPE
Absence of vitreoretinal involvement

IOL, intraocular lens; APMPPE, acute posterior multifocal placoid pigment epitheliopathy.

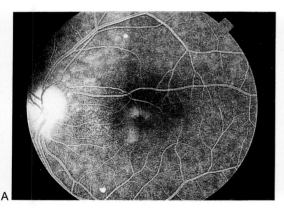
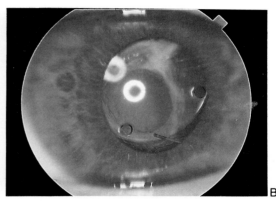

Figure 6.1. Intraocular lens implantation— postoperative uveitis. Intraocular lens implantation in a patient with a past history of anterior uveitis before development of a posterior subcapsular cataract. The uveitis had been quiet for 10 years, and the patient was otherwise healthy before surgery. **A:** The postoperative course was complicated by a return of the anterior uveitis and cystoid macular edema. The inflammation was treated with an 18-month course of topical and regional corticosteroids. **B:** The capsule demonstrates some cocooning and decentration of the intraocular lens.

Even in the ideal patient, IOL implantation carries a higher risk for postoperative complications.[19] Synechiae formation to the IOL, IOL precipitates and fibrin deposition, pupillary membranes, implant decentration, cocooning of the capsular bag, cyclitic membrane formation, recurrence capsular opacification, recurrent inflammation, and persistent CME can occur (Fig. 6.1). Although many of these complications can be managed, explantation of the IOL ultimately may be required.

Pars plana lensectomy and adjunctive vitrectomy should be considered in several clinical situations (Table 6.7).[20–27] Patients with chronic, systemic disorders (e.g., JRA, sarcoidosis), lens-induced uveitis, uveitis with recurrent activity involving the iris and ciliary body, and forms of uveitis with a propensity to form inflammatory membranes and synechiae can often be approached via pars plana techniques. Patients with marked vitreous opacification, retinal pathology, medically unresponsive uveitis, persistent CME, and cyclitic membrane formation will also benefit from vitrectomy and lensectomy procedures. Vitrectomy can be combined with planned ECCE to provide for secondary IOL implantation. It also is often possible to preserve the posterior capsule during pars plana endocapsular lensectomy techniques for secondary IOL implantation as well.

Table 6.7. Indications for pars plana vitrectomy/lensectomy in uveitis.

Lenticular and vitreous opacification
Medically unresponsive inflammation or CME
Cataract and uveitis with:
  Chronic or recurrent activity (JRA, HLA-B27)
  Vitreous debris and/or retinal involvement
  Systemic disease (Behçet's disease, sarcoidosis)
  Severe anterior segment or diffuse inflammation
  Marked synechia formation
  Granulomatous diseases (VKH syndrome, sympathetic ophthalmia)
Lens-induced uveitis
Hypotony with cyclitic membrane

JRA, juvenile rheumatoid arthritis; HLA, human leukocyte antigen; VKH, Vogt-Koyanagi-Harada; CME, cystoid macular edema.

Vitreous Surgery

Pars plana vitrectomy can be helpful in managing several of the complications encountered in uveitis[21-27] (Table 6.7). Vitrectomy surgery can remove vitreous opacities and inflammatory membranes. Removal of the vitreous can often moderate the course of the uveitis and help control medically unresponsive CME. Vitrectomy can be combined with synechialysis, removal of cyclitic and pupillary membranes, and endocapsular lensectomy. Epiretinal membranes can be stripped and internal techniques can be used to repair the often complex retinal detachments associated with severe intraocular inflammation. As mentioned earlier, pars plana lensectomy and vitrectomy is the treatment of choice for cataract and uveitis in patients with certain diseases, such as JRA.

It is unclear how vitrectomy helps moderate uveitis and medically unresponsive forms of CME.[13] It may remove immunocompetent cells or certain autoantigens from the eye such as immunoreactive type II collagen, which is found in the vitreous. The procedure may also change the immunologic milieu of the eye. Converting the eye to a unicameral condition may allow a more immunosuppressive environment to evolve.[31]

Traction on the ciliary body and retina from inflammatory membranes may result in chronic hypotony and CME. Vitrectomy surgery can remove these membranes, thus improving visual prognosis.

Retinal Surgery

Retinal detachment, epiretinal membranes, retinal edema, scarring, retinal ischemia and neovascularization, and subretinal neovascular membrane formation are common complications of uveitis.[32,33] Many of these sequelae can be treated by laser or vitreoretinal surgical techniques. As with anterior segment surgery, active inflammation, media opacities, synechiae, and miosis often challenge the vitreoretinal surgeon. Medical and surgical measures that address these problems can improve the postoperative course.

Laser photocoagulation techniques can be used to repair retinal tears and limit retinal detachments resulting from inflammation and vitreous traction in diseases such as acute retinal necrosis (ARN) syndrome/BARN, toxoplasmosis, and pars planitis. Peripheral retinal neovascularization and secondary vitreous hemorrhage may occur as a result of vaso-occlusion and retinal ischemia in diseases such as systemic lupus erythematosus (SLE) and sarcoidosis. Panretinal photocoagulation can reduce retinal ischemia and cause regression of the retinal neovascularization. Subretinal neovascular membranes have been reported in many forms of posterior uveitis including birdshot retinochoroidopathy, presumed ocular histoplasmosis, Vogt-Koyanagi-Haradas (VKH) syndrome, sympathetic ophthalmia, and tuberculosis. Extrafoveal or juxtafoveal lesions can be directly ablated with laser photocoagulation. Choroiditis may be aggravated by laser therapy, thereby promoting further neovascularization. Controlling the underlying uveitis is essential to treating these membranes successfully.

Vitrectomy can be performed to remove transvitreal, epiretinal, and subretinal membranes. Macular pucker and traction macular detachments can be repaired by delamination and en bloc membrane peeling. New techniques have been developed to permit the removal of submacular scars and neovascular tissue commonly found in patients with histoplasmosis.[34]

Retinal detachment is common in patients with uveitis and may occur in 50% to 75% of certain disorders.[35,36] Successful repair is often compromised by the presence of media opacification, vitreous traction, multiple and posterior tears, retinal necrosis, and subretinal exudation. Scleral buckle, vitrectomy, membranectomy, endolaser photocoagulation, cryoretinopexy,

air/fluid exchanges, retinotomy, retinec-
tomy, and the use of vitreous substitutes
such as silicone oil may be necessary to repair these detachments. Scleral buckle surgery is often impossible in certain settings
and internal approaches via pars plana surgery is often used.[37,38]

Pars plana cryopexy can be performed in
patients with intermediate uveitis.[39] This
procedure can help control medically unresponsive disease and neovascularization of
the vitreous base. The mechanism of action
of pars plana cryopexy is not well understood. It may help reestablish the blood–
eye barrier, delete clones of immunocompetent lymphocytes, or ablate ischemic tissue.
A double freeze-thaw cycle is delivered to
the area of inflammatory debris in the pars
plana. Most patients will have a decrease in
the vitreous base neovascularization and a
moderation of the vitritis and CME.

References

1. Grant WM. New treatment for calcific corneal opacity. *Arch Ophthalmol.* 195;46:681.
2. Breinin GM, DeVoe AG. Chelation of calcium with EDTA in band keratopathy and
corneal calcium affections. *Arch Ophthalmol.*
1954;52:846.
3. Wood TO, Walker GG. Treatment of band
keratopathy. *Am J Ophthalmol.* 1975;80:553.
4. Bokosky JE, Meyer RF, Sugar A. Surgical
treatment of calcific band keratopathy. *Ophthalmic Surg.* 1965;16:645.
5. Michelson JB, Nozik RA. Corneal disease
and surgery associated with uveitis. In: *Surgical Treatment of Ocular Inflammatory Disease.*
Philadelphia: JB Lippincott; 1988.
6. Liesegang TJ. Corneal complications from
herpes zoster ophthalmicus. *Ophthalmology.*
1985;92:316.
7. Panek WC, Holland GN. Glaucoma in patients with uveitis. *Br J Ophthalmol.* 1990;74:
223.
8. Smith RE, Nozik RA. Glaucoma in patients
with uveitis. In: *Uveitis: A Clinical Approach
to Diagnosis and Management.* 2nd ed. Baltimore: Williams & Wilkins; 1989.
9. Lieberman MF, Hoskins HD, Hetherington J.
Laser trabeculoplasty and the glaucomas.
Ophthalmology. 1983;90:790.
10. Robin AL, Pollack IP. Argon laser trabeculoplasty in secondary forms of open-angle
glaucoma. *Arch Ophthalmol.* 1983;3:382.
11. Patitsas CJ, Rockwood EJ, Meisler DM,
Lowder CY. Glaucoma filtering surgery
with postoperative 5-fluorouracil in patients
with intraocular inflammatory disease. *Ophthalmology.* 1992;99:594.
12. Hill RA, Nguyen QH, Baerveldt G, et al.
Trabeculectomy and Molteno implantation
for glaucomas associated with uveitis. *Ophthalmology.* 1993;100:903.
13. Hooper PL, Narsing AE, Smith RE. Cataract
extraction in uveitis patients. *Surv Ophthalmol.* 1990;35:120.
14. Duke-Elder S. Cataracta complicata. In: *System of Ophthalmology, Vol. 11, Diseases of the
Lens and Vitreous; Glaucoma and Hypotony.*
St. Louis: CV Mosby; 1969:210.
15. Smiley WK. The eye in juvenile rheumatoid
arthritis. *Trans Ophthalmol Soc UK.* 1974;94:
817.
16. Wolf MD, Lichter PR, Ragsdale CG. Prognostic factors in the uveitis of juvenile rheumatoid arthritis. *Ophthalmology.* 1987;94:
1242.
17. Foster CS, Fong LP, Singh G. Cataract surgery and intraocular lens implantation in
patients with uveitis. *Ophthalmology.* 1989;
96:281.
18. Kanski JJ, Shun-Shin GA. Systemic uveitis
syndromes in childhood: an analysis of 340
cases. *Ophthalmology.* 1984;91:1247.
19. Michelson JB, Friedlaender MH, Nozik RA.
Lens implant surgery in pars planitis. *Ophthalmology.* 1990;97:1023.
20. Algvere P, Alanko H, Dickhoff K, et al. Pars
plana vitrectomy in the management of intraocular inflammation. *Acta Ophthalmol.*
1981;59:727.
21. Dangel ME, Stark WJ, Michels RG. Surgical
management of cataract associated with
chronic uveitis. *Ophthalmic Surg.* 1983;14:
145.
22. Diamond JG, Kaplan HJ. Uveitis: effect of
vitrectomy combined with lensectomy. *Ophthalmology.* 1979;86:1320.
23. Diamond JG, Kaplan HJ. Lensectomy and
vitrectomy for complicated cataract secondary to uveitis. *Arch Ophthalmol.* 1978;96:1798.
24. Fitzgerald CR. Pars plana vitrectomy for
vitreous opacity secondary to presume toxoplasmosis. *Arch Ophthalmol.* 1980;98:321.
25. Girard LJ, Rodriguez J, Mailman ML, Ro-

mano TJ. Cataract and uveitis management by pars plana lensectomy and vitrectomy by ultrasonic fragmentation. *Retina*. 1985;5: 107.

26. Girard LJ. Managing cataracts in patients with uveitis (letter to the editor). *Ophthalmology*. 1989;96:1574.

27. Nobe JR, Kokoris D, Diddie KR, et al. Lensectomy: vitrectomy in chronic uveitis. *Retina*. 1983;3:71.

28. Green WF. Diagnostic cytopathology of ocular fluid specimens. *Ophthalmology*. 1984;91: 726.

29. Davis JL, Solomon D, Nussenblatt RB, et al. Immunocytochemical staining of vitreous cells. *Ophthalmology*. 1992;99:250.

30. Stulting RD, Leif RC, Clarkson JG, Bobbitt D. Centrifugal cytology of ocular fluids. *Arch Ophthalmol*. 1982;100:822.

31. Streilein JW. Anterior chamber associated immune deviation: the privilege of immunity in the eye. *Surv Ophthalmol*. 1990;35:67.

32. Smith RE, Nozik RA. Retinal detachment and uveitis. In: *Uveitis: A Clinical Approach to Diagnosis and Management*. 2nd ed. Baltimore: Williams & Wilkins; 1989.

33. Nussenblatt RB, Palestine AL. Surgical treatment in uveitis. In: *Uveitis: Fundamentals and Clinical Practice*. Chicago: Year Book Medical Publishers; 1989.

34. Thomas MQ, Grand MG, Williams DF, et al. Surgical management of subfoveal choroidal neovascularization. *Ophthalmology*. 1992;99: 952.

35. Schepens CL. *Retinal Detachment and Allied Diseases*, vol. 2. Philadelphia: WB Saunders; 1983.

36. Clarkson JG, Blumenkranz MS, Culbertson WW, et al. Retinal detachment following the acute retinal necrosis syndrome. *Ophthalmology*. 1984;91:1665.

37. Jabs DA, Enger C, Haller J, de Bustros S. Retinal detachments in patients with cytomegalovirus retinitis. *Arch Ophthalmol*. 1991; 109:794.

38. Freeman WR, Henderly DE, Wan WL, et al. Prevalence, pathophysiology, and treatment of rhegmatogenous retinal detachment in treated cytomegalovirus retinitis. *Am J Ophthalmol*. 1987;103:527.

39. Aaberg TM, Cesarz TJ, Flikinger RR. Treatment of peripheral uveoretinitis by cryotherapy. *Am J Ophthalmol*. 1973;75:685.

Ocular Inflammation Associated with Trauma

7
Traumatic Uveitis

Nonsurgical Trauma

Tissue injury resulting from nonsurgical trauma can produce an exogenous form of ocular inflammation.

Etiology

Cell injury or death can occur after many forms of trauma. Blunt contusion, penetrating and perforating wounds, chemical exposure, and electrical and radiation injury can all cause tissue damage[1-6] (Table 7.1). Certain intraocular metallic foreign bodies (e.g., iron, lead, copper) are toxic and can cause chronic inflammation.[7]

Epidemiology

Nonpenetrating ocular trauma may account for up to 5% of uveitis cases seen at tertiary referral centers.[8] There is no racial predilection. Men are affected more often than women because of occupational exposure and life-style differences.

Pathogenesis

Trauma results in compromise of the normal blood–eye barriers from mechanical injury to the vascular endothelium, non-pigmented ciliary epithelium, and retinal pigment epithelium.[8,9] Serum proteins and leukocytes gain access to the eye, resulting in flare, fibrin formation, and the presence of inflammatory cells.

Injured tissues release arachidonic acid and, in the presence of cyclooxygenase, form prostaglandins and thromboxane. Leukotrienes and hydroperoxy-eicosatetra-enoic acids (HPETES) are generated from arachidonic acid via the lipoxygenase pathway. These arachidonic acid metabolites further promote an inflammatory response and recruit white blood cells to the site of injury for the repair process.[8,9]

Intraocular foreign bodies such as glass, gold, silver, and plastic are well tolerated in the eye. If retained, these materials rarely incite inflammation. Iron, copper, zinc, and lead, however, are toxic and can promote further injury and often chronic or severe inflammation.

Clinical Presentation

General physical examination often supports the diagnosis through other signs of trauma such as facial bruising, burns, localized swelling, or lacerations. Ocular examination verifies the nature of the trauma. Chemical, radiation, or electrical burns may be noted on the conjunctiva and cornea. Corneoscleral lacerations or occult globe rupture may occur after sharp or blunt trauma. Flare, fibrin and inflammatory cells can be seen in the anterior chamber and vitreous cavity. Hyphema and vitreous hemorrhage may be present. The angle structures may be damaged with angle recession or cyclodialysis. A Vossius pigment ring is

Table 7.1. Common causes of traumatic uveitis.

Contusion
Penetration/perforation of the globe
Chemical exposure
Electrical injury
Radiation
Foreign body

Diagnosis

The diagnosis is made on clinical grounds in most cases. The history, physical examination, and ocular examination support the diagnosis. Ultrasonography and radiologic studies should be performed when the presence of a retained intraocular foreign body is suspected.

Differential Diagnosis

Bacterial or fungal endophthalmitis, which may result from perforating or penetrating injuries and from contaminated intraocular foreign bodies, causes severe pain and profound loss of vision.[4,7] Marked lid edema, chemosis, hypopyon, and medically unresponsive inflammation are also indicators of a secondary endophthalmitis. Anterior chamber and vitreous aspirate for microbial cultures should be performed in this clinical setting.

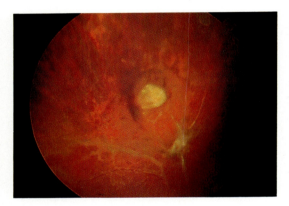

Figure 7.1. Traumatic uveitis—nonsurgical trauma. Medically unresponsive, nongranulomatous, diffuse uveitis and retinal vasculitis in a patient with a retained, iron-containing, intraocular foreign body. The hypopigmented scar is the impact site. Note the posterior vitreous cell and retinal vasculitis. Scleral depression and ultrasound examination demonstrated the presence of the metallic foreign body in the inferior vitreous base.

Treatment

The first goals in treating uveitis associated with nonsurgical trauma are removing the noxious stimuli and assisting with tissue repair. To achieve these goals the clinician may rinse chemical material from the cul-de-sac, repair a laceration, or remove a foreign body. In most injuries such as contusion, penetrating wounds, and electrical or radiation burns, the tissue damage is completed by the time of the ophthalmic examination.

Posttraumatic inflammation can be treated with topical nonsteroidal anti-inflammatory drugs (NSAIDs) and corticosteroid preparations.[8] Mydriasis and cycloplegia help prevent synechia formation and control ocular pain. Systemic or regional corticosteroids may be required in severe trauma or to assist in control of retinal vasculitis, edema, or choroidal effusions. Prophylactic, broad-spectrum topical and oral antibiotics can be prescribed if there is

often noted on the anterior lens capsule from impact with the pigmented iris epithelium. Deeper injuries from radiation burns and retained intraocular foreign bodies often result in secondary retinal vasculitis (Fig. 7.1). Retinal commotio, retinal tears, choroidal detachments, and ruptures may be noted in severe blunt trauma. Intraocular foreign bodies may be noted on biomicroscopic or dilated fundus examination.

risk for infection. Clindamycin should be considered to address anaerobic bacteria frequently isolated in traumatic forms of endophthalmitis.

Prognosis

Visual outcome after trauma is unpredictable. The prognosis is often established at the time of the injury.[4,6,8] Sharp injuries carry the best prognosis. Severe blunt trauma and injury to the optic nerve and retina, including the retina, have a worse prognosis. Cataract formation and corneal scars may be amenable to surgical correction.

Inflammation after trauma is usually self-limiting. It can be medically controlled until the blood–eye barriers are reestablished. Perforating and penetrating injuries have a risk of developing sympathetic ophthalmia (1.9 cases/1000 injuries).

Surgical Trauma and Postoperative Inflammation

Surgical injury to ocular tissues may result in postoperative inflammation.

Etiology

Laser or standard surgical procedures cause tissue damage. The location and amount of trauma are presumably more controlled and less extensive than in nonsurgical trauma. Both standard and laser surgery are designed to enter or address parts of the eye that are "inert," such as the surgical limbus or the pars plana region.

Epidemiology

Any invasive surgical procedure, including laser therapy, produces tissue injury and damage.[10–17] Cataract surgery, retinal detachment repair, laser capsulotomy, argon laser trabeculoplasty, and panretinal photo-coagulation are all accompanied by postoperative uveitis.

Pathogenesis

The mechanism of inflammation is similar to that of nonsurgical trauma.[8,9,17] Damage to the blood–eye barrier and injury to ocular cells result in a nonspecific inflammatory response.

Clinical Presentation

Typically, postsurgical inflammation is accompanied by little pain. Vision can be relatively good. Conjunctival hyperemia and cell and flare can be noted in the anterior chamber and vitreous cavity. Cystoid macular edema (CME) may occur after any surgical procedure as a result of this low-grade inflammation.[10,11,17]

Diagnosis

The diagnosis is made on clinical grounds. Fluorescein angiography can help establish the presence and degree of CME in certain settings.[17]

Differential Diagnosis

The differential diagnosis for severe, chronic, or medically unresponsive postoperative inflammation is often a diagnostic challenge (Table 7.2). Poorly fitted or positioned

Table 7.2. Differential diagnosis for postoperative inflammation.

Surgical trauma
IOL-associated UGH syndrome
Lens-induced uveitis
Acute endophthalmitis
Chronic anaerobic endophthalmitis
Preexisting uveitis
Sympathetic ophthalmia

IOL, intraocular lens; UGH, uveitis, glaucoma, and hemorrhage.

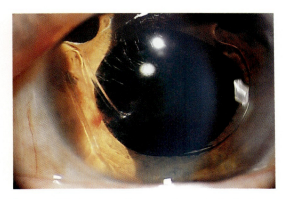

Figure 7.2. Traumatic uveitis—surgical. Uveitis, glaucoma, and hemorrhage in a patient after cataract surgery and placement of an anterior chamber intraocular lens. The patient had 20/400 visual acuity due to medically unresponsive CME. The intraocular lens was explanted, with resolution of the inflammation and cystoid macular edema. Vision returned to 20/25 with an aphakic contact lens.

intraocular lenses can promote chronic inflammation. Anterior chamber, iris-fixated, or ciliary sulcus–located lenses may mechanically irritate the iris and ciliary body. Uveitis, glaucoma, and hemorrhage may occur and has been called the UGH syndrome (Fig. 7.2). Biomicroscopic examination can establish the diagnosis. Often, the intraocular lens needs to be exchanged or explanted.

Retained nuclear material or large amounts of lens cortex can result in a true autoimmune, lens-induced uveitis following cataract surgery (see Chapter 17). Lens remnants can be seen on ophthalmic examination. The diagnosis may be challenging when only small amounts of lens material are present. Anterior chamber and vitreous biopsy help establish the diagnosis through characteristic cytology. Macrophages containing periodic acid–Schiff (PAS)-positive lens material are seen in this disorder.

Postoperative endophthalmitis and chronic anaerobic endophthalmitis also should be considered in the differential diagnosis of postsurgical inflammation. In contrast to postsurgical uveitis, bacterial endophthalmitis (see Chapter 20) is typically associated with severe pain and profound loss of vision.

Chronic anaerobic endophthalmitis is a more indolent process (Chapter 20.2). The eye may be comfortable and have keratic precipitates. Cellular reaction is moderate. The inflammation may be controlled initially with topical corticosteroids but will characteristically return with each taper. Diagnostic aqueous and vitreous biopsy is required to establish the diagnosis.

An important consideration is the presence of an unrecognized, preexisting systemic or ocular inflammatory disease. An underlying uveitis may be the source for persistent or excessive inflammation after ocular surgery. A low-grade or recurrent uveitis may have been the cause for the cataract, glaucoma, or retinal detachment. Surgical trauma may then trigger an exacerbation of the uveitis. Clues to this diagnosis can often be found by examining the contralateral eye. It may show subtle signs of prior inflammation, indicating chronic bilateral disease. As mentioned earlier, sympathetic ophthalmia may occur after surgical (1/10,000 cases) or nonsurgical (1.9/1000 cases) trauma and is discussed further in Chapter 19.

Treatment

The surgeon should strive to minimize postoperative inflammation by limiting the amount of tissue manipulation or destruction during surgery. Proper tissue apposition can further promote wound healing. Suture material should be nontoxic. Intraocular prostheses that are composed of inert material, such as silicon or polymethylmethacrylate (PMMA), should be used.

Treatment of mild postsurgical inflammation is with topical corticosteroids and cycloplegic agents. Prednisolone acetate 1%, four times a day, will control most cases. Aggressive topical, regional, and oral corticosteroids can help eliminate the low-grade inflammation associated with postoperative CME. Oral and topical NSAIDs may also be beneficial in treating postsurgical CME. CME that is resistant to topical therapy may respond to 40 mg triamcinolone given in the sub-Tenon space, either alone or with adjunctive oral NSAIDs.

Prognosis

Postoperative inflammation is typically mild and self-limiting. It responds well to topical corticosteroids and cycloplegic agents. The prognosis is good in most cases. As discussed in Chapter 5, if chronic CME develops, it may limit visual acuity.

References

1. Greenwald MJ, Weiss A, Oesterle CS, Friendly DS. Traumatic retinoschisis in battered babies. *Ophthalmology.* 1986;93:618.
2. Grizzard WS, Kirk NM, Pavan PR, et al. Perforating ocular injuries caused by anesthesia personnel. *Ophthalmology.* 1991;98:1011.
3. Martin DF, Meredith TA, Topping TM, et al. Perforating (through-and-through) injuries of the globe: surgical results with vitrectomy. *Arch Ophthalmol.* 1991;109:951.
4. Sternberg P Jr, de Juan E Jr, Michels RG, Auer C. Multivariate analysis of prognostic factors in penetrating ocular injuries. *Am J Ophthalmol.* 1984;98:467.
5. Tilden M, Rosenbaum JT, Fraunfelder FT. Systemic sulfonamides as a cause of bilateral, anterior uveitis. *Arch Ophthalmol.* 1991;109:67.
6. Opremcak EM, Davidorf FH. Bilateral retinal infarction associated with high dose dopamine. *Ann Ophthalmol.* 1985;17:141.
7. Williams DF, Mieler WF, Abrams GW, Lewis H. Results and prognostic factors in penetrating ocular injuries with retained intraocular foreign bodies. *Ophthalmology.* 1988;95: 911.
8. Rosenbaum JT, Tammaro J, Robertson JE Jr. Uveitis precipitated by nonpenetrating ocular trauma. *Am J Ophthalmol.* 1991;112:392.
9. Makley TA, Opremcak EM. Foreign protein shock therapy in ophthalmology. *J Toxicol Cutan Ocular Toxicol.* 1991;10:27.
10. Yannuzzi LA. A perspective on the treatment of aphakic cystoid macular edema. *Surv Ophthalmol.* 1984;28(suppl):540.
11. Jampol LM. Pharmacologic therapy of aphakic and pseudophakic cystoid macular edema. *Ophthalmology.* 1985;92:807.
12. Karcioglu ZA, Aran AJ, Holmes DL, et al. Inflammation due to surgical glove powders in the rabbit eye. *Arch Ophthalmol.* 1988;106: 808.
13. Bellows AR, Grant WM. Cyclocryotherapy of chronic open-angle glaucoma in aphakic eyes. *Am J Ophthalmol.* 1978;85:615.
14. Foster CS, Fong CP, Singh G. Cataract surgery and intraocular lens implantation in patients with uveitis. *Ophthalmology.* 1989;96: 281.
15. Hampton C, Shields MB, Miller KN, Blasini M. Evaluation of a protocol for transscleral neodymium:YAG cyclophotocoagulation in one hundred patients. *Ophthalmology.* 1990; 97:910.
16. Swartz M. Histology of macular photocoagulation. *Ophthalmology.* 1986;93:959.
17. Cunha-Vaz JG, Travassos A. Breakdown of the blood-retinal barriers and cystoid macular edema. *Surv Ophthalmol.* 1984;28(suppl): 485.

Ocular Inflammation Associated with Infectious Diseases

8
Viral Diseases

Viruses are infectious agents that contain either RNA or DNA. Although they cause a wide variety of disorders systemically, in the eye, viruses may cause keratitis, uveitis, and retinitis.

Viral Diseases Associated with Keratouveitis

Herpes Simplex

Herpes simplex virus (HSV) is a common human pathogen capable of causing a recurrent infectious keratouveitis.

Etiology

HSV is an alphaherpesvirus within the Herpesvirinea family.[1] It is an encapsulated, double-stranded DNA virus (150–200 nm) with an icosahedral nucleocapsid. There are two types of HSV: herpes simplex type 1 (HSV-1) and herpes simplex type 2 (HSV-2).

Epidemiology

HSV-1 and HSV-2 are common human pathogens with worldwide distribution.[1,2] Approximately 500,000 cases of HSV keratouveitis cases are reported per year, with a prevalence of 149 cases per 100,000 population.[3]

Pathogenesis

During primary infection, the HSV capsule fuses with the cell membranes.[1,2] The viral DNA becomes incorporated in the host DNA, resulting in both active and latent viral infection. Localized disease occurs at the site of inoculation. HSV is neurotropic and establishes a latent infection within ganglion cells. Recurrent ocular infection occurs in 25% to 70% of patients.[4,5]

Clinical Presentation

Primary HSV-1 ocular infections occur as a result of contact with a patient shedding virus from oral secretion. This route of infection may occur through kissing on the face and around the eye. HSV-2 ocular infections occur as a result of direct contact with infectious vesicles during childbirth. Primary HSV infection typically results in a vesicular blepharitis or conjunctivitis with minimal corneal disease. Recurrent HSV-1 disease can result in active epithelial disease, stromal keratitis, and/or iridocyclitis.

Recurrent herpetic keratouveitis is painful and is associated with marked photophobia.[6,7] The disease is unilateral, often reducing vision and increasing lacrimation in the affected eye. Iridocyclitis is common with herpetic keratitis and is usually nongranulomatous. When present, keratitic precipitates (KP) are often distributed

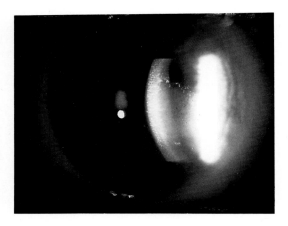

Figure 8.1. Infectious uveitis—herpes simplex keratouveitis. Herpes simplex keratouveitis in a patient with unilateral, nongranulomatous, anterior uveitis. The patient had active epithelial disease before the development of the stromal keratitis and uveitis. Note the distribution of the KP in the region underlying the area of keratitis in a "ring-like" configuration.

under the area of active keratitis (Fig. 8.1). Chronic disease can result in a granulomatous inflammation and "mutton fat" KP.

Diagnosis

Several pathognomonic findings assist in the diagnosis of herpetic keratouveitis: (1) the presence of an active epithelial dendrite, (2) corneal anesthesia, and (3) the presence of a unilateral keratouveitis with elevated intraocular pressure. Although more common with herpes zoster, the iris may become necrotic and develop focal iris atrophy.

Cytology and cultures can be performed to confirm the diagnosis. Multinucleated giant cells and intranuclear eosinophilic inclusion bodies (Cowdry A bodies) can be seen on corneal scrapings.

Differential Diagnosis

Herpes zoster virus can cause a keratouveitis. These patients typically have a history of shingles involving the trigeminal nerve. The iridocyclitis is more severe in zoster and occurs with sector iris atrophy. Syphilis may also cause an interstitial keratitis and uveitis and should be considered in atypical cases.

Treatment

Epithelial disease can be treated with gentle debridement.[4] Topical antiviral agents such as trifluridine 1% (1 gtt every 1–2 hours) should be used to inhibit further viral replication. Other topical antiviral drugs, including idoxuridine and vidarabine, are effective in treating active disease. Cycloplegics can be used to control pain. Topical corticosteroids should be avoided in most cases of mild disease that are limited to the corneal epithelium.

Corticosteroids can be used cautiously in cases of stromal disease, endotheliitis, trabeculitis, and significant uveitis.[4] Unlike with other forms of uveitis, topical corticosteroids can often be used at very low doses with dramatic clinical response. Concurrent antiviral therapy should be used whenever corticosteroids are used. In severe cases oral acyclovir and prednisone may be used to treat refractory disease.

Prognosis

Herpes simplex is a recurrent disease and is the most common cause of corneal blindness in developed nations. Uveitis is often a secondary clinical concern in this disease. Patients often develop visually significant stromal scars, and corneal transplantation is often required.

Herpes Zoster

Varicella-zoster virus (VZV) is a DNA virus known to cause a chronic, necrotizing keratouveitis. It can also cause a severe viral retinitis (see *Acute Retinal Necrosis Syndrome*).

Etiology

VZV or herpes zoster virus is a double-stranded DNA virus in the Alphaherpesvirus family.[8] The virus measures 150 to 200 nm and has icosahedral symmetry.

Epidemiology

VZV causes two separate disease syndromes: Chickenpox and shingles. Chickenpox, or varicella, is an extremely contagious systemic disease of childhood.[8] Spread via droplet transmission, it results in a respiratory illness. After a 14-day incubation and viral prodrome, the characteristic chickenpox rash develops. Approximately 3 million cases of chickenpox are reported in the United States each year. More than 90% of adults have serologic evidence for prior VZV infection.[9,10] Shingles, or zoster, is a secondary manifestation of VZV infection and represents a reactivation of a latent viral infection. It affects both sexes with equal frequency and has no racial predilection.[10]

Pathogenesis

Most cases occur in healthy individuals. VZV establishes a latent infection within sensory ganglion.[8] Zoster, or shingles, results from reactivation of the VZV within the ganglion. The dermatome affected develops a painful, grouped vesicular rash. If the nasociliary division of the fifth cranial nerve is involved the eye may be affected.

Clinical Presentation

A viral prodrome consisting of malaise, fever, and headache often is noted before an outbreak of zoster. A vesicular rash develops, following the distribution of the fifth cranial nerve. Zoster involves the ophthalmic branch in 8% to 56% of cases.[10] Intraocular involvement may be more frequent when the nasociliary branch is infected, as indicated by lesions on the tip of the nose.

The eyelids may have painful vesicular lesions on an erythematous base.[10–12] A watery, follicular conjunctivitis and true scleritis often occur. The cornea may develop a dendritic lesion without terminal bulbs as seen with HSV.[13] Stromal keratitis can be noted and the cornea will have relative anesthesia.

In the acute stage, a severe iridocyclitis with nongranulomatous KP can develop. Sectoral iris atrophy, noted on biomicroscopic transillumination, is a characteristic sign and illustrates the necrotizing nature of the inflammation (see Fig. 2.16). Profound damage to the blood–eye barrier in the iris can result in chronic inflammation with heavy flare, granulomatous KP, and chronic cellular reaction. Intraocular inflammation may last months to years. Posterior synechiae, glaucoma, and cataract are frequent sequelae of VZV uveitis.

Diagnosis

The presence of the characteristic skin lesions, corneal findings, sector iris atrophy, and iridocyclitis establishes the diagnosis.[11] Cytologic study of a scraping taken from the base of a lesion reveals multinucleated giant cells and eosinophilic nuclear inclusion bodies (Lipshitz bodies). The diagnosis is more difficult when the skin lesions are mild or absent. The lesions may be hidden in the scalp or behind the ear. A unilateral, keratouveitis with corneal anesthesia and sector iris atrophy should suggest VZV as the etiology, even in the absence of classic skin lesions.

Differential Diagnosis

Syphilis and HSV may both cause a keratouveitis. Sector iris atrophy and dermatomal skin lesions are not present in these two disorders.

Treatment

Oral acyclovir (800 mg, five times a day) is beneficial in controlling the active infectious phase of the disease.[1,14,15] The drug is often given over a 10- to 21-day course. The presence of iridocyclitis in herpes zoster may indicate active intraocular viral replication. As with HSV keratouveitis, oral acyclovir (800 mg orally, five times a day) should be administered when significant iridocyclitis is noted with zoster to inhibit further viral replication and cytolysis. Acyclovir does not seem to reduce the severity of postherpetic neuralgia with eye disease.[14] In one series, the use of high-dose oral acyclovir reduced the rate of long-term complications from 21% to 4%.[15] Topical cycloplegia and corticosteroids should be used to moderate the inflammation. Oral prednisone (40–60 mg, four times a day) may be required if the patient is not immunocompromised and is on oral antiviral therapy.

Patients should be followed closely for several months to monitor intraocular pressure and to direct the slow tapering off of the medication. Postherpetic neuralgia can occur in up to 20% of patients and may last months to years. Severe insomnia, depression, and anorexia can be associated with postherpetic, chronic pain. These symptoms can be managed with adjunctive nonnarcotic or narcotic analgesics, amitriptyline (25–75 mg every hour), or cimetidine (400 mg four times a day).[11–14] Capsaicin cream (Zostrix) is a neuropeptide active agent that can reduce postzoster neuralgia in some patients.[16]

Prognosis

VZV-associated uveitis may be chronic and difficult to control. Patients may require long-term, low dose topical therapy. Viral infection, secondary inflammation, and steroid therapy all contribute to the development of glaucoma and cataract. The glaucoma may be difficult to control with topical beta-blockers and oral carbonic anhydrase inhibitors and often requires filtration surgery. Corneal anesthesia and low-grade inflammation make standard cataract extraction and intraocular lens (IOL) implantation challenging. Lens-induced uveitis may develop with intumescent lens changes, and pars plana lensectomy and vitrectomy may be required.

Viral Diseases Associated with Retinitis and Uveitis

Our ability to diagnose viral infections of the retina has improved greatly during the last decade.[17] Advances in vitreoretinal sur-

gery and the development of techniques for chorioretinal/retinal biopsy have provided fresh tissue for study in cases of sight-threatening retinal disease.[18–21] Through the use of light and electron microscopy, immunohistochemistry, newer microbial culture techniques, and molecular biologic probes, specific infectious agents have been identified in several disorders.[3,4]

The most important family of viruses capable of infecting the retina are the herpesviruses. HSV-1, HSV-2, cytomegalovirus (CMV), and VZV are responsible for the vast majority of cases of viral retinitis in the United States. Both immunocompromised persons and those with intact immune systems are susceptible to this family of viruses. For example, the acute retinal necrosis syndrome (ARN/BARN) typically occurs in healthy adults and is the result of retinal infection with HSV-1, HSV-2, or VZ viruses.[9–12] In contrast, CMV retinitis affects immunosuppressed patients such as those on chemotherapy, neonates, and persons with acquired immunodeficiency syndrome (AIDS). These viral diseases are discussed separately.

In addition to these herpesviruses, herpes B virus, Epstein-Barr virus (EBV), coxsackievirus B, rubella, Rift Valley fever virus, influenza A, mumps, measles, and subacute sclerosing panencephalitis viruses, and the virus causing Creutzfeldt-Jakob disease have all been shown to be agents of infectious retinitis in humans (Table 8.1). Other retinal disorders, such as acute posterior multifocal placoid pigment epitheliopathy (APMPPE), acute retinal pigment epitheliitis (ARPE), multiple evanescent white dot syndrome (MEWDS), and Leber's idiopathic stellate neuroretinitis often begin with a viral prodrome and may be manifestations of a viral illness as well.[5–8]

Herpes B Virus

Herpes B virus can cause a necrotizing retinitis and panuveitis.

Table 8.1. Viral diseases associated with retinitis and uveitis—summary of clinical features

Virus	Vitreous	Vessels	Sensory retina	RPE	Choroid	Optic nerve
HV-B	Hemorrhage Scar Vitritis	—	RD Multifocal necrotizing retinitis	Scar	Chorioretinal scarring	Atrophy
EBV	Vitritis	—	Macular edema Hemorrhage Multifocal outer retinitis Multifocal choroiditis and panuveitis Chorioretinitis	Scar Pigment changes	Multifocal choroiditis Subretinal neovascular membrane	Edema
Coxsackievirus	—	—	Multifocal chorioretinitis	Scar	—	—
Rubella						
Aquired	Vitritis	—	Gray lesions Exudative RD	Exudative RPE detachment	—	—
Congenital	—	—	Salt and pepper Dull foveal reflex	SRNVM	—	
RVFV	Vitritis	Occlusion	Macular lesions Exudative RD Hemorrhage Fibrosis	Scarring	—	—
Influenza A	—	Leakage	Submacular hemorrhage Macular star CME Inner retinitis	—	—	Edema
Mumps	Vitritis	—	White retinitis	Scarring	—	Edema
Measles						
Aquired	—	Attenuated arterioles	Macular star	—	—	Edema
Congenital	—	Attenuated	CME Macular star	Pigment changes	—	—
SSPE	—	—	Macular edema White infiltrates Hemorrhage Serous detachment	Scarring	Chorioretinitis	Edema Atrophy
CJD	—	—	—	—	—	Atrophy

HV-B, Herpes B virus; EBV, Epstein-Barr virus; RVFV, Rift Valley fever virus; RD, retinal detachment; CME, cystoid macular edema; RPE, retinal pigment epithelium; SRNVM, subretinal neovascular membrane; SSPE, subacute sclerosing panencephalitis; CJD, Creutzfeldt-Jakob disease.

Etiology

Herpes B virus (HV-B), or herpesvirus simiea, an alphaherpesvirus within the Herpesvirinea family, is an encapsulated, double-stranded DNA virus (100 nm) with an icosahedral nucleocapsid.[20] Other alphaherpesviruses include HSV-1, HSV-2, and VZV.

Epidemiology

HV-B is endemic among macaque monkeys; 30% to 80% of animals are seropositive. Transmission to humans occurs through bites or scratches from infected monkeys.[20,21] Human infections have also occurred by puncture wounds from contaminated objects.[22]

Pathogenesis

HV-B gains access to the blood via direct inoculation. Similar to the other alphaherpesviruses, HV-B is neurotropic and inoculation may result in severe encephalomyelitis and retinitis.[20–22] One patient who died from culture-proven HV-B encephalomyelitis was found on autopsy to have a vitritis, panuveitis, optic neuritis, and multifocal necrotizing retinitis.[22] Electron microscopy demonstrated herpesvirus in the retina. Vitreous cultures obtained postmortem were positive for HV-B.

Clinical Presentation

HV-B causes a rapidly progressive ascending meningitis and encephalitis.[20,22] The infection can be severe and is often fatal despite antiviral therapies. Asymptomatic or latent HV-B infections have not been reported.

Two cases of HV-B encephalomyelitis in monkey handlers have been reported with associated ocular complications and viral retinitis.[21,22] In one case, a 29-year-old handler noted sudden loss of vision due to a vitreous hemorrhage.[21] With resolution of the hemorrhage, vitreous organization and widespread chorioretinal scarring were noted throughout the fundus. The patient went on to develop an irreparable retinal detachment. In a second case of fatal HV-B encephalitis, a multifocal, necrotizing retinitis and panuveitis were identified at autopsy.[22] These reports suggest that all four alphaherpesviruses appear to be able to infect the retina and cause an ARN/BARN-like syndrome with multifocal, necrotizing retinitis and panuveitis in immunocompetent hosts.[9–12]

Diagnosis

Encephalomyelitis that develops in monkey handlers after a bite, scratch, or contaminated puncture wound should suggest HV-B infection. In this clinical setting, the presence of an acute retinal necrosis, vitritis, and subsequent retinal detachment would support a clinical diagnosis of HV-B retinitis. Serologic studies demonstrating a fourfold rise in complement fixation (CF) or enzyme-linked immunoadsorbent assay (ELISA) antibodies toward HV-B would confirm the diagnosis.[20] Vitreous cultures may isolate HV-B.[22]

Differential Diagnosis

Other viral infections may produce a fundus appearance similar to that in HV-B. Specifically, HSV-1, HSV-2, and VZV can cause an acute, multifocal necrotizing retinitis, which would be difficult to distinguish by fundus examination alone.[9–12] The history of exposure to monkeys is important in establishing the diagnosis. Retinal biopsy may help with the differential diagnosis in severe, sight-threatening, or medically unresponsive cases of suspected viral retinitis.[1,2,9–12] Other diseases that can affect both the retina and central nervous system (CNS) include Lyme disease, rickettsial infections, sarcoidosis, and Behçet's disease. These conditions are discussed in detail elsewhere in the text.

Treatment

Antiviral agents may play a role in treating HV-B retinitis. Acyclovir is effective in treating ARN syndrome secondary to HSV and VZV when given intravenously at a dose of 1500 mg/m^2 per day.[18] In one fatal case of HV-B encephalitis and retinitis, the use of both acyclovir and ganciclovir failed to halt the CNS disease. The role of oral corticosteroids is not clear, but there may be a theoretical advantage to using systemic corticosteroids to minimize the vigorous intraocular inflammation that accompanies herpesvirus infections of the retina.[23]

Prognosis

As with other forms of necrotizing retinitis, HV-B infection can result in retinal breaks and vitreous traction. Vitreoretinal surgical repair may be required in cases of tractional detachment with multiple, posterior retinal breaks as observed in viral infection of the retina.[24-26]

Epstein-Barr Virus

EBV is a herpes family virus that has been associated with several retinal and chorioretinal inflammatory disorders.

Etiology

EBV is a member of the *Gammaherpesvirinae* genus in the Herpesviridae family.[27] First identified in 1964 by Epstein and Barr with the aid of electron microscopy, EBV is a double-stranded DNA virus (100–200 nm) with an encapsulated, icosahedral nucleocapsid.

Epidemiology

EBV is ubiquitous, with as high as 90% of the population demonstrating antibodies to the virus by the third decade of life.[27,28] Asymptomatic shedding of virus in saliva is the primary mode of transmission. The virus can be isolated from the oropharynx in 15% to 25% of all seropositive individuals in the absence of clinical disease. Infectious mononucleosis (IM), or the "kissing disease," peaks during adolescence, that is, 14 to 16 years in girls and 16 to 18 years in boys.[29]

Pathogenesis

Initial viral replication occurs within the oropharyngeal mucosal epithelium. EBV has surface receptors for the C3d marker found on B lymphocytes. This B-cell tropism plays an important role in the pathogenesis of EBV-mediated diseases.[28,29] During an infection, up to 20% of circulating B cells demonstrate EBV-encoded gene products. Once inside the B-cell, EBV may cause B-cell activation or B-cell lysis, or it may establish a latent viral infection. Nonspecific B-cell activation and mononuclear

cell proliferation result in a relative lymphocytosis and polyclonal secretion of immunoglobulin. Heterophil antibodies noted in 50% to 95% of patients with IM are a result of this nonspecific B-cell activation.

Antibodies to several EBV-specific antigens develop during the primary infection and are diagnostically helpful.[27,28] IgM antibodies to the viral capsid antigen (VCA) indicate recent infection. IgG antibodies directed toward this same antigen develop later and persist for life. EBV nuclear antigens (EBNA) can be detected in the nucleus of B cells within 24 hours of infection and can stimulate anti-EBNA antibody production. These lifelong antibodies are detectable within the first 6 to 8 weeks after infection. Antibodies directed toward diffuse and restricted early viral antigens (EA-D and EA-R) occur in 70% of patients with IM, peak at 3 to 4 weeks, and become undetectable with resolution of disease. A fourfold rise in IgG and the presence of IgM and EA-D/EA-R antibodies indicate recent infection.

Resolution of the disease occurs with the development of viral neutralizing antibodies that can inactivate extracellular virus.[28,29] In addition, an EBV-specific, T cell–mediated immune response controls B-cell proliferation and immunoglobulin production. This cell-mediated immune response appears to be directed at unique lymphocyte-determined membrane antigens (LYDMA) induced on the surface of EBV-infected B cells.

Clinical Presentation

EBV may produce an acute, recurrent, or chronic disorder as a result of a primary, persistent, or latent viral infection.[27-29] Infection may be asymptomatic (childhood infections), self-limiting (IM), or result in neoplastic disorders. IM, nasopharyngeal carcinoma, Burkitt's lymphoma, and Sjögren's syndrome have all been associated with EBV.[29-34] Recently, the EBV genome has been detected in Reed-Sternberg cells of Hodgkin's disease through in situ DNA hybridization.[35,36]

Ocular involvement with EBV has been reported primarily in patients with IM. These patients develop sore throat, fever, lymphadenopathy, and hepatosplenomegaly. A follicular conjunctivitis can be noted in 2% to 40% of patients with IM.[37] Stromal keratitis, iritis, episcleritis, optic neuritis, and ophthalmoplegia have been reported during the acute phases of IM.[37,38]

IM and EBV are associated with several retinal presentations: (1) macular edema, (2) retinal hemorrhages, (3) chorioretinitis, (4) punctate outer retinitis, and (5) a multifocal chorioretinitis and panuveitis (MCP) syndrome.[39–49] A severe macular edema and optic neuritis in a 20-year-old patient with IM and loss of central acuity was reported.[39] The macula developed extensive pigmentary changes, but acuity returned to normal. In another report, one of three patients with chronic EBV infection developed bilateral macular edema with an associated vitritis, uveitis, and disc edema.[41]

A patient with IM was reported with diplopia and intraretinal hemorrhages.[42] Others have reported a similar fundus presentation. The retinal hemorrhages may be associated with disc and macular edema.[43,44]

A patient with acute IM was reported to develop multiple, gray-white, outer retinal punctate lesions (50–75 μm) in the midperipheral retina, which were associated with a mild vitritis.[45] The macula developed mild pigment epithelial changes. A group of patients with idiopathic MCP syndrome (see Fig. 2.34) was compared to both normal subjects and patients with other forms of uveitis.[47] Patients with MCP had a serologic pattern indicating either recent or chronic EBV infection. In contrast to normal persons and patients with other forms of uveitis, patients with idiopathic MCP had immunoglobulin M (IgM) antibodies against EBV capsid antigens and antibodies to EBV early antigens. A role for chronic EBV infection was postulated.

Other investigators have not found this strong association.[48]

It is possible that MCP and progressive subretinal fibrosis and uveitis syndrome (SFU) are different stages of the same disease. A chorioretinal biopsy of one patient with SFU demonstrated a predominance of subretinal B cells.[49] We have tested six patients with SFU for EBV serology and have found EA and IgM antibodies to EBV in all of them. These two conditions appear to be related and have serologic and histologic findings compatible with EBV infection.

A case of bilateral retinochoroiditis was reported in a 17-year-old boy with acute IM.[50] The patient had a granulomatous iritis, vitritis, and a disc diameter area of discrete retinitis in the macula of both eyes, which resembled toxoplasmosis. A chorioretinal scar developed 7 days after resolution of the active retinitis.

Diagnosis

Retinal involvement is uncommon in most cases of IM. Fundus lesions that develop during acute IM would support the diagnosis of EBV. Serologic testing for heterophile antibodies, IgM antibodies directed against VCA, and antibodies to early viral antigens would help confirm the diagnosis.[27,28]

Differential Diagnosis

The differential diagnosis of retinal edema, retinal hemorrhages, multifocal outer retinitis, and MCP is expansive. Sarcoidosis, tuberculosis, syphilis, toxoplasmosis, histoplasmosis, retinal vascular disorders, and idiopathic retinal white dot syndromes can all present with similar fundus findings. These disorders are discussed in other sections. Characteristic systemic symptoms and serologic studies in IM distinguish EBV retinitis from these conditions.

Treatment

Retinal involvement in IM is typically mild and self-limiting and therapy is chiefly supportive. Systemic corticosteroids and acyclovir may be useful in cases with sight-threatening complications of chronic intraocular inflammation.

Prognosis

Retinal edema, intraretinal hemorrhages, and the punctate outer retinal lesions gradually resolve.[39–45,47] One patient with more severe retinochoroiditis developed loss of central vision due to a macular scar.[50] The prognosis for patients with EBV-associated MCP is more guarded.[46,47] Intraocular inflammation tends to be chronic, and retinal sequelae such as chronic cystoid macular edema and subretinal neovascular membranes are frequent.

Coxsackievirus

Coxsackievirus, an enterovirus, is a rare etiologic agent for conjunctivitis, keratitis, and retinitis.

Etiology

The coxsackieviruses groups A and B are enteroviruses belonging to the Picornaviridae family.[51] Polioviruses and echoviruses are related to coxsackievirus and are in this same enterovirus subfamily. First isolated in 1948, in Coxsackie, New York, by Dalldorf and Sickles, the coxsackieviruses are a small, single-stranded RNA virus (25–35 nm) with an unencapsulated, icosahedral nucleocapsid. They are called enteroviruses because of their common isolation in the gastrointestinal (GI) tract.

Epidemiology

Human beings are the only natural host for coxsackievirus.[51] Epidemics of coxsackievirus-mediated diseases have been reported in the United States (1963 coxsackievirus B1, 1972 coxsackievirus B5). The virus is able to tolerate gastric acids and intestinal enzymes and can survive for long periods in untreated sewage.[51] These features play an important role in the epidemiology of enterovirus diseases. Fecal-oral routes of infection are the most common mode of viral transmission. The virus also may be spread by respiratory or insect vectors. Coxsackieviruses occur more frequently in children and during the summer months.

Pathogenesis

Initial viral replication occurs within the GI tract.[51] End-organ infection results from a secondary viremia. The respiratory tract, heart, liver, brain, and GI tract are primarily affected in coxsackievirus-mediated disease. Histopathology of infected tissues reveal focal areas of necrosis and cellular infiltration.

Clinical Presentation

Systemic infections with coxsackieviruses range from subclinical to potentially fatal diseases. Common presentation for coxsackievirus infection include herpangina, hand-foot-and-mouth disease, pharyngitis, gastroenteritis, aseptic meningitis, encephalitis, myocarditis, hepatitis, and pneumonia.[51]

Coxsackievirus has a unique role in the acute hemorrhagic conjunctivitis syndrome (AHC),[52] a tropical disease that appears to have evolved from an animal strain of enterovirus. Enterovirus 70 has been the dominant agent of AHC since the first epidemics in 1969. More recently, coxsackievirus type A24 has been isolated during epidemics of AHC. These separate strains of enterovirus appear to produce an identical ocular picture characterized by a sudden, painful, follicular conjunctivitis, which is often accompanied by superficial keratitis.

One case of bilateral chorioretinitis associated with coxsackievirus B4 infection has been reported.[53] An 11-year-old boy developed high fever, fatigue, and abdominal pain. Examination revealed an aseptic meningitis and hepatitis due to coxsackievirus B4. He had no ocular complaints. Visual acuity was 20/20. Biomicroscopic and fundus examination revealed bilateral chorio-retinitis. White lesions along the retinal vessels throughout the midperipheral fundus measured 0.25 to 1.5 disc diameters. The macula and optic nerve were not involved. The lesions resolved spontaneously but left a chorioretinal scar.

Diagnosis

Coxsackievirus retinitis appears to be rare, and ocular involvement may be asymptomatic.[53] The diagnosis depends on ophthalmic examination during the course of the systemic viral illness.

The virus can be isolated from the conjunctiva, nasopharyngeal secretions, and stool specimens during active disease. Acute and convalescent titers of viral neutralizing antibodies (VNA) have been used extensively during epidemics of coxsackievirus-mediated diseases.[52] A fourfold rise in VNA indicates a recent infection.

Differential Diagnosis

The differential diagnosis for a multifocal chorioretinitis occurring in children with an acute systemic illness should include Lyme disease and Rocky Mountain spotted fever (RMSF). Serologic testing can help differentiate these conditions, but is not useful during the acute phase.

Lyme disease is a tick-borne, spirochetal systemic infection caused by *Borrelia burgdorferi*.[54] This disease occurs during the summer months and can present with fever, malaise, and fatigue. A characteristic annular skin lesion (erythema chronicum migrans) can be found before the onset of CNS, cardiac, and joint involvement. Conjunctivitis, iritis, vitritis, and chorioretinitis have been reported in Lyme disease.[55,56]

RMSF is another tick-borne disease caused by *Rickettsia rickettsii*, which has been associated with chorioretinitis.[57] Fever, malaise, and headache occur with a characteristic skin rash. The skin lesions are small erythematous macules associated with petechial hemorrhages and occur initially on the extremities.

Treatment

Therapy for coxsackievirus infections is primarily supportive. Coxsackievirus retinitis appears to improve spontaneously with resolution of the disease.[53]

Prognosis

Visual prognosis is good. Asymptomatic peripheral retinal scars may develop as a sequela of the disease.

Rubella Virus

Congenital and acquired rubella can cause conjunctivitis, keratitis, uveitis, and retinitis.

Etiology

Rubella virus belongs to the *Rubivirus* genus within the Togaviridae family.[58] The virus is an enveloped, single-stranded RNA virus (50–70 nm) with an icosahedral nucleocapsid. In addition to a viral hemagglutinin, the capsule has a viral antigen (V-antigen) and an S-antigen.

Epidemiology

Rubella virus is species-specific, human beings being the natural host. Rubella (German measles) is endemic and before widespread vaccination, epidemics occurred in 6- to 9-year cycles.[58] Rubella is spread by droplets expelled from an infected host. It is only moderately contagious and typically occurs in children. Approximately 10% to 25% of pregnant women may be nonimmune.[59]

Pathogenesis

The virus replicates in the upper respiratory tract epithelium before a more disseminated infection and viremia develop.[58,59]

Viral neutralizing antibodies appear coincident with the rash and may play a role in producing the skin lesions. Rubella may involve the retina in both congenital and acquired forms. Autopsy reports from congenital rubella have shown retinal pigment epithelial degeneration with an occasional phagocytic cell.[60,61] The contiguous choroid and choriocapillaris are uninvolved.

The virus may establish a lifelong, persistent infection.[58] Rubella virus has been isolated from cataracts in children 3 years of age. It has also been cultured from the brain as long as 12 years after congenital infection.

Clinical Presentation

Rubella can cause both acquired and congenital infections.[59,62] Acquired rubella begins with a mild prodrome of fever, headache, malaise, and conjunctivitis. Lymphadenopathy and splenomegaly may occur.[58,59] The skin rash develops 1 to 3 days after the initial prodrome. Consisting of discrete maculopapular lesions, it begins on the trunk and spreads toward the extremities. The rash lasts 3 to 5 days (3-day measles). Complications of rubella infection include encephalitis, arthritis, and hemorrhage. Ocular manifestations of acquired rubella include conjunctivitis (70%), superficial keratitis, and iritis.[62]

Two cases of acquired rubella retinitis have been reported.[63,64] A bilateral retinitis and associated exudative detachment of the retina were noted, as well as retinal pigment epithelium.[63] The retinal lesions were in the posterior pole and were described as dark gray with atrophy. The optic nerve and retinal vessels were not involved. Fluorescein angiography demonstrated multifocal punctate hyperfluorescent lesions at the level of the choroid. The retinal detachments resolved with oral corticosteroid therapy.

Congenital rubella syndrome was first recognized by Gregg in 1941.[65] This syndrome consists of congenital cataracts, deafness, cardiac malformation, and mild mental retardation.[62,65] The disease is caused by a maternal infection with rubella during the first trimester. Fetal outcome depends on the timing of the transplacental infection. Spontaneous abortion may occur with infections early in the first trimester. Infections in the second or third trimester typically result in normal offspring. Ocular manifestations of congenital rubella include cataract (2–15%), glaucoma (10%), iritis, and microphthalmia.[62,66–70]

Rubella retinitis is perhaps the most common manifestation of infection.[35,67] Fundus examination reveals a diminished foveal light reflex and a widespread fine mottling of the retinal pigment epithelium (RPE) which is most prominent within the posterior pole. The optic nerve and retinal vessels are normal. This fundus picture has been called a "salt and pepper fundus" because of the alternating hypopigmented and hyperpigmented changes (Fig. 8.2). The "salt and pepper fundus" changes are life long. Rarely, rubella retinitis may result in disciform macular scar formation.[68]

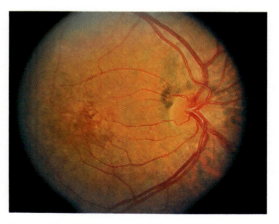

Figure 8.2. Infectious uveitis—rubella retinopathy. Fundus photograph of a patient with congenital rubella retinopathy. The fundus has a "salt and pepper" appearance. Despite the widespread disturbance in the RPE, visual acuity was 20/25.

Diagnosis

Acquired rubella retinitis can be diagnosed in the presence of active German measles. Viral culture and the diagnostic fourfold rise in hemagglutination inhibition, CF, or ELISA antibodies confirm the clinical diagnosis.[58] Congenital rubella syndrome can be diagnosed with a history of maternal rubella and the characteristic congenital findings. Viral isolation from the oropharynx and the presence of IgM antibodies in the newborn support the diagnosis.[58,59]

Differential Diagnosis

Serology studies can assist in the diagnosis. Bilateral exudative retinal detachments noted in the acquired form of rubella retinitis may also occur in syphilis and Vogt-Koyanagi-Haradas (VKH) syndrome. The skin rash in syphilis typically involves the palms and soles of the feet.[69] VKH syndrome can manifest constitutional symptoms including headache and fatigue.[70] Hearing loss, vitiligo, poliosis, and a panuveitis are also noted. The "salt and pepper fundus" observed in congenital rubella may be similar to that seen in luetic retinitis and hereditary retinal degenerations.

Treatment

There is no specific therapy for rubella. Acquired rubella is a self-limiting disease. If severe, acquired rubella retinitis may be treated with oral corticosteroids.[63]

Prognosis

The visual prognosis for congenital rubella retinitis is good. Despite widespread RPE changes, patients typically enjoy 20/20 to 20/40 visual acuities with full visual fields.

Glaucoma and cataract may be problematic in congenital rubella. Glaucoma therapy is often unsuccessful. Early cataract extraction may be required to prevent severe amblyopia.

Rift Valley Fever Virus

Rift Valley fever virus (RVFV) can cause a febrile, systemic illness associated with conjunctivitis, uveitis, and an exudative and hemorrhagic retinitis.

Etiology

RVFV, an insect-borne virus in the Bunyaviridae family,[71,72] is an encapsulated RNA virus (100 nm) with a coiled circular nucleocapsid. The viruses associated with this endemic disease are named for the regions of eastern Africa and for South Africa, where they originate.[73,74]

Epidemiology

RVFV is an infectious disease of animals and livestock.[73,74] Goats, cattle, and sheep are the primary host and reservoir for the virus. Mosquitos are thought to be the primary vector for transmission of both between animals and human beings.

Pathogenesis

The arthropod vector directly inoculates the virus within the bloodstream. The viremia results in end-organ infection, including the retina.

Clinical Presentation

RVFV causes an acute febrile illness with malaise, chills, myalgias, and headache.[71,73] Incubation is 2 to 7 days. GI involvement is common later in the disease course. The fever can be high and is characteristically relapsing. The disease is usually self-limiting with rapid recovery. In one recent epidemic, a 1% mortality rate was noted as a result of encephalitis, hepatitis, and hemorrhagic complications.

Conjunctivitis and uveitis can develop during the acute phases of the disease.[72-74] A viral retinitis has been described during several outbreaks. Typically, patients present with loss of central vision 7 to 21 days after the onset of the fever. Unilateral or bilateral macular, paramacular, and mid-peripheral retinal exudates and intraretinal hemorrhages are noted on dilated fundus examination. Fluorescein angiography demonstrates retinal vasculitis and vascular occlusion. The retinal lesions resolve over several months.

Diagnosis

In endemic areas, the diagnosis should be suspected during outbreaks of RVFV. The characteristic fundus findings help establish a clinical diagnosis. The virus can be isolated and cultured in mice to confirm the diagnosis.[71] In addition, a fourfold rise in CF and hemagglutination inhibition (HI) antibodies toward RVFV can support a recent RVFV infection. Fluorescein angiography may assist in determining the mechanism for the loss of central acuity.

Differential Diagnosis

Lyme disease, rickettsial diseases, and sarcoidosis may present as a febrile, systemic illness.[54–57] History, physical examination, and laboratory testing can help differentiate these disorders, as discussed in other chapters.

Treatment

Rift Valley fever is a self-limiting disease, and therapy is typically supportive. A small percentage of patients (1%) develop serious complications from the virus, including encephalitis, hepatitis, and visceral hemorrhage.[71] RVFV retinitis, if mild and outside the posterior pole, can be observed, with no further treatment required. In severe sight-threatening cases, corticosteroid therapy can be considered to minimize inflammatory damage.

Prognosis

In one series of 80 patients, 50% of patients with severe disease had residual loss of central vision as a result of macular scar formation, epiretinal membrane, ischemic maculopathy, or retinal detachment.[72,74]

Influenza A

Influenza A is a respiratory viral illness associated with worldwide epidemics. It can cause conjunctivitis, iritis, interstitial keratitis, and retinitis.

Etiology

Influenza A virus (IAV) is one type of influenzavirus in the Orthomyxoviridae family.[75] First isolated in 1933, IAV is a single-stranded RNA virus (80–120 nm) with an outer lipoprotein envelope and a helical nucleocapsid. Neuraminidase and hemagglutinin, surface glycoproteins within this envelope, are important for viral adherence and entry into cells.

Epidemiology

Epidemics of IAV are cyclic (every 2–4 years) and occur as a result of major and minor antigenic variations in the surface glycoproteins ("antigenic shifts").[75] These shifts play an important role in the severity of the outbreaks. Epidemics and pandemics of IAV occur typically in the winter months, with an overall attack rate of 40%.

Pathogenesis

Influenza A is a pneumotropic virus with affinity to the tracheobronchial epithelial cells. The virus is transmitted by droplets, which are exhaled from an infected person.[75] Once in the respiratory tract, the virus causes cell lysis and desquamation of the ciliated epithelium.

Clinical Presentation

Influenza is an acute febrile illness characterized by malaise, headache, and myalgias. The illness lasts 2 to 7 days. Recovery is complete unless secondary bacterial infections occur. Influenza can be serious and may cause cardiopulmonary complications or death in elderly or debilitated patients.

Ocular involvement with influenza includes conjunctivitis, a mild iritis, interstitial keratitis, and dacryoadenitis during the acute illness. Several authors have reported cases of influenza A retinitis.[76–80]

A 21-year-old woman with influenza A and bilateral submacular hemorrhages was described.[76] On examination, she had 20/20 vision with annular central scotomas. Fundus examination revealed a quiet vitreous and normal optic nerve and retinal vessels. Both maculae had small subretinal hemorrhages. The hemorrhages resolved over several weeks and the patient maintained 20/20 vision. A persistent ring-shaped scotomas was noted despite a normal fundus examination 2 years later.

A 23-year-old man with active influenza A, decreased vision, and central scotomas has been reported.[77] Dilated fundus examination revealed bilateral macular lipid star formation without hemorrhage. Fluorescein angiography demonstrated retinal capillary leakage in the posterior pole. The fundus lesions cleared and visual acuity returned to normal 6 weeks later. Three years later the macula exhibited subtle RPE changes.

More recently, a case of serologically proven IAV was reported that was associated with a bilateral posterior microvasculopathy and secondary macular and disc edema.[78] Vision was reduced to 20/400 bilaterally. Fundus examination demonstrated multifocal white patches in the inner retina. The vitreous was quiet. Fluorescein angiography revealed perifoveal capillary leakage and both diffuse and cystoid macular edema. Visual acuities improved over several days, and repeat angiography documented complete resolution of the retinal vascular leakage. Convalescent serum showed a fourfold rise in influenza A titers. At follow-up examination, the patient had 20/20 acuities and decreased foveal reflexes bilaterally.

Diagnosis

Submacular hemorrhages, macular star formation, or retinal capillary microvasculopathy with multifocal inner retinitis that occurs in the setting of an influenza epidemic suggest the clinical diagnosis of IAV retinitis. Serologic testing that documents a fourfold rise in IAV titers by ELISA, CF, or HI can help confirm the diagnosis.[75]

Differential Diagnosis

Several disorders can present with submacular hemorrhages. Age-related macular degeneration, ocular histoplasmosis, trauma, and angioid streaks can all result in subretinal neovascular membranes and subretinal macular hemorrhage.[81] These disorders do not typically occur with systemic flu-like symptoms, and spontaneous resolution is rare. Macular lipid stars can occur in measles and mumps virus infections, diabetic retinopathy, hypertension, anterior ischemic optic neuropathy, and Leber's idiopathic stellate neuroretinitis.[8]

Treatment

Influenza A retinitis appears to be self-limiting. Patients reported in the literature had complete resolution of their retinopathy and return of 20/20 vision. One patient had a persistent subjective annular scotoma, and another had reduced foveal light reflexes.[76,78]

Vaccination for IAV is recommended for those at higher risk for contracting the disease, such as health care workers. Others at high risk for complications include the elderly and patients with chronic pulmonary disease, cardiovascular disease, or other debilitating disorders.

Prognosis

Although most patients recover from influenza, it can be fatal in debilitated patients. Visual prognosis is variable.

Mumps Virus

Mumps virus (MV) causes a characteristic parotitis and has been associated with conjunctivitis, iridocyclitis, keratitis, optic neuritis, and retinitis.

Etiology

MV belongs to the Paramyxoviridae family of viruses.[82] It is an enveloped RNA virus (85–300 nm) with a helical nucleocapsid.

Epidemiology

Human beings are the only natural host for the MV, although close contact between infected children and their pets has been associated with isolated cases of canine mumps parotitis.[83] Transmission is by direct contact with droplets expelled by an infected host.[82] Most cases of mumps (90%) occur in children. The virus is endemic and can produce epidemics in 2- to 4-year cycles.

Pathogenesis

MV may replicate directly in the salivary glands or in the epithelial cells of the upper respiratory tract.[82] Secondary viremia disseminates the MV throughout the body. The virus can infect the testes, meninges, brain, pancreas, heart, and kidneys.

Clinical Presentation

Onset of disease occurs 14 to 21 days after initial exposure to the virus. A viral prodrome of fever, myalgias, headache, and anorexia can occur 1 to 2 days before salivary gland and other organ involvement. Typically, the parotid and submandibular glands develop massive swelling and become tender for 1 to 2 weeks.

Ocular involvement with mumps includes dacryoadenitis, conjunctivitis, iritis, optic neuritis, and keratitis.[82] A case of unilateral mumps neuroretinitis in a 15-year-old boy was recently reported.[84] Visual acuity was 20/200 in the involved eye with an afferent pupillary defect. A mild posterior vitritis was noted on biomicroscopy. Fundus examination revealed marked disc edema and hyperemia. A star exudate was noted in the posterior pole. Two small white intraretinal lesions were noted in the midperipheral retina. Intravenous methylprednisolone was administered because of progressive loss of vision. The lesions stabilized, and 5 months later vision had improved to 20/40. The two areas of retinitis evolved into a chorioretinal scar.

Diagnosis

Mumps have a characteristic clinical picture, which is sufficient for diagnosis in most cases. Serologic testing can be performed detecting a fourfold rise in CF antibodies toward S and V mumps antigens, as well as a fourfold rise in antibodies using standard HI neutralization or hemolysis-in-gel assays.[82] IgM antibodies also indicate recent infection.

Differential Diagnosis

Macular lipid stars can be found in IAV and measles virus infections, diabetes, hypertension, anterior ischemic optic neuropathy, and Leber's idiopathic stellate neuroretinitis.[85] Sarcoidosis can cause parotid swelling and intraocular inflammation (uveoparotid fever, Heerfordt's syndrome). The inflammation is often bilateral, with a chronic granulomatous uveitis, vasculitis, and retinitis.[86]

Treatment

Systemic treatment of mumps is supportive with administration of fluids and analgesics. One case of mumps neuroretinitis required intravenous methylprednisolone therapy because of severe optic nerve and macular involvement.[84] Visual acuity improved to 20/40 with resolution of the acute process. Children older than 1 year routinely receive a live attenuated mumps vaccination to limit the spread of this virus. A controlled study suggests that hyper-immune gammaglobulin may modify the course of mumps in selected cases.[85]

Prognosis

Recovery and visual prognosis is good.

Measles Virus

Measles virus causes congenital and acquired disease that has been associated with retinitis and neuroretinitis.

Etiology

Measles virus is a morbillivirus in the Paramyxoviridae family.[87] The virus is an enveloped, RNA virus (120–250 nm) with a coiled helical nucleocapsid core.

Epidemiology

Measles is one of the most common infectious diseases worldwide. Human beings and monkeys are the only hosts for measles or rubeola virus.[87,88] The virus is extremely contagious (90% attack rate) and can be spread by either contaminated fomites or direct droplet transmission. Measles is endemic and, before widespread immunization, occurred in cyclic pandemics of 2 to 3 years.

Pathogenesis

Measles virus replicates in the upper respiratory tract and produces a viremia within the first few days, which causes infection of the lymphoid tissues. A second, larger viremia occurs, resulting in disseminated infection.[87,22] Multinucleated giant cells can be found in the skin lesions, mucous membranes, and respiratory tract.

Clinical Presentation

Measles virus can cause both congenital and acquired infections.[87,89] Congenital measles is transmitted through the placenta and can cause fetal demise and serious congenital malformations, including deafness and cardiac and skeletal anomalies. Cataracts have been reported in several cases of congenital measles.[89] Congenital measles retinitis has been observed in two cases, in which visual acuity was normal.[89,90] Fundus examination revealed a bilateral fine pigmentary change throughout the retina. Associated retinal edema, macular star formation, and mild arteriolar attenuation were reported in one patient.

Acquired measles presents with a prodrome of persistent cough, conjunctivitis, and fever.[87,91] Koplik's spots can be found on the oral mucosa. A pink macular rash appears on the face and trunk and spreads toward the extremities over several days. Complications of measles include encephalitis and myocarditis.[88] Acquired measles retinitis is characterized by macular edema, neuroretinitis, macular star formation, attenuated arterioles, and disc edema.[92,93] One report of pigmented paravenous dystrophy associated with measles infection was reported.[94] Immunosuppressed patients may develop a more severe clinical course.[95] Fundus examination in one patient on chemotherapy for testicular carcinoma revealed annular depigmented retinal lesions, fine pigmentary changes, and a central serous chorioretinopathy (CSR-like) lesion.

Diagnosis

Acquired measles has a characteristic clinical picture. A fourfold rise in HI, CF, or ELISA antibodies confirms the diagnosis.[87] Congenital measles retinopathy may be more difficult to diagnose. A history of maternal measles and the presence of other congenital malformations would suggest the diagnosis.

Differential Diagnosis

Other forms of viral retinitis (mumps and influenza A) discussed earlier may present

with retinal edema, macular star formation, and widespread pigmentary changes
in the fundus. History, clinical examination, and serology testing may assist in differentiating these conditions in atypical
presentations. Central serous retinopathy
and Leber's idiopathic stellate neuroretinitis may also have a similar fundus picture,
but may present without the systemic manifestations.

Treatment

The treatment of measles is supportive. No
therapy has been described for measles retinitis. Passive immunization in nonimmune
pregnant women and debilitated patients
may be considered after exposure.

Prognosis

Visual prognosis is variable.

Subacute Sclerosing Panencephalitis Virus

Subacute sclerosing panencephalitis (SSPE)
is a slow, viral, CNS disease that can cause
optic neuritis and a distinct maculopathy.

Etiology

SSPE, or Dawson's inclusion body encephalitis, is caused by a variant of the measles
virus.[96] A morbillivirus within the Paramyxoviridae family, it differs from the
wild-type measles virus by alterations or
absence of viral M protein and possibly
other envelope components.[97-99]

Epidemiology

SSPE virus is a slow virus that involves the
CNS of school-aged children (5–14 years
of age).[96] In rare cases, adults develop
SSPE.[100] The frequency of SSPE after measles is 1 to 10 per million cases of measles.
Boys are involved more often than girls
(4:1). Symptoms of SSPE begin 6 to 7 years
after the initial measle virus infection. Most

children who develop SSPE contracted
measles at an early age (younger than 2
years).

Pathogenesis

In contrast to the acute febrile illness of
wild-type measles, SSPE is a persistent,
slow viral infection of the central nervous
system including the cerebrum, cerebel-
lum, spinal cord, and eye. The virus causes
a true panencephalitis. On autopsy, inflammatory foci in both the gray and white matter of the brain are noted. Intranuclear, eosinophilic inclusion bodies are found in the
lesions and contain paramyxovirus on electron microscopy. Immunohistochemical
techniques have identified the presence of
the measles virus within the brain tissue.[101,102] High titers of measles antibodies
are found in the blood and cerebrospinal
fluid.[103]

In the retina, focal areas of photoreceptor
loss and periretinal fibrosis are noted on
histopathologic examination.[104,105] Measles
virus has also been localized in the retina
at the ganglion and inner nuclear layers.

Clinical Presentation

The first stage of the disease begins with be-
havioral changes and intellectual deterioration. In the second stage, progressive neurologic deficits, extrapyramidal signs, and
cortical blindness develop. Dementia occurs in the last stage of the disease, with
death typically occurring within 1 to 3
years after disease onset.[106,107]

Patients with SSPE have ocular findings
in 30% to 75% of cases.[108,109] Disc edema,
papillitis, and optic atrophy are commonly
noted. The most consistent finding is a maculopathy. The contiguous vitreous and
choroid are not involved. Retinitis begins
as focal macular edema,[110,111] which may
evolve into a white retinal infiltrate and, in
rare cases, may be associated with intraretinal hemorrhage. Later in the course of the
disease, macular gliosis is noted. Retinal

pigmentary changes are often noted on fluorescein angiography. One patient was noted to have serous retinal detachment associated with SSPE.[110] In another series, two patients presented with a focal chorioretinitis.[111]

Diagnosis

SSPE should be considered in any school-aged child with slowly progressive deterioration in mental function and emotional behavior. The diagnosis requires a high level of clinical suspicion. SSPE retinitis does not necessarily coincide with any specific stage of the disease and may actually precede the onset of CNS symptoms and signs.[112,113] High titers of measles antibody can be found in patients with SSPE and can assist in the diagnosis.[103] Brain biopsy is the most accurate way to confirm the diagnosis.

Differential Diagnosis

Neurologic complaints and macular edema can be found in children with multiple sclerosis–associated intermediate uveitis.[114] Children present with pars planitis and progressive neurologic signs. Multiple sclerosis is not a panencephalitis, and the focal demyelination and neurologic findings differentiate this condition from SSPE. Inflammatory cystoid macular edema is noted on clinical examination and fluorescein angiography in cases of multiple sclerosis, and magnetic resonance imaging (MRI) demonstrates focal areas of demyelination.

Treatment

Treatment of SSPE is supportive. Isoprinosine delays the neurologic deterioration.[115,116] No therapy has been described for SSPE retinitis.

Prognosis

The visual and overall prognosis is grave.

Creutzfeldt-Jakob Disease

Creutzfeldt-Jakob disease (CJD) is a virus-like agent that can cause a slow virus-like disease associated with optic atrophy and retinal degeneration.

Etiology

CJD is a rare illness caused by a yet unnamed agent, which is a transmissible particle with several unique properties. It is extremely small (100 nm), lacks nucleic acids, and does not induce an immunologic response.[117] This "unconventional virus" or prion is very resistant to inactivation by formaldehyde, proteases, nucleases, heat to 80°C, ultraviolet light, and gamma irradiation.[117]

Epidemiology

With a worldwide distribution, CJD has a prevalence of 1 per million population.[118] Most cases occur in persons between the ages of 50 and 70 years.[117] A cluster of cases of CJD among Libyan Jews was associated with a dietary custom of eating sheep's eyeballs.[119]

Pathogenesis

CJD can be transmitted via corneal transplantation and by direct inoculation of tissues from infected patients.[120,121] It can be transmitted to monkeys, mice, hamsters, and other animals. CJD causes spongiform degeneration of the gray matter of the brain, loss of neurons, and astrocytic proliferation. Remarkably, little inflammation is noted in the tissues.

Clinical Presentation

Patients with CJD present with a progressive dementia, ataxia, and myoclonic jerking. The disease may progress rapidly over 6 months to stupor, coma, and eventual death.

The most common ocular manifestations in CJD is cortical blindness.[122–124] Patients may note a rapid loss of vision. Most patients have a normal fundus examination except for optic atrophy. On histopathologic examination, these patients were found to have optic atrophy with degeneration of the nerve fiber layer and loss of the ganglion cell layer.[122-124]

Diagnosis

CJD should be suspected in patients with cortical blindness, optic atrophy, and a rapidly progressing dementia. Radiologic studies, computed tomography (CT), and MRI may depict cerebral atrophy. Brain biopsy confirms the clinical diagnosis by demonstrating the characteristic spongiform degeneration.

Differential Diagnosis

The differential diagnosis for dementia is expansive. Kuru is another slow virus-like illness with associated dementia that can cause this characteristic spongiform degeneration of the brain.[117]

Treatment

Treatment is supportive.

Prognosis

The prognosis is poor.

Acute Retinal Necrosis Syndrome

The acute retinal necrosis syndrome (ARN) or the bilateral ARN (BARN) was first described in Japan by Kirisawa.[125] It is a fulminant, necrotizing viral infection of the retina.[126]

Etiology

ARN/BARN is not an etiologic diagnosis. It appears to be a bimodal disease, with one peak occurring at age 20 years and a second peak at age 50 years. Serologic, histologic, and culture information suggests HSV-2 and VZV as causes of the syndrome.[127-131] CMV has been reported in one case.[132] ARN has been reported to follow herpes zoster dermatitis and chickenpox infections.[133-135]

Epidemiology

Patients diagnosed with ARN/BARN range in age from 13 to 78 years, with an average age of 43 years.[136] This syndrome occurs typically in healthy patients, with a 2:1 male/female ratio. Patients who are immunosuppressed and persons with AIDS may also develop ARN. ARN/BARN is unilateral in 66% of cases.[136] An association with HLA-DQw7 and Bw62,DR4 has been reported.[137]

Pathogenesis

The virus is thought to spread to the eye via hematogenous or neuronal spread.[131] In the eye it causes a necrotizing retinitis, retinal arteriolitis, and vitritis.[131,138,139] A secondary granulomatous choroiditis and optic neuritis are noted on pathologic studies. In several reports viral agents have been seen enucleated with or in retinal biopsy.[130-132,138]

Clinical Presentation

Initially, patients describe an acute loss of vision and pain.[125,126,136] Early in the course, an episcleritis and a granulomatous anterior uveitis with mutton fat KP can be seen. As with many herpetic diseases, the intraocular pressure may be elevated. Within 2 weeks, the classic triad of occlusive retinal arteriolitis, prominent vitritis, and a multifocal, deep, yellow-white peripheral retinitis is noted in 100% of patients (Fig. 8.3). The retinal lesions have been called "thumbprint" lesions and have discrete margins. Macular lesions are uncommon but may be present as well. Other

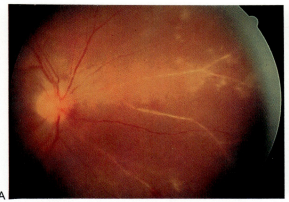
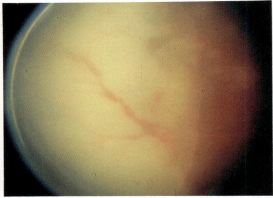

A   B

Figure 8.3. Infectious uveitis—ARN syndrome. Vitritis, retinal vasculitis (**A**), and peripheral necrotizing retinitis (**B**) in an immunocompetent adult with BARN syndrome.

findings at this stage include disc edema, choroidal thickening, retinal hemorrhage, and vein occlusion.[140,141] Retinal lesions advance rapidly and coalesce to form a confluent, peripheral, "creamy" retinitis. There is minimal hemorrhage and the posterior pole may be spared.

Later in the course, the vitreous becomes organized and the retina develops multiple, large atrophic tears. Traction/rhegmatogenous retinal detachments occur in up to 75% of patients[131,142] (see Fig. 2.31). ARN/BARN may also evolve into a chronic, granulomatous uveitis. Healed lesions may develop surrounding hyperpigmentation.

The disease is bilateral in 33% of patients. The contralateral eye can be affected immediately or up to 26 years after the initial infection.[143]

Diagnosis

The diagnosis is established clinically (Table 8.2). The triad of an acute vitritis, retinal vasculitis, and peripheral necrotizing retinitis should suggest the diagnosis.

Fluorescein angiography demonstrates optic disc staining and an ischemic retinal vasculitis. Laboratory testing is normal. Vitreous aspirate or retinal biopsy can be performed in atypical cases to confirm the diagnosis.

Differential Diagnosis

Other infectious agents such as toxoplasmosis, CMV, syphilis, and tuberculosis can cause vitritis, retinitis, and retinal vasculitis. Toxoplasmosis typically causes a focal retinitis adjacent to an older pigmented "mother" lesion. CMV retinitis occurs in immunocompromised hosts and is characterized by minimal vitritis. CMV spreads in a brushfire fashion and is often associated with retinal hemorrhage. Syphilis and tuberculosis can present with vitritis, retinitis, and retinal vasculitis. The clinical course is less fulminant than in ARN/BARN.

Autoimmune diseases such as sarcoidosis and Behçet's disease may also present with a vitritis and a retinal vasculitis but are not typically associated with confluent peripheral retinitis. Patients have other systemic manifestations in these more generalized diseases.

Treatment

Intravenous acyclovir (1500 mg/m² per day in three doses) is the treatment of choice to halt further viral replication.[144] Antiviral therapy can reduce the incidence of bilateral disease.[145] Response to therapy may be slow. Corticosteroids can be used with

Table 8.2. American Uveitis Society criteria diagnosis of the acute retinal necrosis syndrome and other necrotizing herpetic retinopathies.

Criteria for use of the term *acute retinal necrosis syndrome*:
1. A designation of acute retinal necrosis syndrome should be based solely on clinical appearance and course of infection. Clinical characteristics that must be seen:
    a. One or more foci of retinal necrosis with discrete borders located in the peripheral retina (primarily involving the area adjacent to, or outside of, the major temporal vascular arcades). Macular lesions, although less common, do not preclude a diagnosis of acute retinal necrosis syndrome if they occur in the presence of peripheral lesions
    b. Rapid progression of disease (advancement of lesion borders or development of new foci of necrosis) if antiviral therapy has not been given
    c. Circumferential spread of disease
    d. Evidence of occlusive vasculopathy, with arteriolar involvement
    e. A prominent inflammatory reaction in the vitreous and anterior chamber
2. Characteristics that support, but are not required for, a diagnosis of acute retinal necrosis syndrome:
    a. Optic neuropathy/atrophy
    b. Scleritis
    c. Pain
3. The definition of acute retinal necrosis syndrome does not depend on the extent of necrosis. As long as the criteria in 1 (a–e) are met, the disease can be designated acute retinal necrosis syndrome and modifiers such as *limited* are not necessary.
4. The definition of acute retinal necrosis syndrome does not depend on the sex, age, race, or immunologic status of the host.
5. Because it is based on the clinical appearance and course of disease only, the designation of acute retinal necrosis syndrome is not influenced by isolation of any virus or other pathogen from ocular tissues of fluid. If lesions do not meet the criteria outlined in 1 (a–e) above, the disease should not be referred to as acute retinal necrosis syndrome, whether or not varicella-zoster virus is isolated from the eye.

From Holland GN, Executive Committee of the American Uveitis Society, 1993.

antiviral therapy. Prednisone should be given after an initial 24 to 48 hours of acyclovir therapy. Aspirin (300 mg twice a day) has been administered to treat the hypercoaguable state reported in this condition.[146]

Prophylactic laser photocoagulation may help prevent retinal detachment, which develops in 75% of patients with ARN/BARN. Holes are surrounded and, in severe cases, a "new ora serrata" is created in the healthy retina to limit detachment. Once a detachment has occurred, surgical repair is complicated by the multiple, large, and often posterior retinal breaks. Inflammation and vitreous opacification present other challenges. Scleral buckle procedures alone are not as successful as internal approaches.[147,148] Pars plana vitrectomy, membranectomy, internal drainage, and endolaser photocoagulation with gas tamponade are often required in these cases.

Prognosis

The visual prognosis in ARN/BARN is poor, with 65% of patients having worse than 20/200 acuity.[131,149] The retina becomes atrophic after the acute infection. The macula often is spared in this disease, and early aggressive medical and surgical treatment can preserve central vision in the fortunate patient.

Ocular Manifestations of Infection with HIV and AIDS

AIDS is a collection of specific opportunistic infections or malignancies in a young, previously healthy person caused by infection with HIV-1.[149,150]

Etiology

HIV is an RNA virus with reverse transcriptase (retrovirus). HIV has several important envelope glycoproteins (gp). GP-120 is the ligand for the CD-4 receptor on helper T cells; gp-41 is responsible for the fusion of the virus with the host cell wall. Viral core proteins include p-24, which is currently the antigen tested for in AIDS screening.[149,150]

Epidemiology

HIV-1 has worldwide distribution and affects all races.[149-154] In the United States during the early stage of the epidemic, AIDS affected primarily young adult homosexual or bisexual men between 20 and 49 years of age. Over time intravenous (IV) drug abusers were included in the affected group.[151-154] Recently, as a result of modification in behavior, the spread of HIV has slowed in the homosexual and bisexual community. The most rapid rise today is among heterosexuals.[151,152] As a blood-borne pathogen, HIV can be transmitted through needle sticks in health care workers and through transfusion of infected blood.[149,155]

In the United States, 365,000 cases of AIDS have been reported as of 1993,[15] but the Public Health Service estimates that 1.5 million persons are infected with HIV. All those infected are thought ultimately to develop AIDS.

Pathophysiology

HIV is found in blood, semen, saliva, and urine. It has also been found in tears and in ocular tissues including the conjunctiva, cornea, and retina.[156-159] The presence of the virus in saliva, urine, and tears does not implicate these fluids in disease transmission.[149] Studies of families with nonsexual contact with an HIV-infected member have demonstrated no transmission of disease. The reasons for such lack of infectivity may be the small amount of HIV found in these fluids, the presence of inactivating substances, the absence of tissue trauma, and the low number of infected T cells found in these fluids. The median incuba-

tion period from time of infection to development of AIDS is 10 years.

HIV-1 has a predilection for cells with the CD4+ receptor. Infection of this population of cells can result in both lytic and latent infection.[150,160] T-helper cells have this receptor and are the lymphocyte population responsible for coordinating and promoting the cellular immune events and T cell–dependent antibody production. These cells are selectively and progressively depleted in HIV infection. T-cell lysis may occur through a variety of mechanisms, including the accumulation of unintegrated HIV DNA.

Clinical Presentation

The systemic manifestations of AIDS are protean.[161] Early in the course of the disease, many nonspecific symptoms can be noted including malaise, fatigue, and fevers. When the T-cell count falls below 500, specific opportunistic infections and malignancies develop, including Kaposi's sarcoma, *Pneumocystis*, CNS toxoplasmosis, and CMV retinitis (Table 8.3).[162]

Ocular findings are present in 75% of patients with AIDS.[163-167] The incidence of eye findings reported varies according to whether the series is from an ambulatory population or autopsy results. The eyelids and conjunctiva may be involved with Kaposi's sarcoma. Giant molluscum contagiosum lesions and trigeminal shingles may develop. Herpes zoster in young, healthy persons may suggest an underlying immunodeficiency. Neuroophthalmologic manifestations can be found in 8% of patients and include orbital lymphoma, cranial nerve palsies, CMV papillitis, and papilledema from cryptococcal meningitis.[163]

The retina is most often involved in AIDS; 65% to 70% of patients have retinal findings, which can be divided into microvascular or occlusive findings and opportunistic infections (Table 8.4).[163,164] Microvascular changes noted in the fundus are thought to be related to circulating immune complexes and secondary capillary

Table 8.3. CDC surveillance case definition for AIDS.

Diseases diagnosed definitively without confirmation of HIV infection in patients without other causes of immunodeficiency

Candidiasis of the esophagus, trachea, bronchi, or lungs

Cryptococcosis, extrapulmonary

Cryptosporidiosis >1 month duration

CMV infection of any organ except the liver, spleen, or lymph nodes in patients >1 month old

Herpes simplex infection, mucotaneous (>1 month duration) or of the bronchi, lungs, or esophagus in patients >1 month duration

Kaposi's sarcoma in patients <60 years old

Primary CNS lymphoma in patients <60 years old

Lymphoid interstitial pneumonitis (LIP) and/or pulmonary lymphoid hyperplasia (PLH) in patients <13 years old

Mycobacterium avium complex or *M. kansasii* disseminated

Pneumocystis carinii pneumonia

Progressive multifocal leukoencephalopathy

Toxoplasmosis of the brain in patients >1 month old

Diseases diagnosed definitively with confirmation of HIV infection

Multiple or recurrent pyogenic bacterial infections in patients <13 years old

Coccidioidomycosis, disseminated

Histoplasmosis, disseminated

Isopsoriasis >1 month duration

Kaposi's sarcoma, any age

Primary CNS lymphoma, any age

Non-Hodgkin's lymphoma (small, noncleaved lymphoma; Burkitt or non-Burkitt type; or immunoblastic sarcoma)

Mycobacterial disease other than *M. tuberculosis,* disseminated

M. tuberculosis, extrapulmonary

Salmonella septicemia, recurrent

Diseases diagnosed presumptively with confirmation of HIV infection

Candidiasis of the esophagus

CMV retinitis

Kaposi's sarcoma

LIP/PLH in patients <13 years old

Disseminated mycobacterial disease (not cultured)

Pneumocystis carinii pneumonia

Toxoplasmosis of the brain in patients >1 month old

HIV encephalopathy

HIV wasting syndrome

From Centers for Disease Control. Revision of the CDC surveillance case definition for acquired immunodeficiency syndrome. *MMWR* 1987;36(suppl):1.
HIV, human immunodeficiency virus; CNS, central nervous system; CMV, cytomegalovirus; AIDS, acquired immunodeficiency syndrome.

Table 8.4. Retinal manifestations of AIDS.

Microvascular/occlusive findings
  Cotton-wool spots
  Hemorrhages
  Perivascular sheathing
  Microaneurysms/telangiectasis
Infectious retinopathy
  Viral:
    CMV retinitis
    VZV retinitis
    Herpes simplex
    ARN/BARN
  Bacterial:
    Syphilis
    Tuberculosis
    Metastatic endogenous endophthalmitis
  Fungal:
    Candida
    Histoplasmosis
  Protozoa:
    Toxoplasmosis
    Pneumocystis

CMV, cytomegalovirus; VZV, varicella-zoster virus; ARN, acute retinal necrosis; BARN, bilateral acute retinal necrosis; AIDS, acquired immunodeficiency syndrome.

injury.[164,165] These findings include cotton-wool spots and intraretinal hemorrhages, which are not specific for HIV infection and can be found in many disorders affect-

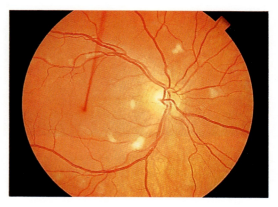

Figure 8.4. AIDS retinopathy—microvascular. Cotton-wool spots in the fundus of a patient with HIV infection. The patient had not developed opportunistic infections or AIDS-defining malignancy.

ing the small blood vessels such as diabetes, hypertension, and lupus erythematosus (Fig. 8.4). Cotton-wool spots and small hemorrhages are not typically symptomatic and may be confused for small areas of CMV retinitis.

The retina can become involved, with several microorganisms able to infect both immunocompetent and immunosuppressed patients. These diseases are described else-

where and include VZV retinitis, syphilis and tuberculosis (Chapter 9), ocular histoplasmosis and *Candida* (Chapter 10), and toxoplasmosis (Chapter 11). CMV retinitis and *Pneumocystis* choroiditis (Chapter 11) infections are typically found only in immunocompromised hosts and are opportunistic infections that can define AIDS.

Although these infectious diseases can result in a characteristic clinical presentation

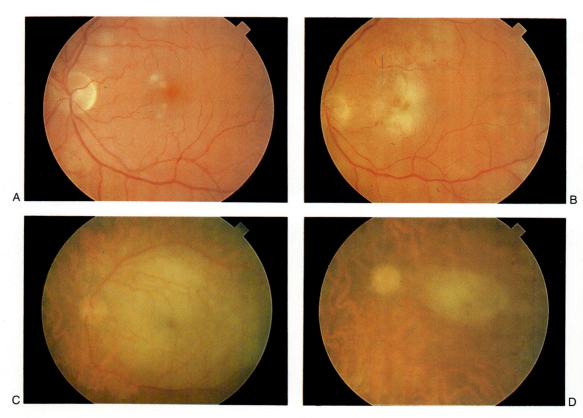

Figure 8.5. AIDS retinopathy—varicella-zoster retinitis. VZV retinitis in patients with AIDS. In contrast to ARN syndrome, the vitritis is mild and retinal vasculitis is minimal. The retinitis often begins in the posterior pole and progresses rapidly. Prognosis for visual acuity is poor. **A** and **B** show the rapid progression of the retinitis over 3 days. Central acuity fell to 20/400. **C** and

D show another patient with sudden loss of vision due to VZV retinitis. The retinitis progressed over 9 days and resulted in destruction of the posterior pole. Note the "cherry red spot" occurring with the opacification of the macula. The disease was unresponsive to high-dose IV acyclovir in both cases.

in persons with AIDS, the profound immunosuppression can greatly modify the clinical picture. For example, patients with AIDS can develop typical ARN/BARN syndrome that parallels the clinical course in immunocompetent hosts.[166,167] In AIDS, VZV appears to cause a unique form of retinitis as well (Fig. 8.5). In contrast to ARN/BARN, VZV retinitis syndrome in immunocompromised hosts begins as a rapidly progressing retinitis in the posterior pole and involves the optic nerve and macula early in the clinical course.[168,169] The posterior pole often develops a "cherry red spot." Unlike in ARN/BARN, there is minimal vitritis and no retinal vasculitis. The disease is fulminant, does not respond to routine antiviral regimens, and causes a profound loss of vision.

Syphilis, tuberculosis, and atypical mycobacterial organisms can cause retinitis and uveitis in patients with AIDS.[170-173] Because of the profound immunosuppression, diagnosis can be difficult. Skin testing for cellular hypersensitivity to tuberculin protein and testing for antibody production toward treponemal antigens may be altered. Prolonged courses of antibiotic and retreatment may be necessary because of an impaired ability of the host's immune

system to clear the microorganism. Drug-resistant strains of bacteria are emerging rapidly in these patients as well. Because of the high bacterial load, antibiotic treatment for syphilis can result in a systemic and ocular Herxheimer-like reaction, with marked worsening of the uveitis and exudative retinal detachment (Fig. 8.6). This reaction may result from the release of endotoxin and bacterial antigen associated with the death of the microorganism.

Remarkably, fungal infections of the retina are not common in AIDS. Only occasional cases of metastatic histoplasmosis or *Candida* have been reported.[174,175] In these cases, the fundus develops bilateral, multifocal, creamy subretinal lesions, which on biopsy demonstrate the presence of fungus.

Toxoplasmosis has several unique presentations in AIDS.[176-179] De novo lesions may arise that are not associated with congenital "mother" lesions typically noted in healthy persons. Multifocal areas of toxoplasmosis can also occur.[177] A severe, fulminant form of toxoplasmosis retinitis has been reported.[178] On autopsy, the retina was necrotic and hemorrhagic with active trophozoites found on histologic examination. A final form of toxoplasmosis-associated retinitis appears similar to CMV retini-

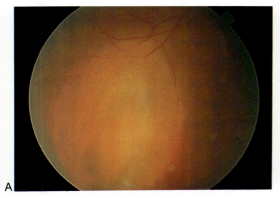 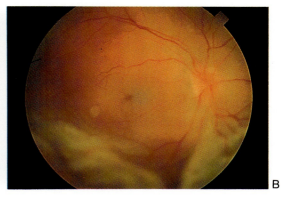

A   B

Figure 8.6. AIDS retinopathy—syphilis. Retinitis in a patient with AIDS and secondary syphilis. **A:** Note the area of subtle retinal opacification and mild vitritis. **B:** With high-dose IV penicillin, the patient developed more severe vitritis and bilateral exudative retinal detachments.

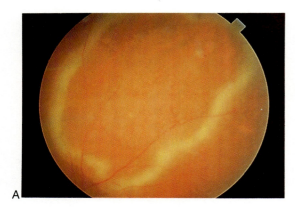

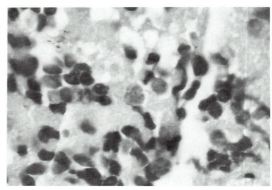

Figure 8.7. AIDS retinopathy—toxoplasmosis. Atypical toxoplasmosis may develop in immunocompromised patients. **A:** An expanding area of retinitis, vitritis, and minimal hemorrhage was unresponsive to antiviral agents. **B:** The disease progressed and a retinal biopsy was performed, showing the characteristic tissue cysts of toxoplasmosis. The retinitis responded to trimethoprim-sulfamethoxazole.

tis[179] (Fig. 8.7). Biopsy-proven cases have documented toxoplasmosis organisms in the advancing, "brushfire-like" edge of retinitis. In contrast to CMV retinitis, this form of toxoplasmosis is characterized by more vitritis, less hemorrhage, and a "creamier" appearance.

Pneumocystis carinii is an opportunistic protozoan that commonly causes pneumonia in persons with AIDS.[162] A rare characteristic form of choroiditis has been recently associated with *Pneumocystis* infection.[180,181] The organism is metastatic to the choroid. The fundus lesions are large, creamy white, and well demarcated. They occur in the posterior pole and are not associated with significant vitritis.

Diagnosis

The presence of HIV-1 infection can be determined by ELISA and Western Blot testing for anti–core protein (p24) and antiglycoprotein (gp41) antibodies.[182] Antibodies may be detected 6 weeks after primary infection. Total T-cell and helper T-cell counts can parallel the clinical disease course. The transition from HIV-1 infection to AIDS is a clinical diagnosis and is associated with a CD_4 count of less than 200. CMV retinitis is an opportunistic infection that defines AIDS.

Differential Diagnosis

The differential diagnosis for AIDS is large and includes other congenital and acquired forms of immunosuppression. Cytotoxic drugs can predispose patients to opportunistic infections and secondary malignancies.

Treatment

Prevention is an important public health priority.[149] The use of condoms can help prevent disease transmission. Health care workers and others with potential exposure to blood-borne pathogens should use universal precautions to prevent exposure.[183] The risk of HIV infection after a stick with a contaminated needle is 1 per 300 incidents. Tonometers and diagnostic contact lenses should be sterilized after each use with alcohol, heat, or 10% bleach solution.

Supportive care, treatment of opportunistic infections, and antiretroviral agents can improve the quality of life in persons with AIDS.[184] Currently, zidovudine (AZT) and dideoxynosine (DDi) are used to inhibit HIV-1 replication and slow progression of the disease.

Prognosis

HIV-1 establishes a latent infection and is incorporated in the host DNA, making a true cure improbable. At the present time, HIV infection is 100% fatal. A 1-year, median survival rate of less than 45% is reported once patients develop AIDS.[185] Opportunistic infections account for more than 90% of deaths in AIDS. Further vaccination strategies must prevent both HIV infection and disease development. Vaccines have been ineffective.

CMV Retinitis

CMV retinitis is a necrotizing, viral retinitis that occurs in immunocompromised hosts.

Etiology

CMV is a ubiquitous, double-stranded DNA virus in the Herpesvirus family.[186] Infection with CMV causes cytomegalic and cytopathologic changes and cytolysis in infected cells. CMV is species specific.

Epidemiology

The infection rate for CMV in the general population is high: 40% to 100% of adults are seropositive.[187] Clinical disease occurs in neonates and immunosuppressed patients with leukemia, lymphoma, patients on immunosuppressive chemotherapy, kidney transplant recipients, and patients with AIDS.[188] Approximately 30% of patients with AIDS develop CMV retinitis.[163] Rarely, CMV retinitis is the initial manifestation of AIDS.[189,190]

Pathophysiology

CMV is an endothelial and neurotropic virus that can cause focal retinal infections.[186] Retinal infection with CMV results in cell lysis and subsequent cell-to-cell or "brushfire-like" spread. The retina becomes opacified and hemorrhagic from ischemia and necrosis. The choroid can develop a secondary granulomatous reaction.

Similar to other herpes family viruses, CMV causes a latent viral infection. Unless the immunodeficiency is corrected, the viral retinitis reactivates in most patients when antiviral therapy is discontinued.

Clinical Presentation

Patients with CMV retinitis typically have a comfortable, "white and quiet" eye.[163,191–195] If the lesions are small and involve the peripheral retina, the disease may go unrecognized. On biomicroscopic examination, the eye may exhibit a mild vitritis. Early in the course, the lesions are small, white, and granular (Fig. 8.8). The retinitis may evolve to a more geographic, "creamy" lesion. The retinal vessels are usually involved, and intraretinal hemorrhage is a common finding. Over time, the retina becomes necrotic and may develop multiple atrophic breaks, which may lead to rhegmatogenous retinal detachment. The RPE becomes mottled, with scarring after the sensory retinitis. Subretinal deposits of whitish material can be found in the wake of the viral retinitis.

Diagnosis

CMV retinitis usually can be diagnosed on clinical grounds alone. Cultures and serology are not helpful, as most adults have antibodies to this virus.

Differential Diagnosis

The differential diagnosis for CMV retinitis includes other forms of viral retinitis such as ARN/BARN, VZV retinitis, and herpes

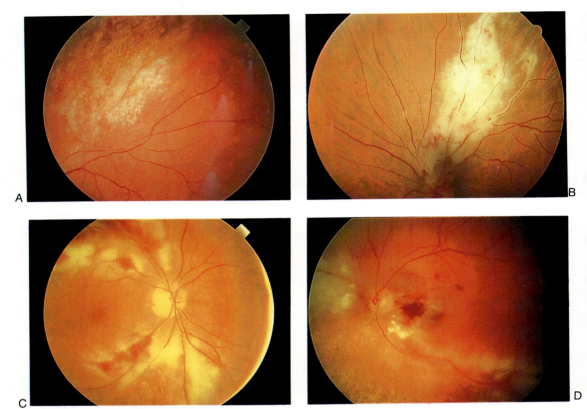

Figure 8.8. AIDS retinopathy—CMV retinitis. A: A small area of retinal opacification in a patient with early CMV retinitis and AIDS. **B:** With disease progression, the viral retinitis can appear "creamy." Intraretinal hemorrhage is often present (**C**), and the viral retinitis will spread in a "brushfire-like" fashion (**D**). Retinal detachment can occur as a result of the retinal necrosis and formation of multiple retinal breaks.

simplex retinitis. These other forms typically have more vitreous reaction and retinal vasculitis and are usually much more rapidly progressing and fulminant. Syphilis, tuberculosis, toxoplasmosis, and retinal vascular events such as branch retinal vein occlusion also should be considered in the working diagnosis.

Treatment

Small peripheral lesions (zone III) may be watched. These lesions have been known to resolve spontaneously with fluctuations in the immune status. The presence of retinal CMV, however, may be an indicator of more widespread infection and often requires antiviral therapy to prevent and treat systemic manifestations of CMV.

Disease progression or lesions that threaten the macula or optic nerve (zone 1) are ophthalmic indications for prompt treatment. Multiple reports have demonstrated effective treatment of CMV with ganciclovir.[196–201] In a controlled retrospective study of ganciclovir treatment for CMV retinitis, disease progression occurred in 94% of untreated patients over a 22-day period compared with a 43% progression in patients treated with ganciclovir.[201] Ganciclovir, 15 mg/kg per day IV, should be administered in divided doses every 8 hours for 2 weeks, followed by daily maintenance doses of 2.5 to 7.5 mg/kg per day. This drug causes leukopenia in 36% of treated patients and compromises the use of AZT therapy. Intravitreal ganciclovir can be given at a dose of 200 to 400 μg/ 0.1 ml for severe myelosuppression and for delays in induction.[202,203] A single injection has an ID_{50} of approximately 60 hours.[204] Long-term, weekly intervitreal injections of ganciclovir can be administered safely in patients who cannot tolerate systemic antiviral drugs.[205,206] Contralateral retinitis and systemic CMV disease are to be expected with intravitreal treatments.

Devices are being designed and have been used to provide a sustained release of ganciclovir after intravitreal implantation.[207,208] Complications include hemorrhage, inflammation, and retinal detachment.

Foscarnet is an effective antiviral agent for the treatment of CMV.[209] It can be given at a dose of 60 mg/kg per day every 8 hours for 14 days followed by a maintenance dose of 90 to 120 mg/kg per day. Foscarnet has been shown to have a beneficial effect on survival rate.[210] In a multicenter trial, patients treated with foscarnet lived longer than those treated with ganciclovir, although both agents were effective in treating viral retinitis. After 19 months of therapy, 51% of patients treated with ganciclovir had died compared with 34% of those treated with foscarnet.[210] AZT was discontinued more often in the ganciclovir arm of this study.

Prognosis

The prognosis for survival after the development of CMV retinitis is poor. Untreated CMV retinitis is associated with a 2-month life expectancy.[211] With antiviral therapy, survival has improved to 7 months. In most patients (80–97%), the retinitis responds to antiviral therapy. A favorable clinical response results in halting of disease progression, diminishing of the active "creamy" retinitis, and clearing of the intraretinal hemorrhage. This response may not be noted for several weeks after therapy. If the antiviral drugs are discontinued for any reason, CMV retinitis will recur in close to 100% of patients. Maintenance therapy is essential to limit reactivation. Even on maintenance therapy, however, 50% of patients experience a relapse within 6 months. Drug resistance can arise with prolonged treatment.[212,213] Patients can be switched from one agent to another if they fail a reinduction course of antiviral drug.

Retinal detachment occurs in 15% to 50% of eyes treated for CMV retinitis.[214–216] A cumulative probability of detachment may be as high as 50%.[217] Multiple posterior breaks, retinal atrophy, and active viral retinitis compromise standard laser and scleral buckle repair. Internal repair via vitrectomy and silicone oil tamponade result in the highest reattachment rates (70–100%).[216–218] Visual outcome is often poor as a result of underlying retinopathy and CMV progression. Median survival after retinal detachment is 6 to 9 months.[217]

References

1. Straus SE. Introduction to Herpesviridae. In: Mandell GL, Douglas RG, Bennett JE, eds. *Principles and Practice of Infectious Diseases.* 3rd ed. New York: Churchill Livingstone; 1990:1139.
2. Hirsch MS. Herpes simplex V. In: Mandell GL, Douglas RG, Bennett JE, eds. *Principles and Practice of Infectious Diseases.* 3rd ed. New York: Churchill Livingstone; 1990.
3. Liesegang TJ, Melton LJ III, Daly PJ, Ilstrup DM. Epidemiology of ocular herpes simplex. Incidence in Rochester, Minn, 1950 through 1982. *Arch Ophthalmol.* 1989;107: 1155.
4. Pavan-Langston D. Viral disease: herpetic infections. In: Smolin G, Thoft RA, eds. *The*

Cornea: Scientific Foundations and Clinical Practice. 2nd ed. Boston: Little, Brown; 1987.

5. Green MT, Dunkel EC. Herpes simplex virus infections: latency and reactivation. In: Darrell RW, ed. *Viral Diseases of the Eye.* Philadelphia: Lea & Febiger; 1985:9.

6. Dawson CR, Togni B. Herpes simplex eye infections: clinical manifestations, pathogenesis and management. *Surv Ophthalmol.* 1976;21:121.

7. Nahmias AJ, Visintine AM, Caldwell DR, Wilson LA. Eye infections with herpes simplex viruses in neonates. *Surv Ophthalmol.* 1976;21:100.

8. Whitley RJ. Varicella-zoster virus. In: Mandell GL, Douglas RG, Bennett JE, eds. *Principles and Practice of Infectious Diseases.* 3rd ed. New York: Churchill Livingstone; 1990.

9. Straus SE, Ostrove JM, Inchauspé G, et al. NIH conference varicella-zoster virus infections. Biology, natural history, treatment, and prevention. *Ann Intern Med.* 1988;108:221.

10. Ostler HB, Thygeson P. The ocular manifestations of herpes zoster, varicella, infectious mononucleosis, and cytomegalovirus disease. *Surv Ophthalmol.* 1976;21:148.

11. Liesegang TJ. Diagnosis and therapy of herpes zoster ophthalmicus. *Ophthalmology.* 1991;98:1216.

12. Liesegang TJ. Corneal complications from herpes zoster ophthalmicus. *Ophthalmology.* 1985;92:316.

13. Pavan-Langston D, McCulley JP. Herpes zoster dendritic keratitis. *Arch Ophthalmol.* 1973;89:25.

14. Cobo IM, Foulks GN, Liesegang T, et al. Oral acyclovir in the treatment of acute herpes zoster ophthalmicus. *Ophthalmology.* 1986;93:763.

15. Herbort CP, Buechi ER, Piguet B, et al. High-dose oral acyclovir in acute herpes zoster ophthalmicus: the end of the corticosteroid era. *Curr Eye Res.* 1991;10(suppl): 171.

16. Bernstein JE, Bickers DR, Dahl NV, Roshal JY. Treatment of chronic postherpetic neuralgia with topical capsaicin. A preliminary report. *J Am Acad Dermatol.* 1987;17: 93.

17. Opremcak EM. Viral infections of the retina. In: Pepose JS, Holland GN, Wilhelmus KR, eds. *Ocular Infection and Immunity.* St Louis: Mosby–Year Book; 1994.

18. Pepose JS. Infectious retinitis: diagnostic modalities. *Ophthalmology.* 1986;93:570.

19. Freeman WR, Stern WH, Gross JG, et al. Pathologic observations made by retinal biopsy. *Retina.* 1990;10:195.

20. Peyman GA, Fishman GA, Sanders DR, et al. Biopsy of human scleralchorioretinal tissue. *Invest Ophthalmol Vis Sci.* 1975;14:707.

21. Fujikawa LS, Haugen JP. Immunopathology of vitreous and retinochoroidal biopsy in posterior uveitis. *Ophthalmology.* 1990;97: 1644.

22. Nanda M, Curtin VT, Hilliard JK, et al. Ocular histopathologic findings in a case of human herpes B virus infection. *Arch Ophthalmol.* 1990;108:713.

23. Liesegang TJ. Diagnosis and therapy of herpes zoster ophthalmicus. *Ophthalmology.* 1991;98:1216.

24. Orellana J, Teich SA, Lieberman RM, et al. Treatment of retinal detachments in patients with the acquired immune deficiency syndrome. *Ophthalmology.* 1991;98: 939.

25. Sidikaro Y, Silver L, Holland GN, Kreiger AE. Rhegmatogenous retinal detachments in patients with AIDS and necrotizing retinal infections. *Ophthalmology.* 1991;98:129.

26. Jabs DA, Enger C, Haller J, de Bustros S. Retinal detachments in patients with cytomegalovirus retinitis. *Arch Ophthalmol.* 1991;109:794.

27. Schooley RT, Dolin R. Epstein-Barr virus (infectious mononucleosis). In: Mandell GL, Douglas RG, Bennett JE, eds. *Principles and Practices of Infectious Diseases.* 3rd ed. New York: Churchill Livingstone; 1990:1172.

28. Schooley RT. Epstein-Barr virus infections including infectious mononucleosis. In: Braunwald E, Isselbacher KJ, Petersdorf RG, et al., eds. *Harrison's Principles of Internal Medicine.* 11th ed. New York: McGraw-Hill Book Company; 1987:699.

29. Henle W, Henle G. Epstein-Barr virus and infectious mononucleosis. *N Engl J Med.* 1973;288:263.

30. Henle G, Henle W. Epstein-Barr virus-specific IgA serum antibodies as an outstanding feature of nasopharyngeal carcinoma. *Int J Cancer.* 1976;17:1.

31. Lenoir GM. Role of the virus, chromosomal translocations and cellular oncogens in the etiology of Burkitt's lymphoma. In: Epstein MW, Achong BG, eds. *The Epstein-*

Barr Virus: Recent Advances. New York: John Wiley and Sons; 1986:184.

32. Pflugfelder SC, Roussel TJ, Culbertson WW. Primary Sjögren's syndrome after infectious mononucleosis. *JAMA*. 1987;257:1049.

33. Alspaugh MA, Jensen PC, Rabin H, Tan EM. Lymphocytes transformed by Epstein-Barr virus. Induction of nuclear antigens reactive with antibody in rheumatoid arthritis. *J Exp Med*. 1978;147:1018.

34. Jones JF, Williams M, Schooley RT, et al. Antibodies to Epstein-Barr virus-specific DNase and DNA polymerase in the chronic fatigue syndrome. *Arch Intern Med*. 1988;148:1957.

35. Mueller N, Evens A, Harris NL, et al. Hodgkin's disease and Epstein-Barr virus. *N Engl J Med*. 1989;320:689.

36. Weiss LM, Movahed LA, Warnkee RA, Sklar J. Detection of Epstein-Barr viral genomes in Reed-Sternberg cells of Hodgkin's disease. *N Engl J Med*. 1989;320:502.

37. Gardner BP, Margolis TP, Mondino BJ. Conjunctival lymphocytic nodule associated with Epstein-Barr virus. *Am J Ophthalmol*. 1991;112:567.

38. Pinnolis M, McCulley JP, Urman JD. Nummular keratitis associated with infectious mononucleosis. *Am J Ophthalmol*. 1980;89:791.

39. Karpe G, Wising P. Retinal changes with acute reduction of vision as initial symptoms of infectious mononucleosis. *Acta Ophthalmol*. 1948;26:19.

40. Tanner OR. Ocular manifestations of infectious mononucleosis. *Arch Ophthalmol*. 1954;51:229–41.

41. Wong KW, D'Amico DJ, Hedges TR, et al. Ocular involvement with chronic Epstein-Barr virus disease. *Arch Ophthalmol*. 1987;105:788.

42. Peil JJ, Thelander HE, Shaw EB. Infectious mononucleosis of the central nervous system with bilateral papilledema. *J Pediatr*. 1950;37:661.

43. Blaustein A, Caccavo A. Infectious mononucleosis complicated by bilateral papilloretinal edema. *Arch Ophthalmol*. 1950;43:853.

44. Boynge TW, Von Hagen KO. Severe optic neuritis in infectious mononucleosis. Report of a case. *JAMA*. 1952;148:933.

45. Raymond LA, Wilson CA, Linnemann CC.

Punctate outer retinitis in acute EBV infection. *Am J Ophthalmol*. 1987;104:424.

46. Nozik RA, Dorsch W. A new chorioretinopathy associated with anterior uveitis. *Am J Ophthalmol*. 1973;76:758.

47. Tiedeman JS. Epstein-Barr viral antibodies in multifocal choroiditis and panuveitis. *Am J Ophthalmol*. 1987;104:659.

48. Spaide RF, Sugin S, Yannuzzi LA, DeRosa JT. Epstein-Barr virus antibodies in multifocal choroiditis and panuveitis. *Am J Ophthalmol*. 1991;112:410.

49. Palestine AG, Nussenblatt RB, Chan C-C, et al. Histopathology of subretinal fibrosis and uveitis syndrome. *Ophthalmology*. 1985;92:838.

50. Kelly SP, Rosenthal AR, Nicholson KG, Woodward CG. Retinochoroiditis in acute Epstein-Barr virus infection. *Br J Ophthalmol*. 1989;73:1002.

51. Modlin JF. Coxsackieviruses, echoviruses, and newer enteroviruses. In: Mandell GL, Douglas RG, Bennett JE, eds. *Principles and Practice of Infectious Diseases*. 3rd ed. New York: Churchill Livingstone; 1990:1367.

52. Heirholzer JC, Hatch MH. Acute hemorrhagic conjunctivitis. In: Darrell RW, ed. *Viral Diseases of the Eye*. Philadelphia: Lea & Febiger; 1985:165.

53. Hirakata K, Oshima T, Azuma N. Chorioretinitis induced by coxsackievirus B4 infection. *Am J Ophthalmol*. 1990;109:225.

54. Steere AC. *Borrelia burgdorferi* (Lyme disease, Lyme borreliosis). In: Mandell GL, Douglas RG, Bennett JE, eds. *Principles and Practice of Infectious Diseases*. 3rd ed. New York: Churchill Livingstone; 1990:1819.

55. Aaberg TM. The expanding ophthalmologic spectrum of Lyme disease. *Am J Ophthalmol*. 1989;107:77.

56. Lang GE, Schonherr U, Naumann GOH. Retinae vasculitis with proliferative retinopathy in a patient with evidence of *Borrelia burgdorferi* infection. *Am J Ophthalmol*. 1991;111:243.

57. Raoult D, Walker DH. *Rickettsia rickettsii* and other spotted fever group rickettsiae (Rocky Mountain spotted fever and other spotted fevers). In: Mandell GL, Douglas RG, Bennett JE, eds. *Principles and Practice of Infectious Diseases*. 3rd ed. New York: Churchill Livingstone; 1990:1465.

58. Gershon AA. Rubella virus (German measles). In: Mandell GL, Douglas RG, Bennett

JE, eds. *Principles and Practice of Infectious Diseases*. 3rd ed. New York: Churchill Livingstone; 1990:1242.

59. Ray CG. Rubella ("German measles") and other viral exanthems. In: Braunwald E, Isselbacher KJ, Petersdorf RG, et al., eds. *Principles and Practice of Medicine*. 11th ed. New York: McGraw-Hill Book Company; 1987:684.

60. Kresky B, Nauheim JS. Rubella retinitis. *Am J Dis Child*. 1967;113:305.

61. Zimmerman LE. Histopathologic basis for ocular manifestations of congenital rubella syndrome. *Am J Ophthalmol*. 1968;65:837.

62. Wolf SM. The ocular manifestations of congenital rubella. *J Pediatr Ophthalmol*. 1973; 10:101.

63. Hayashi M, Yoshimura N, Kondo T. Acute rubella retinal pigment epitheliitis in an adult. *Am J Ophthalmol*. 1982;93:285.

64. Gerstle C, Zinn KM. Rubella-associated retinitis in an adult: report of a case. *Mt Sinai J Med*. 1976;43:303.

65. Gregg NM. Congenital cataract following German measles in the mother. *Trans Ophthalmol Soc Aust*. 1942;3:35.

66. Matoba A. Ocular viral infections. *Pediatr Infect Dis*. 1984;3:358.

67. Blankstein SS, Feiman LH. Macular pigmentation following maternal rubella. *Am J Ophthalmol*. 1952;35:408.

68. Frank KE, Purnell EW. Subretinal neovascularization following rubella retinopathy. *Am J Ophthalmol*. 1978;86:462.

69. Tramont EC. *Treponema pallidum* (syphilis). In: Mandell GL, Douglas RG, Bennett JE, eds. *Principles and Practice of Infectious Diseases*. 3rd ed. New York: Churchill Livingstone; 1990:1794.

70. Rubsamen PE, Gass JDM. Vogt-Koyanagi-Harada syndrome: clinical course, therapy and long-term visual outcome. *Arch Ophthalmol*. 1991;109:682.

71. Johnson KM. California encephalitis and bunyaviral hemorrhagic fevers. In: Mandell GL, Douglas RG, Bennett JE, eds. *Principles and Practice of Infectious Diseases*. 3rd ed. New York: Churchill Livingstone; 1990:1326.

72. Deutman AF, Klomp HJ. Rift Valley fever retinitis. *Am J Ophthalmol*. 1981;92:38.

73. Van Velden DJ, Meyer JD, Olivier J, et al. Rift Valley fever affecting humans in South Africa: a clinicopathologic study. *S Afr Med J*. 1977;51:867.

74. Siam AE, Gharbawi KF, Meegan JM. Ocular complications of Rift Valley fever. *J Egyptian Public Health Ass*. 1978;53:185.

75. Betts RF, Douglas RG. Influenza virus. In: Mandell GL, Douglas RG, Bennett JE, eds. *Principles and Practice of Infectious Diseases*. 3rd ed. New York: Churchill Livingstone; 1990:1306.

76. Winberg RJ, Nerney JJ. Bilateral submacular hemorrhages with an influenza syndrome. *Ann Ophthalmol*. 1983;15:710.

77. Kovacs B. Alterations of the blood-retina barriers in cases of viral retinitis. *Int Ophthalmol*. 1985;8:159.

78. Rabon RJ, Louis GJ, Zegarra H, Gutman FA. Acute bilateral posterior angiopathy with influenza A viral infection. *Am J Ophthalmol*. 1987;103:289.

79. Mathur SP. Macular lesions after influenza. *Br J Ophthalmol*. 1958;42:702.

80. Knapp A. Optic neuritis after influenza with changes in the spinal fluid. *Arch Ophthalmol*. 1916;45:247.

81. Bressler NM, Bressler SB, Fine SL. Age-related macular degeneration. *Surv Ophthalmol*. 1988;32:375.

82. Baum SG, Litman N. Mumps virus. In: Mandell GL, Douglas RG, Bennett JE, eds. *Principles and Practice of Infectious Diseases*. 3rd ed. New York: Churchill Livingstone; 1990:1260.

83. Noice F, Bolin FM, Eveleth PF. Incidence of viral parotitis in the domestic dog. *Am J Dis Child*. 1959;98:350.

84. Foster RE, Lowder CY, Meisler DM, et al. Mumps neuroretinitis in an adolescent. *Am J Ophthalmol*. 1990;110:92.

85. Gellis SS, McGuiness AC, Peters M. A study of the prevention of mumps orchitis by gammaglobulin. *Am J Med Sci*. 1945; 210:661.

86. Jabs DA, Johns CJ. Ocular involvement in chronic sarcoidosis. *Am J Ophthalmol*. 1986; 102:297.

87. Gershon AA. Measles virus (rubeola). In: Mandell GL, Douglas RG, Bennett JE, eds. *Principles and Practice of Infectious Diseases*. 3rd ed. New York: Churchill Livingstone; 1990:1279.

88. Johnson RT, Griffin DE, Hirsch RL, et al. Measles encephalomyelitis—clinical and

immunologic studies. *N Engl J Med.* 1984; 310:137.

89. Metz HS, Harkey ME. Pigmentary retinopathy following maternal measles (morbilli) infection. *Am J Ophthalmol.* 1968;66:1107.

90. Guzinati GC. Suula possibilita de lesion oculari congenita da morbillo e da epatite gridemica. *Bull Ocul.* 1954;3:833.

91. Suringa DWR, Bank LJ, Ackerman AB. Role of measles virus in skin lesions and Koplik's spots. *N Engl J Med.* 1970;283:1139.

92. Bedrossian RH. Neuroretinitis following measles. *J Pediatr.* 1955;46:329.

93. Scheie HG, Morse PH. Rubeola retinopathy. *Arch Ophthalmol.* 1972;88:341.

94. Foxman SG, Heckenlively JR, Sinclair SH. Rubeola retinopathy and pigmented paravenous retinochoroidal atrophy. *Am J Ophthalmol.* 1985;99:605.

95. Haltia M, Paetau A, Vaheri A, et al. Fatal measles encephalopathy with retinopathy during cytotoxic chemotherapy. *J Neurosci.* 1977;32:323.

96. Lehrich JR. Measles-like virus (subacute sclerosing panencephalitis). In: Mandell GL, Douglas RG, Bennett JE, eds. *Principles and Practice of Infectious Diseases.* 3rd ed. New York: Churchill Livingstone; 1990: 1286.

97. Katz M, Rorke LB, Masland WS. Transmission of an encephalitogenic agent from brains of patients with subacute sclerosing panencephalitis to ferrets: preliminary report. *N Engl J Med.* 1969;279:793.

98. Chen TT, Watanabe I, Zeman W. Subacute sclerosing panencephalitis: propagation of measles virus form brain biopsy in tissue culture. *Science.* 1967;163:1193.

99. Payne FE, Baublis JV, Itashi HH. Isolation of measle virus in subacute sclerosing panencephalitis. *N Engl J Med.* 1969;281:585.

100. David P, Maurizio E, Mariotti P, Macchi G. Adult onset of subacute sclerosing panencephalitis: a case report. *Rivist Neurol.* 1990;60:83.

101. Dawson JR Jr. Cellular inclusions in cerebral lesions of lethargic encephalitis. *Am J Pathol.* 1933;9:7.

102. Dawson JR Jr. Cellular inclusions in cerebral lesions of epidemic encephalitis: second report. *Arch Neurol Psychiatry.* 1933;31: 685.

103. Connolly JH, Allen I, Hurwitz LJ. Measles-like antibody and antigen in subacute sclerosing panencephalitis. *Lancet.* 1967;1: 542.

104. Delaey JJ, Hanssens M, Colette P, et al. Subacute sclerosing panencephalitis: fundus changes and histopathologic correlations. *Doc Ophthalmol.* 1983;56:11.

105. Font RL, Jenis EH, Tuck KD. Measles maculopathy associated with subacute sclerosing panencephalitis: immunofluorescent and immuno-ultrastructural studies. *Arch Pathol.* 1973;96:168.

106. Obenour LC. Subacute sclerosing panencephalitis. *Int Ophthalmol Clin.* 1972;12:215.

107. Salib EA. Subacute sclerosing panencephalitis presenting at the age of 21 as a schizophrenic-like state with bizarre dysmorphic features. *Br J Psychiatry.* 1988;152:709.

108. Robb RM, Watters GW. Ophthalmic manifestations of subacute sclerosing panencephalitis. *Arch Ophthalmol.* 1970;83:426.

109. Green SH, Wirtschafter JD. Ophthalmoscopic findings in subacute sclerosing panencephalitis. *Br J Ophthalmol.* 1932;57:780.

110. Andriola M. Maculopathy in subacute sclerosing panencephalitis. *Am J Dis Child.* 1972;124:187.

111. Zagami AS, Lethleean AK. Chorioretinitis as a possible very early manifestation of subacute sclerosing panencephalitis. *Aust N Z J Med.* 1991;21:350.

112. Gravina RF, Nakanishi AS, Faden A. Subacute sclerosing panencephalitis. *Am J Ophthalmol.* 1978;86:106.

113. Gilden DH, Rorke LB, Tanaka R. Acute SSPE. *Arch Neurol.* 1975;32:644.

114. Giles CL. Peripheral uveitis in patients with multiple sclerosis. *Am J Ophthalmol.* 1970; 70:17.

115. DuRant RH, Dyken PR, Swift AV. The influence of inosoplex treatment on the neurologic disability of patients with subacute sclerosing panencephalitis. *J Pediatr.* 1982; 101:288.

116. Jones CE, Dyken PR, Huttenlocker PR. Inosoplex therapy in subacute sclerosing panencephalitis. *Lancet.* 1982;1:1034.

117. Lehrich JR, Tyler KL. Slow infections of the central nervous system. In: Mandell GL, Douglas RG, Bennett JE, eds. *Principles and Practice of Infectious Diseases.* 3rd ed. New York: Churchill Livingstone; 1990:769.

118. Gajdusek DC. Unconventional viruses and

the origin and disappearance of kuru. *Science.* 1977;197:943.

119. Zlotnik I, Rennie JC. Experimental transmission of mouse passaged scrapie to goats, sheep, rats and hamsters. *J Comp Pathol.* 1965;75:147.

120. Duffy P, Wolf J, Collin G, et al. Person-to-person transmission of Creutzfeldt-Jakob disease. *N Engl J Med.* 1974;299:692.

121. Rapidly progressive dementia in a patient who received a cadaveric dura mater graft. *MMWR.* 1987;36:49.

122. Lesser RL, Albert DM, Bobowick AR, O'Brien FH. Creutzfeldt-Jakob disease and optic atrophy. *Am J Ophthalmol.* 1979;87:317.

123. Tsutsui J, Kawashima S, Kajikawa I, et al. Electrophysiological and pathological studies on Creutzfeldt-Jakob disease with retinal involvement. *Doc Ophthalmol.* 1986;63:13.

124. Kitagawa Y, Gotoh F, Koto A, et al. Creutzfeldt-Jakob disease: a case with extensive white matter degeneration and optic atrophy. *J Neurol.* 1983;229:97.

125. Urayama A, Yamada N, Sasaki T, et al. Unilateral acute uveitis with retinal periarteritis and detachment. *Jpn J Clin Ophthalmol.* 1971;25:607.

126. Young NJA, Bird AC. Bilateral acute retinal necrosis. *Br J Ophthalmol.* 1978;62:581.

127. Lewis ML, Culbertson WW, Post MJD, et al. Herpes simplex virus type 1: a cause of the acute retinal necrosis syndrome. *Ophthalmology.* 1989;96:875.

128. Duker JS, Nielsen JC, Eagle RC Jr, et al. Rapidly progressive acute retinal necrosis secondary to herpes simplex virus, type 1. *Ophthalmology.* 1990;97:1638.

129. Margolis T, Irvine AR, Hoyt WF, Hyman R. Acute retinal necrosis syndrome presenting with papillitis and arcuate neuroretinitis. *Ophthalmology.* 1988;95:937.

130. Freeman WR, Thomas EL, Rao NA, et al. Demonstration of herpes group virus in acute retinal necrosis syndrome. *Am J Ophthalmol.* 1986;102:701.

131. Culbertson WW, Blumenkranz MS, Pepose JS, et al. Varicella zoster virus is a cause of the acute retinal necrosis syndrome. *Ophthalmology.* 1986;93:559.

132. Rungger-Brändle E, Roux L, Leuenberger PM. Bilateral acute retinal necrosis (BARN). Identification of the presumed infectious agent. *Ophthalmology.* 1984;91:1648.

133. Yeo JH, Pepose JS, Stewart JA, et al. Acute retinal necrosis syndrome following herpes zoster dermatitis. *Ophthalmology.* 1986;93:1418.

134. Browning DJ, Blumenkranz MS, Culbertson WW, et al. Association of varicella zoster dermatitis with acute retinal necrosis syndrome. *Ophthalmology.* 1987;94:602.

135. Culbertson WW, Brod RD, Flynn HW Jr, et al. Chickenpox-associated acute retinal necrosis syndrome. *Ophthalmology.* 1991;98:1641.

136. Fisher JP, Lewis ML, Blumenkranz M, et al. The acute retinal necrosis syndrome. Part 1. Clinical manifestations. *Ophthalmology.* 1982;89:1309.

137. Holland GN, Cornell PJ, Park MS, et al. An association between acute retinal necrosis syndrome and HLA-DQw7 and phenotype Bw62, DR4. *Am J Ophthalmol.* 1989;108:370.

138. Culbertson WW, Blumenkranz MS, Haines H, et al. The acute retinal necrosis syndrome. Part 2: histopathology and etiology. *Ophthalmology.* 1982;89:1317.

139. Topilow HW, Nussbaum JJ, Freeman HM, et al. Bilateral acute retinal necrosis. Clinical and ultrastructural study. *Arch Ophthalmol.* 1982;100:1901.

140. Sergott RC, Belmont JB, Savino PJ, et al. Optic nerve involvement in the acute retinal necrosis syndrome. *Arch Ophthalmol.* 1985;103:1160.

141. Margolis T, Irvine AR, Hoyt WF, Hyman R. Acute retinal necrosis syndrome presenting with papillitis and arcuate neuroretinitis. *Ophthalmology.* 1988;95:937.

142. Clarkson JG, Blumenkranz MS, Culbertson WW, et al. Retinal detachment following the acute retinal necrosis syndrome. *Ophthalmology.* 1984;91:1665.

143. Martinez J, Lambert HM, Capone A, et al. Delayed bilateral involvement in the acute retinal necrosis syndrome [letter to the editor]. *Am J Ophthalmol.* 1992;113:103.

144. Blumenkranz MS, Culbertson WW, Clarkson JG, Dix R. Treatment of the acute retinal necrosis syndrome with intravenous acyclovir. *Ophthalmology.* 1986;93:296.

145. Palay DA, Sternberg P Jr, Davis J, et al. De-

crease in the risk of bilateral acute retinal necrosis by acyclovir therapy. *Am J Ophthalmol.* 1991;112:250.

146. Ando F, Kato M, Goto S, et al. Platelet function in bilateral acute retinal necrosis. *Am J Ophthalmol.* 1983;96:27.

147. Peyman GA, Goldberg MF, Uninsky E, et al. Vitrectomy and intravitreal antiviral drug therapy in acute retinal necrosis syndrome. *Arch Ophthalmol.* 1984;102:1618.

148. Carney MD, Peyman GA, Goldberg MF, et al. Acute retinal necrosis. *Retina.* 1986;6:85.

149. Chamberland ME, Curran JW. Epidemiology and prevention of AIDS and HIV infection. In: Mandell GL, Douglas RG, Bennett JE, eds. *Principles and Practice of Infectious Diseases.* 3rd ed. New York: Churchill Livingstone; 1990.

150. Pantaleo G, Graziosi C, Fauci AS. The immunopathogenesis of human immunodeficiency virus infection. *N Engl J Med.* 1993; 328:327.

151. Redfield RR, Markham PD, Salahuddin SZ, et al. Heterosexually acquired HTLV-III/LAV disease (AIDS-related complex and AIDS). Epidemiologic evidence for female-to-male transmission. *JAMA.* 1985;254:2094.

152. Leads from the MMWR. Heterosexual transmission of human T-lymphotropic virus type III/lymphadenopathy-associated virus. *JAMA.* 1985;254:2051.

153. Weiss SH, Saxinger WC, Rechtman D, et al. HTLV-III infection among health care workers. *JAMA.* 1985;254:2089.

154. Report of the Second Public Health Service AIDS Prevention and Control Meeting. *Public Health Rep.* 1989;103:10.

155. Human immunodeficiency virus infection in the United States. A review of current knowledge. *MMWR.* 1987;36(suppl 6):1.

156. Fujikawa LS, Salahuddin SZ, Ablashi D, et al. HTLV-III in the tears of AIDS patients. *Ophthalmology.* 1986;93:1479.

157. Fujikawa LS, Salahuddin SZ, Ablashi D, et al. Human T-cell leukemia/lymphotropic virus type III in the conjunctival epithelium of a patient with AIDS. *Am J Ophthalmol.* 1985;100:507.

158. Salahuddin SZ, Palestine AG, Heck E, et al. Isolation of the human T-cell leukemia/lymphotropic virus type III from the cornea. *Am J Ophthalmol.* 1986;101:149.

159. Pomerantz RJ, Kuritzkes DR, de la Monte SM, et al. Infection of the retina by human immunodeficiency virus type I. *N Engl J Med.* 1987;317:1643.

160. Hamburg MA, Koenig S, Fauci AS. Immunology of AIDS and HIV infection. In: Mandell GL, Douglas RG, Bennett JE, eds. *Principles and Practice of Infectious Diseases.* 3rd ed. New York: Churchill Livingstone; 1990.

161. Chaisson RE, Volberding PA. Clinical manifestations of HIV infection. In: Mandell GL, Douglas RG, Bennett JE, eds. *Principles and Practice of Infectious Diseases.* 3rd ed. New York: Churchill Livingstone; 1990.

162. Centers for Disease Control. Revision of the CDC surveillance case definition for acquired immunodeficiency syndrome. *MMWR.* 1987;36(suppl):1.

163. Jabs DA, Green WR, Fox R, et al. Ocular manifestations of acquired immune deficiency syndrome. *Ophthalmology.* 1989;96: 1092.

164. Pepose JS, Holland GN, Nestor MS, et al. Acquired immune deficiency syndrome. Pathogenic mechanisms of ocular disease. *Ophthalmology.* 1985;92:472.

165. Newsome DA, Green WR, Miller ED, et al. Microvascular aspects of acquired immune deficiency syndrome retinopathy. *Am J Ophthalmol.* 1984;98:590.

166. Jabs DA, Schachat AP, Liss R, et al. Presumed varicella zoster retinitis in immunocompromised patients. *Retina.* 1987;7:9.

167. Chambers RB, Derick RJ, Davidorf FH, et al. Varicella-zoster retinitis in human immunodeficiency virus infection. *Arch Ophthalmol.* 1989;107:960.

168. Forster DJ, Dugel PU, Frangieh GT, et al. Rapidly progressive outer retinal necrosis in the acquired immunodeficiency syndrome. *Am J Ophthalmol.* 1990;110:341.

169. Margolis TP, Lowder CY, Holland GN, et al. Varicella-zoster virus retinitis in patients with the acquired immunodeficiency syndrome. *Am J Ophthalmol.* 1991;112:119.

170. Margo CE, Hamed LM. Ocular syphilis. *Surv Ophthalmol.* 1992;37:203.

171. McLeish WM, Pulido JS, Holland S, et al. The ocular manifestations of syphilis in the human immunodeficiency virus type 1-infected host. *Ophthalmology.* 1990;97:196.

172. Passo MS, Rosenbaum JT. Ocular syphilis

in patients with human immunodeficiency virus infection. *Am J Ophthalmol.* 1988;106:1.

173. Becerra LI, Ksiazek SM, Savino PJ, et al. Syphilitic uveitis in human immunodeficiency virus-infected and noninfected patients. *Ophthalmology.* 1989;96:1727.

174. Specht CS, Mitchell KT, Bauman AE, Gupta M. Ocular histoplasmosis with retinitis in a patient with acquired immune deficiency syndrome. *Ophthalmology.* 1991;98:1356.

175. Macher A, Rodrigues MM, Kaplan W, et al. Disseminated bilateral chorioretinitis due to *Histoplasma capsulatum* in a patient with the acquired immunodeficiency syndrome. *Ophthalmology.* 1985;92:1159.

176. Holland GN, Engstrom RE, Glasgow BJ, et al. Ocular toxoplasmosis in patients with the acquired immunodeficiency syndrome. *Am J Ophthalmol.* 1988;106:653.

177. Heinemann M-H, Gold JM, Maisel J. Bilateral toxoplasma retinochoroiditis in a patient with acquired immune deficiency syndrome. *Retina.* 1986;6:224.

178. Parke DW, Font R. Diffuse toxoplasmic retinochoroiditis in a patient with AIDS. *Arch Ophthalmol.* 1986;104:571.

179. Elkins BS, Holland GN, Opremcak EM, et al. Ocular toxoplasmosis misdiagnosed as cytomegalovirus retinopathy in immunocompromised patients. *Ophthalmology.* In press. 1994;101:499–507.

180. Freeman WR, Gross JG, Labelle J, et al. *Pneumocystis carinii* choroidopathy. A new clinical entity. *Arch Ophthalmol.* 1989;107:863.

181. Shami MJ, Freeman W, Friedberg D, et al. A multicenter study of *Pneumocystis* choroidopathy. *Am J Ophthalmol.* 1991;112:15.

182. Schleupner CJ. Detection of HIV-1 infection. In: Mandell GL, Douglas RG, Bennett JE, eds. *Principles and Practice of Infectious Diseases.* 3rd ed. New York: Churchill Livingstone; 1990.

183. Oritz R, Aaberg TM. Human immunodeficiency virus disease epidemiology and nosocomial infection. *Am J Ophthalmol.* 1991;112:335.

184. Masur H. Therapy for AIDS. In: Mandell GL, Douglas RG, Bennett JE, eds. *Principles and Practice of Infectious Diseases.* 3rd ed. New York: Churchill Livingstone; 1990.

185. Rothenberg R, Woelfel M, Stoneburner R, et al. Survival with the acquired immunodeficiency syndrome: experience with 5833 cases in New York City. *N Engl J Med.* 1987;317:1297.

186. Ho M. Cytomegalovirus. In: Mandell GL, Douglas RG, Bennett JE, eds. *Principles and Practice of Infectious Diseases.* 3rd ed. New York: Churchill Livingstone; 1990.

187. Krech U. Complement-fixing antibodies against cytomegalovirus in different parts of the world. *Bull WHO.* 1973;49:103.

188. Fiala M, Payne JE, Berne TV, et al. Epidemiology of cytomegalovirus infection after transplantation and immunosuppression. *J Infect Dis.* 1975;132:421.

189. Sison RF, Holland GN, MacArthur LJ, et al. Cytomegalovirus retinopathy as the initial manifestation of the acquired immunodeficiency syndrome. *Am J Ophthalmol.* 1991;112:243.

190. Henderly DE, Freeman WR, Smith RE, et al. Cytomegalovirus retinitis as the initial manifestation of the acquired immune deficiency syndrome. *Am J Ophthalmol.* 1987;103:316.

191. Freeman WR, Lerner CW, Mines JA, et al. A prospective study of the ophthalmologic findings in the acquired immune deficiency syndrome. *Am J Ophthalmol.* 1984;97:133.

192. Palestine AG, Rodrigues MM, Macher AM, et al. Ophthalmic involvement in acquired immunodeficiency syndrome. *Ophthalmology.* 1984;91:1092.

193. Holland GN, Pepose JS, Pettit TH, et al. Acquired immune deficiency syndrome. *Ophthalmology.* 1983;90:859.

194. Rosenberg PR, Uliss AE, Friedland GH, et al. Acquired immunodeficiency syndrome. Ophthalmic manifestations in ambulatory patients. *Ophthalmology.* 1983;90:874.

195. Jabs DA, Enger C, Bartlett JG. Cytomegalovirus retinitis and acquired immunodeficiency syndrome. *Arch Ophthalmol.* 1989;107:75.

196. Felsenstein D, D'Amico DJ, Hirsch MS, et al. Treatment of cytomegalovirus retinitis with 9-[2-hydroxy-1-(hydroxymethyl) ethoxymethol] guanine. *Ann Intern Med.* 1985;103:377.

197. Palestine AG, Stevens G Jr, Lane HC, et al. Treatment of cytomegalovirus retinitis with dihydroxy propoxymethyl guanine. *Am J Ophthalmol.* 1986;101:95.

198. Holland GN, Sidikaro Y, Kreiger AE, et al. Treatment of cytomegalovirus retinopathy with ganciclovir. *Ophthalmology.* 1987;94: 815.

199. Jabs DA, Newman C, de Bustros S, Polk BF. Treatment of cytomegalovirus retinitis with ganciclovir. *Ophthalmology.* 1987;94:824.

200. Holland GN, Sakamoto MJ, Hardy D, et al. Treatment of cytomegalovirus retinopathy in patients with acquired immunodeficiency syndrome. *Arch Ophthalmol.* 1986; 104:1794.

201. Holland GN, Buhles WC Jr, Mastre B, Kaplan HJ. A controlled retrospective study of ganciclovir treatment for cytomegalovirus retinopathy. *Arch Ophthalmol.* 1989; 107:1759.

202. Ussery FM III, Gibson SR, Conklin RH, et al. Intravitreal ganciclovir in the treatment of AIDS-associated cytomegalovirus retinitis. *Ophthalmology.* 1988;95:640.

203. Cochereau-Massin I, Lehoang P, Lautier-Frau M, et al. Efficacy and tolerance of intravitreal ganciclovir in cytomegalovirus retinitis in acquired immune deficiency syndrome. *Ophthalmology.* 1991;98:1348.

204. Henry K, Cantrill H, Fletcher C, et al. Use of intravitreal ganciclovir (dihydroxy propoxymethyl guanine) for cytomegalovirus retinitis in a patient with AIDS. *Am J Ophthalmol.* 1987;103:17.

205. Cantrill HL, Henry K, Melroe H, et al. Treatment of cytomegalovirus retinitis with intravitreal ganciclovir. *Ophthalmology.* 1989;96:367.

206. Heinemann M-H. Long-term intravitreal ganciclovir therapy for cytomegalovirus retinopathy. *Arch Ophthalmol.* 1989;107:1767.

207. Smith TJ, Pearson A, Blandford DL, et al. Intravitreal sustained-release ganciclovir. *Arch Ophthalmol.* 1992;110:255.

208. Sanborn GE, Anand R, Torti RE, et al. Sustained-release ganciclovir therapy for treatment of cytomegalovirus retinitis. *Arch Ophthalmol.* 1992;110:188.

209. Palestine AG, Polis MA, de Smet MD, et al. A randomized controlled trial of foscarnet in the treatment of cytomegalovirus retinitis in patients with AIDS. *Ann Intern Med.* 1991;115:665.

210. Studies of Ocular Complication of AIDS Research Group, in collaboration with the AIDS Clinical Trials Group. Mortality in patients with the acquired immunodeficiency syndrome treated with either foscarnet or ganciclovir for cytomegalovirus retinitis. *N Engl J Med.* 1992;326:213.

211. Holland GN, Sison RF, Jatulis DE, et al. Survival of patients with the acquired immune deficiency syndrome after development of cytomegalovirus retinopathy. *Ophthalmology.* 1990;97:204.

212. Erice A, Chou S, Biron KK, et al. Progressive disease due to ganciclovir-resistant cytomegalovirus in immunocompromised patients. *N Engl J Med.* 1989;320:289.

213. Chatis PA, Miller CH, Schrager LE, Crumpacker CS. Successful treatment with foscarnet of an acyclovir-resistant mucocutaneous infection with herpes simplex virus in a patient with acquired immunodeficiency syndrome. *N Engl J Med.* 1989;320: 297.

214. Sidikaro Y, Silver L, Holland GN, Kreiger AE. Rhegmatogenous retinal detachments in patients with AIDS and necrotizing retinal infections. *Ophthalmology.* 1991;98:129.

215. Freeman WR, Henderly DE, Wan WL, et al. Prevalence pathophysiology and treatment of rhegmatogenous retinal detachment in treated cytomegalovirus retinitis. *Am J Ophthalmol.* 1987;103:527.

216. Orellana J, Teich SA, Lieberman RM, et al. Treatment of retinal detachments in patients with the acquired immune deficiency syndrome. *Ophthalmology.* 1991;98: 939.

217. Jabs DA, Enger C, Haller J, de Bustros S. Retinal detachments in patients with cytomegalovirus retinitis. *Arch Ophthalmol.* 1991;109:794.

218. Regillo CD, Vander JF, Duker JS, et al. Repair of retinitis-related retinal detachments with silicone oil in patients with acquired immunodeficiency syndrome. *Am J Ophthalmol.* 1992;113:21.

9
Bacterial Diseases

Treponema pallidum—Syphilis

Syphilis is a sexually transmitted or blood-borne bacterial infection that is associated with myriad ocular manifestations.

Etiology

Treponema pallidum belongs to the Spirochaetaceae family and is the causative agent in syphilis. *Borrelia* and *Leptospira* are also memebers of this family.[1] Other members of the *Treponema* genus include *T. carateum* (pinta) and *T. pertenue* (yaws). The bacteria is a tightly coiled, helical organism with a 30-hour replication cycle.

Epidemiology

Syphilis can be congenital or acquired. Congenital syphilis occurs as a result of transplacental transmission. As a blood-borne pathogen, syphilis can also be transmitted by exposure to contaminated bodily fluids. Most cases of syphilis are acquired as a venereal disease through sexual intercourse. Syphilis accounts for approximately 1% to 3% of all cases of uveitis; 5% to 10% of patients with secondary syphilis develop uveitis.[2,3]

A dramatic rise in the number of cases of syphilis has occurred since the acquired immunodeficiency syndrome (AIDS) epidemic.[1,4,5] Although the adoption of safer sexual practices has slowed the spread among homosexuals and bisexuals, a rapid increase in syphilis has been reported in the heterosexual population.

Pathogenesis

T. pallidum enters the body through a break in the epidermis or mucous membranes. A spirochetemia results in widespread dissemination throughout the body, including the brain and the eye.[6] Cell-mediated immune responses play a role in limiting the spread and the eradication of the organism.[7] Antibodies do not appear to be effective in controlling the disease. The alterations and dysfunction noted in T cells in patients infected with human immunodeficiency virus (HIV) explain the altered clinical course observed with syphilis in AIDS.[8]

Clinical Presentation

Systemic manifestations of syphilis are variable and protean. In congenital syphilis, 25% of babies die, 25% are stillborn, and 40% develop neonatal lues.[1] Skin rash, notched incisor teeth, interstitial keratitis, frontal bossing, and saddle nose deformity are signs of congenital syphilis. Interstitial keratitis typically occurs in the second decade of life and is the result of antigen-antibody interaction and subsequent activation of complement.

In acquired, primary syphilis, the bacteria invade breaks in the skin or mucous membranes.[1,9] A painless chancre occurs at the site of invasion, with associated lymph node swelling 2 weeks after exposure. Multiple chancres may develop with HIV infection. With bacterial dissemination, secondary syphilis may result with widespread systemic disease. The skin, central nervous system (CNS), blood vessels, and eye are all involved. A characteristic skin rash including the palms and soles of the feet can occur. Generalized adenopathy, alopecia, and pharyngitis can also be present with low-grade fever and general malaise. Any organ system may be involved at this stage.

Tertiary syphilis occurs in 8% to 40% of patients.[1] This stage of the disease is characterized by marked debilitation, gumma formation, and severe cardiovascular and CNS manifestations. In neurosyphilis, tabes dorsalis and paresis represent meningeal inflammation and parenchymal degeneration, respectively.

Ocular manifestations in congenital syphilis include interstitial keratitis, "salt and pepper fundi," and chorioretinal scarring.[10] Visual acuity is often good in congenital forms, although optic atrophy may be present. Interstitial keratitis may be treated with penicillin but requires topical corticosteroids for control of the uveitis and neovascularization.

Secondary syphilis can involve all layers of the eye and is the "great imitator."[2,3,10–14] Patients may develop an episcleritis or true scleritis.[15,16] Keratitis linearis migrans is a slowly migrating line of inflammation in the deep corneal stroma that is unique to syphilis and is often associated with underlying keratitic precipitates (KP). Iridocyclitis in secondary syphilis may be acute, chronic, or recurrent (see Fig. 2.11).[2,3,10–14] The inflammation may be either granulomatous or nongranulomatous. Iris roseata, (areas of iris capillary dilation), vascular papules called iris papulosa, and inflammatory nodules called iris nodosa have all been observed in this stage of the disease. Posterior synechiae and vitritis are common.[10,12,14] Choroiditis, chorioretinitis, retinitis, and retinal vasculitis also may be present[17–20] (Fig. 9.1). None of these findings are characteristic or specific for syphilis. In

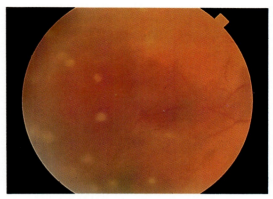

Figure 9.1. Infectious uveitis—syphilis. Vitritis, retinitis, retinal vasculitis, and multifocal choroiditis in a patient with secondary syphilis.

contrast to viral and protozoal infections, active syphilitic retinitis is often more subtle and ill defined (see Fig. 8.6). Retinal edema, segmental retinal vasculitis, and papillitis may be present.[21–24] Exudative retinal detachments have been reported.[25] With resolution of the active chorioretinitis, large areas of pigmentary disruption and retinal pigment epithelial scarring can be noted.

The ocular manifestations of secondary and neurosyphilis are more fulminant with concurrent HIV infection.[22–30] Serologic diagnosis may be impaired by the immune alterations noted in AIDS. Disease recurrences occur more frequently after appropriate courses of antibiotics.[26] Optic neuritis and neuroretinitis may occur more often in immunocompromised patients and may be the initial manifestation.[31–36]

Tertiary syphilis may have associated gumma of the iris and an Argyll Robertson pupil.[10] Intraocular inflammation is uncommon at this stage.

Diagnosis

Syphilis can be diagnosed directly by identifying the organism in specimens taken from active lesions or indirectly through the detection of antibodies.[37] The Venereal

Disease Research Laboratory test (VDRL) detects nonspecific reagin antibodies found in syphilis.[37] The fluorescent treponemal antibody absorption test (FTA-Abs) and the microhemagglutination test for syphilis (MHA-TP) are bacteria-specific assays. Blood, cerebrospinal fluid (CSF), and aqueous and subretinal fluids can all be used to diagnose the presence of these *Treponema*-associated antibodies. These tests may be negative with coexisting HIV infection.[38]

Early congenital syphilis may not be associated with positive serologies. Darkfield examination of blood or mucus confirms the presence of spirochetes. Later, 60% of patients with congenital syphilis test positive for VDRL and FTA-Abs. Primary syphilis can be diagnosed via darkfield scraping from the chancre.[1,37] At this stage of the disease, 76% of patients have a positive VDRL, and 86% are positive for FTA-Abs. All patients with active secondary syphilis have positive VDRL and FTA-Abs serology. In latent and tertiary syphilis, VDRL is positive in 70% of the cases, and the FTA-Abs is positive in 97% of cases. Neurosyphilis can be confirmed via CSF analysis for VDRL and FTA-Abs. The VDRL titer should fall in the CSF with effective therapy.

Nontreponemal serologies (VDRL and RPR) decline to undetectable levels after effective antibiotic therapy, but *Treponema*-specific antibodies (FTA-Abs and MHA-TP) are detectable throughout life. Many authors have suggested that both VDRL and *Treponema*-specific antibody testing should be performed in patients with uveitis to reduce false-negative results.[2,12–14,39]

Differential Diagnosis

Syphilis should be included in the differential diagnosis of all forms of uveitis because of its protean ocular manifestations. Scleritis, retinal vasculitis, optic neuritis, interstitial keratitis, neuroretinitis, chorioretinitis, and nonspecific uveitis may all be caused by syphilis and appropriate screening should be initiated.

Treatment

Because of its embryologic development, anatomic relationships, and analogous blood–eye barriers, ocular inflammation secondary to syphilis should be considered and treated as neurosyphilis.[10,13,14,39] Penicillin is the drug of choice.[40] Patients who are allergic to penicillin should be skin tested and, if found positive, desensitized to provide for adequate therapy.[41]

Penicillin G, 2 to 5 million units given intravenously every 4 hours for 10 to 14 days, or penicillin G procaine, 2 to 4 million units given intramuscularly every day with oral probenecid, 500 mg given every 4 hours for 10 to 14 days, are the only proven effective therapies for ocular syphilis and neurosyphilis and in both normal and immunosuppressed patients. Doxycycline, 200 mg given orally twice a day for 21 days, and other drug regimens have been used in neurosyphilis, but increased treatment failures have been reported.[42,43]

The ophthalmologist is often the physician who makes the diagnosis in ocular, secondary, and neurosyphilis. Consultation with the patient's primary care physician and, in most cases, with an infectious disease specialist can be valuable. Antibiotic therapy can be challenging; inadequate therapy results in recurrent or persistent disease.

Topical or regional corticosteroids are sometimes required to assist in the control of ocular inflammation associated with syphilis.[10,33] Several authors have also reported a worsening of the visual acuity and ocular inflammation with penicillin therapy.[44–47] A Jarisch-Herxheimer–like reaction in the eye has been proposed.[44–46]

Prognosis

With appropriate antibiotic therapy, ocular inflammation typically resolves rapidly. Failure to diagnose and treat ocular syphilis can result in permanent tissue damage and blindness. The relative sanctuary offered by the eye can result in recurrent disease from poor antibiotic penetration.

Risk factors and behaviors for acquiring syphilis are similar to those for HIV infection and other blood-borne infectious diseases. All patients with syphilis should be offered HIV testing. Patients with AIDS may have an altered clinical course with syphilis. A suppressed cell-mediated and humoral immune response can result in an increased infectious period, probability of infection, and susceptibility to infection. The diagnosis of syphilis in AIDS may be difficult, as detection relies on the development of antibodies. Because of the massive treponemal load that can develop in the absence of an effective immune response, the clinical course may be more malignant. A Herxheimer-like reaction can be noted in the eye with aggressive antibiotic therapy. Rapid death of large numbers of bacteria can result in the release of endotoxin and bacterial antigens and worsening of the clinical picture.

Borrelia burgdorferi—Lyme Disease

Lyme disease is a multisystem disorder caused by the spirochete *Borrelia burgdorferi*. It is a tick-borne disease with dermatologic, rheumatologic, neurologic, and cardiac manifestations. Lyme disease was named for a cluster of patients who developed an inflammatory arthropathy and characteristic skin rash in Old Lyme, Connecticut, in 1975.[48]

Etiology

B. burgdorferi is a tick-transmitted spirochete. Along with *Treponema* and *Leprospira*, it is a member of the Spirochaetaceae family.[49]

Epidemiology

Lyme disease is transmitted via a tick vector *Ixodes scapularis* in the American Northeast and upper Midwest and by *Ixodes pacificus* in the West.[49,50] More than 90% of cases occur in the eastern coastal United States, the upper Midwest, and nothern California.[51] Recently, dog ticks have been found to carry the bacteria. Nymphal and adult ticks prefer the white-tailed deer; human beings are accidental hosts. In the United States, 9600 cases were reported in 1992.[52]

Pathogenesis

A primary infection occurs at the site of the tick bite. A spirochetemia with bacterial dissemination can occur after primary infection.[49,52]

Clinical Presentation

The first stage of the disease begins with malaise, fatigue, headache, fever, and arthralgias.[48,52] The clinical hallmark is a distinctive expanding erythematous skin, erythema chronicum migrans, that begins at the site of the tick bite and extends outward in a circular pattern. The second stage of the disease begins the fourth week after inoculation. Neurologic involvement may result in meningitis, peripheral radiculopathy, and cranial nerve palsies. Cardiovascular symptoms and signs occur at this stage of the disease as well. The third stage occurs months to years later, with severe arthritis and chronic neurologic syndromes.

Ocular involvement may occur in all late stages of disease. A mild conjunctivitis occurs in approximately 11% of stage-1 patients.[53,54] During the second and third stages, neuroophthalmic manifestations can be noted, including cranial neuropathy, optic neuritis, and Bell's palsy. Other findings include bilateral keratitis, bilateral granulomatous iridocyclitis, bilateral diffuse choroiditis, retinal vasculitis, and intermediate uveitis.[53–60] Exudative retinal detachments have been reported in a patient with active Lyme disease.[61,62] A keratitis and diplopia also have been described in stage 3.[48,63–65] Retinal vascular occlusion and secondary, proliferative retinopathy have also been observed.

Diagnosis

Ocular findings are nonspecific and by themselves do not establish the diagnosis. As in other spirochetal diseases, many parts of the eye may be involved. Patients with ocular inflammation and a history of travel to an endemic area for Lyme disease should be tested for infection. A history of a tick bite, characteristic skin rash, and neurologic, cardiovascular, and joint symptoms further support the diagnosis. Serologic testing via enzyme-linked immunoadsorbent assay (ELISA) for immunoglobulin M (IgM) and immunoglobulin G (IgG) for *B. burgdorferi* and Western Blot testing confirm exposure to the bacteria.[49,52] In endemic areas, the presence of erythema chronicum migrans (ECM) or the confirmation of at least one organ system (e.g., eye) with positive serology is diagnostic.[65] In nonendemic regions, EMC with positive serology or ECM with two-organ system disease are the diagnostic requirements.

False-positive and false-negative testing is not uncommon.[66–68] Antibodies to *B. burgdorferi* cross-react with other spirochetes, including *T. pallidum*.[49]

Differential Diagnosis

Syphilis, tuberculosis, and sarcoidosis may all have multiorgan system involvement with constitutional, arthritic, and neurologic symptoms. History, physical examination, and laboratory testing can help distinguish these conditions.

Treatment

Treatment with antibacterial agents can be challenging.[49,52,59,67] Recurrence has been reported. The organism may take sanctuary in the blood–eye and blood–brain barriers. Treatment in men, nonpregnant women, and children older than 8 years consists of 21 days of oral tetracycline, 250 mg, four times a day or oral doxycycline, 100 mg, twice a day.[69] Penicillin V or amoxicillin in pediatric doses are effective for children. Patients with neurologic symptoms or prolonged disease may require treatment for 4 to 6 weeks. In resistant cases, a second course of oral antibiotics can be given or, alternatively, intravenous ceftriaxone, 2 g/day, for 14 days may be tried. Intravenous penicillin, 10 to 20 IU/day, has also been used in some resistant cases.[70] Topical treatment of uveitis with steroids and cycloplegics is recommended, but only in conjunction with antibacterial agents.

Prognosis

Antibiotic treatment early in the course of the disease carries a better prognosis than therapy initiated at later stages. Chronic inflammation, arthritis, and permanent neurologic and ocular damage may result form long-standing infection.

Leptospira species— Leptospirosis

Leptospirosis is a generalized bacterial disease that can cause an anterior uveitis.

Etiology

Leptospira species are members of the Spirochaetaceae family.[71] There are 170 serotypes of pathogenic bacteria in this genus.

Epidemiology

Disease by any type of *Leptospira* species is called leptospirosis.[71] The disease is a zoonosis; humans acquire the infection from exposure to infected animals or their secretions.

Pathogenesis

Leptospira species gain entry through breaks in skin or mucous membranes. Leptospiremia occurs with dissemination to all parts of the body, including the brain and eye.

Clinical Presentation

Systemic symptoms and signs of leptospirosis include headache, chills, fever, and muscle aches.[71] Kidney and liver involvement may occur and patients may develop jaundice with scleral icterus. Leptospirosis infection can be severe with azotemia, hemorrhage, and hypotension (Weil's disease). Ocular involvement has been reported to occur months after the acute infection.[72,73] Affected patients can develop bilateral iritis with nongranulomatous KP.

Diagnosis

A high degree of clinical suspicion needs to be maintained in the diagnosis of leptospirosis. A patient with iritis, exposure to sick animals, and significant systemic complaints compatible with leptospirosis should be tested serologically for antibodies toward the organisms.

Differential Diagnosis

Brucellosis and rickettsial disease can present with an acute febrile illness with multisystem involvement and an anterior uveitis after exposure to sick animals.

Treatment

Penicillin, 2.4 to 3.6 million units/day given intravenously, or tetracycline (2g/day given orally in four divided doses) have been used to treat this disease.

Prognosis

The prognosis is good with treatment. Severe forms of the disease have been fatal.

*Mycobacterium tuberculi—*Tuberculosis

Tuberculosis is a multisystemic infectious disease caused by *Mycobacterium tuberculi*.

Etiology

M. tuberculi is an acid-fast bacillus belonging to the family Mycobacteriaceae. It is a slow-growing, obligate parasite in humans and primates.[74]

Epidemiology

Worldwide, tuberculosis is endemic. It is thought to infect half the world's population and account for 3 million deaths per year.[75] In the United States, the rate of tuberculin skin test positivity has been declining as a result of public health measures and effective antibiotic chemotherapy. An increase in the number of cases, especially multidrug-resistant cases, has been noted in association with the AIDS epidemic.[74,76] In 1990, 25,701 new cases of tuberculosis were reported, or almost 10,000 more cases than predicted.[77]

Tuberculosis has been thought to be responsible for <1% to 52% of all uveitis[78,79]; most studies report a 1% incidence.[80]

Pathogenesis

Tuberculosis is acquired by inhalation of viable bacteria.[75] Prolonged exposure to an infected person increases the likelihood of infection. Cell-mediated immune responses are required to halt the disease. Once the organism is in the lung, bacterial replication occurs. The organism may then spread to other extrapulmonary sites through infected macrophages. The cell wall proteins of mycobacteria are potent stimulators of the immune system and promote an inflammatory response, with caseating granuloma formation.[75] The granuloma is comprised of lymphocytes, macrophages, Langhans' giant cells, and fibroblasts. This hypersensitivity can be documented by tuberculin skin tests.

Clinical Presentation

Tuberculosis is a multisystemic disease.[75] Patients complain of low-grade fever,

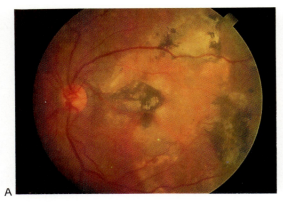
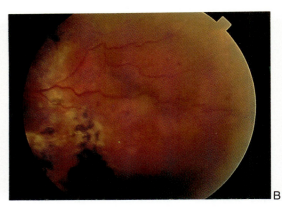

Figure 9.2. **Infectious uveitis—tuberculosis.** Multifocal chorioretinitis (**A**), choroidal nodules (**B**), and bilateral, diffuse, granulomatous uveitis in a patient with active pulmonary tuberculosis. The bacteria were cultured from the sputum and were multidrug resistant.

fatigue, weight loss, and night sweats. Patients with active pulmonary disease exhibit a productive cough and dyspnea.

Any structure in the eye can be affected in tuberculosis. Scleritis, keratitis, and chronic iridocyclitis have all been reported.[81,82] The uveitis may be granulomatous or nongranulomatous. Vitritis, retinochoroiditis, and choroidal nodules are other manifestations of active tuberculosis[83–87] (Fig. 9.2). Orbital infections and optic neuritis have also been reported.[88] Multidrug-resistant strains of tuberculosis can cause severe, medically unresponsive chorioretinitis.[89]

Diagnosis

Induced sputum cultures and gastric washings can be obtained to confirm the diagnosis.[75] Acid-fast bacilli can often be seen on the smears. The bacteria are slow growing and may take several weeks of culture for positive identification. In active pulmonary forms, chest radiographs demonstrate signs suggestive of tuberculosis.

Tuberculin skin testing is useful in screening patients for exposure to tuberculosis. More than 95% of patients with tuberculosis respond to the 5 TU (standard Mantoux) skin test with a 10-mm or greater area of induration. The second-strength skin test has 250 TU and can be used when the first strength fails in suspected cases. Serum lysozyme and angiotensin-converting enzyme (ACE) are often elevated during active disease.

Differential Diagnosis

Tuberculosis can affect any part of the eye and should be considered in the differential diagnosis of all forms of ocular inflammation. Both sarcoidosis and syphilis can cause a similar clinical picture with multiple ocular manifestations. Patients with sarcoidosis also exhibit changes on chest radiograph and elevated levels of serum ACE and lysozyme. Skin testing can help differentiate tuberculosis from sarcoidosis. Patients with sarcoidosis will be anergic to a panel of common antigens and will not react to tuberculin testing.

Treatment

There is little controversy regarding the need for treatment in a patient with uveitis, a skin test that has recently converted to positive, a suggestive chest radiograph and positive bacterial cultures. Standard regimens combine isoniazid (INH), 300 mg/day, with rifampin (RMP), 600 mg/day, for 9 months.[75,90] Various protocols are available for multidrug-resistant strains.[91] The addition of a third antibiotic is indicated early in the course of therapy while waiting for sensitivity reports or in areas endemic for drug-resistant strains. Pyrazinamide (PZA), 25 to 35 mg/kg, streptomycin (STM), 1 g, or ethambutol, 15 to 25 mg/kg, can be added to the standard regimen in these situations.[75,91] Short-term (6 months) courses have been effective when combining INH and RMP regimens with PZA.[92,93] Patients with uveitis who are known to convert from negative to positive on tuberculin skin test should also receive a course of antibiotics. As a result of increasing drug resistance among strains of tuberculosis, culture and sensitivities may be required to direct therapy or assist in patients who fail to respond to initial empiric therapy. Directly observed treatment protocols have been proposed based on public health issues.

It is less clear how to approach a patient with uveitis and a positive skin test of unknown duration and without recent conversion.[82,94,95,96] A thorough assessment of other clinical symptoms and signs, radiologic studies, and laboratory tests such as ACE and lysozyme elevation can help support a presumptive diagnosis. Efforts to obtain cultures from gastric washings or sputum should be made. In this setting, a 3-month trial of antituberculosis therapy has been advised as empiric therapy.[96]

Adjunctive corticosteroid therapy is sometimes required in the treatment of tuberculosis-associated uveitis. Dead organisms have cell wall components that are potent stimulators of the immune response. These proteins may even promote an autoimmune response toward ocular autoantigens.[94] Experimental animal models of autoimmune uveitis use autoantigens combined with an adjuvant comprised of these cell wall proteins (Freund's adjuvant) to induce the uveitis.[97] Any patient who requires oral corticosteroid therapy for any disease and who has a history of tuberculosis should be treated with prophylactic antibiotic therapy as well to prevent recurrent disease.

As a result of liver toxicity, patients on INH and RMP require liver function testing. Ethambutol has been associated with optic neuropathy.

Prognosis

The prognosis may be guarded. Recurrences can occur years after primary infection and even after apparently well-designed antibiotic therapy. New antibiotic-resistant strains have been associated with a high morbidity and mortality.[76] Visual prognosis depends on the location of ocular infection and subsequent scar formation. Macular lesions can result in blindness with extensive chorioretinal scarring.

Mycobacterium leprae—Leprosy

Leprosy is a bacterial disease caused by *Mycobacterium leprae*, which can cause a keratouveitis.

Etiology

M. leprae is an obligate intracellular bacterium with a tropism for nervous tissue. It grows best at cooler temperatures[98] and is acid-fast on staining.

Epidemiology

An estimated 12 million cases of leprosy exist worldwide, with 75,000 blinded by ocular complications. Disease transmission is person to person by either direct contact or through respiratory secretions. Some authors have reported ocular involvement in 50% of patients with leprosy.[82]

Pathogenesis

M. leprae spreads along nerves and secondarily infects the contiguous tissues. Macrophages ingest the bacterium with subsequent granuloma formation. The two forms of leprosy are the lepromatous and the tuberculoid patterns.[98] Patients with strong cell-mediated immunity develop the more favorable tuberculoid form of the disease; patients with absent cellular responses tend to develop the lepromatous form.

Clinical Presentation

M. leprae grows best at lower temperatures. Lepromatous forms of the disease, therefore, have a predilection for the skin and cornea.[99–103] Corneal infection is associated with a prominence of the corneal nerves, interstitial keratitis, and corneal anesthesia. Secondary spread to the contiguous iris and ciliary body causes an anterior uveitis with characteristic iris leproma known as pearls.[103] The tuberculoid form has less skin involvement and the infection typically remains confined to nervous tissues. Orbital disease with granuloma formation is more common with tuberculoid forms of leprosy.

Diagnosis

Diagnosis is based largely on clinical findings.[98] Lepromin skin testing can be positive in tuberculoid leprosy but is negative in lepromatous forms. Serum lysozyme and ACE can be elevated. Skin biopsy of affected areas demonstrates perineural infiltration of the organism on special and acid-fast staining.

Differential Diagnosis

Tuberculosis, sarcoidosis, and syphilis can cause a granulomatous iridocyclitis and keratitis. Herpetic disease should be considered in the differential diagnosis of any keratouveitis.

Treatment

Treatment of leprosy is prolonged and challenging. A combination of dapsone, 50 to 100 mg/day, rifampin, 600 mg/day, and clofazimine, 500 mg/day, is standard therapy. Multidrug therapy is recommended for 2 years.[104] Intermittent therapy can be administered, but is associated with increased risk of drug resistance.[98] Ansamycin has also been used to treat leprosy.[106,107]

Prognosis

The prognosis is worse for the lepromatous form of leprosy.

Brucella species—Brucellosis

Brucella species are a rare cause of a systemic bacterial disease in human beings that has been associated with uveitis.

Etiology

Brucella species is a zoonosis of domestic animals.[108] It is a gram-negative coccobacilli.

Epidemiology

Brucella is transmitted by exposure to sick or wild animals. Direct contact with infected tissues or fluids can result in infection in humans through abraded skin or mucous membranes.

Pathogenesis

The bacteria spread throughout the reticuloendothelial system, including the spleen and bone marrow.[108] The organism replicates and provokes a granulomatous reaction with epithelioid cell formation and noncaseating granulomas. Langhans' cells can be seen on pathologic specimen.

Clinical Presentation

Malaise, arthralgias, headache, and fever are constitutional complaints in the early phases of the disease.[108] Patients may exhibit osteomyelitis and hepatosplenomegaly on examination. The acute toxic phase may evolve into a subacute or chronic disease. Ocular manifestations are rare but include a nongranulomatous iritis and focal nodular choroiditis, as well as a severe panophthalmitis and metastatic endophthalmitis.[109,110]

Diagnosis

A high degree of suspicion is required in the diagnosis of brucellosis. Specific agglutinating antibodies develop slowly and are often too late to assist in the diagnosis during the acute phase of the disease. *Brucella* skin tests are available but not widely used. Rarely, blood cultures can provide evidence for *Brucella* sepsis.

Differential Diagnosis

Acute febrile illness with uveitis may suggest Lyme disease or rickettsial disease such as Rocky Mountain spotted fever.

Exposure to sick animals may suggest the diagnosis.

Treatment

Tetracycline, 30 mg/kg per day, in four divided doses for 4 weeks is the treatment of choice.[108] This regimen is often combined with rifampin, 600 mg/day. Sulfa antibiotics may be used in patients allergic to tetracycline derivatives.

Prognosis

Brucellosis may be fatal if not recognized and treated early with appropriate antibiotics.

Whipple's Disease

Whipple's disease is a multisystem, recurrent disease that is presumed to be infectious.

Etiology

Whipple's organisms have not been isolated or cultured, but they appear to be rod-shaped bacilli.[111] The organism can be

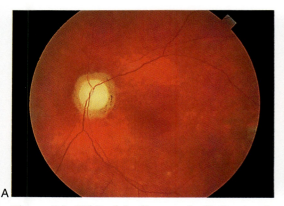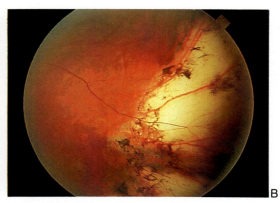

Figure 9.3. Whipple's disease. A, Optic atrophy, and **B**, peripheral chorioretinal scars in a patient with Whipple's disease.

seen within macrophages throughout the body and in the intestinal epithelial cells. The Whipple's bacillus may be an intracellular bacterium.[112]

Epidemiology

The disease is more common in men; the average age of onset is 50 years.

Pathogenesis

Granules [periodic acid–schiff (PAS) positive] and rod-shaped bacilli can be seen within macrophages of the intestinal villi on jejunal biopsy and in the central nervous system (CNS).

Clinical Presentation

Patients with Whipple's disease experience a recurrent, multisystem illness.[111,113] Pneumonia, pleurisy, tonsillitis, sinusitis, cystitis, and arthralgia are common. Patients often have a chronic fever and weight loss. Abdominal pain, diarrhea, and malabsorption are other gastrointestinal (GI) features.[113,114] CNS complaints include seizure, psychosis, mental deterioration, and ophthalmoplegia. Patients with Whipple's disease complain of progressive loss of vision and floaters. Ocular findings include chemosis, vitritis, chorioretinitis, papilledema, retinal vasculitis, and vitreous hemorrhage[115–118] (Fig. 15.1).

Diagnosis

Patients with uveitis, retinal vasculitis, and systemic complaints of abdominal pain, diarrhea, arthralgia, and weight loss should be suspected of having Whipple's disease. Jejunal biopsy demonstrates the bacilliform organism and PAS-positive granules within macrophages.[111,113] Vitrectomy may be diagnostic.[118] Fluorescein angiography has demonstrated disc edema, vasculitis, and multifocal hyperfluorescent areas corresponding to areas of subretinal lesions.[117]

Differential Diagnosis

Systemic lupus erythematosus, polyarteritis nodosa, and Behçet's disease can have multisystemic involvement, retinal vasculitis, and uveitis.

Treatment

Intravenous penicillin followed by a year of tetracyclin or trimethoprim sulfametroxazole is the treatment of choice.[111,113,114] Intraocular inflammation can be controlled with topical, regional, or oral corticosteroids.

Prognosis

Whipple's disease can be progressive, recurrent, and resistent to therapy.[111] CNS involvement is a serious complication and can be fatal.

References

1. Tramont EC. *Treponema pallidum* (syphilis). In: Mandell GL, Douglas RG Jr, Bennett JE, eds. *Infectious Diseases*. 3rd ed. New York: Churchill Livingstone; 1990:1794.
2. Ross WH, Sutton HFS. Acquired syphilitic uveitis. *Arch Ophthalmol*. 1980;98:496.
3. Schlaegel TF Jr, Kao SF. A review (1970–1980) of 28 presumptive cases of syphilitic uveitis. *Am J Ophthalmol*. 1982;93:412.
4. Schmidt H, Jorgensen AS, Petersen HO. An epidemic of syphilis among homosexuals and bisexuals. *Acta Derm Venereol*. 1994; 120(suppl):56.
5. Mindel A, Tovey SJ, Williams P. Primary and secondary syphilis, 20 years' experience. 1. Epidemiology. *Genitourin Med*. 1987;63:361.
6. Lukenhart S, Hook EW, Baker-Zander SH, et al. Invasion of the central nervous system by *Treponema pallidum*. Implications for diagnosis and therapy. *Ann Intern Med*. 1988;109:855.
7. Musher DM, Schell RF. The immunology of syphilis. *Hosp Pract*. December, 1975, p 45.
8. Bowen DL, Lane HC, Fauci AS. Immunopathogenesis of the acquired immunode-

ficiency syndrome. *Ann Intern Med.* 1985; 103:704.

9. Mindel A, Tovey SJ, Timmins DJ, Williams P. Primary and secondary syphilis, 20 years' experience. 2. Clinical features. *Genitourin Med.* 1989;65:1.

10. Margo CE, Hamed LM. Ocular syphilis. *Surv Ophthalmol.* 1992;37:203.

11. Zierhut M, Kreissig I, Pickert A. Panuveitis with positive serological tests for syphilis and Lyme disease. *J Clin Neuro Ophthalmol.* 1989;9:71.

12. Spoor TC, Wynn P, Hartel WC, Bryan CS. Ocular syphilis: acute and chronic. *J Clin Neuro Ophthalmol.* 1983;3:197.

13. Tamesis RR, Foster CS. Ocular syphilis. *Ophthalmology.* 1990;97:1281.

14. Deschenes J, Seamone CD, Baines MG. Acquired ocular syphilis: diagnosis and treatment. *Ann Ophthalmol.* 1992;24:134.

15. Watson PG, Hayreh SS. Scleritis and episcleritis. *Br J Ophthalmol.* 1976;60:163.

16. Wilhelmus KR, Yokoyama CM. Syphilitic episcleritis and scleritis. *Am J Ophthalmol.* 1987;104:595.

17. de Souza EC, Jalkh AE, Trempe CL, et al. Unusual central chorioretinitis as the first manifestation of early secondary syphilis. *Am J Ophthalmol.* 1988;105:271.

18. Gass JDM, Braunstein RA, Chenoweth RG. Acute syphilitic posterior placoid chorioretinitis. *Ophthalmology.* 1990;97:1288.

19. Halperin LS, Lewis H, Blumenkranz MS, et al. Choroidal neovascular membrane and other chorioretinal complications of acquired syphilis. *Am J Ophthalmol.* 1989;108:554.

20. Crouch ER, Goldberg MF. Retinal periarteritis secondary to syphilis. *Arch Ophthalmol.* 1975;93:384.

21. Weinstein JM, Lexow SS, Ho P, Spickards A. Acute syphilitic optic neuritis. *Arch Ophthalmol.* 1981;99:1392.

22. Arruga J, Valentines J, Mauri F, et al. Neuroretinitis in acquired syphilis. *Ophthalmology.* 1985;92:262.

23. Halperin LS, Berger AS, Grand MG. Syphilitic disc edema and periphlebitis. *Retina.* 1990;10:223.

24. Folk JC, Weingeist TA, Corbett JJ, et al. Syphilitic neuroretinitis. *Am J Ophthalmol.* 1983;95:480.

25. de Luise VP, Clark SW III, Smith JL, Collart

P. Syphilitic retinal detachment and uveal effusion. *Am J Ophthalmol.* 1982;94:757.

26. Passo MS, Rosenbaum JT. Ocular syphilis in patients with human immunodeficiency virus infection. *Am J Ophthalmol.* 1988;106:1.

27. McLeish WM, Pulido JS, Holland S, et al. The ocular manifestations of syphilis in the human immmunodeficiency virus type 1–infected host. *Ophthalmology.* 1990;97:196.

28. Becerra LI, Ksiazek SM, Savino PJ, et al. Syphilitic uveitis in human immunodeficiency virus-infected and noninfected patients. *Ophthalmology.* 1989;96:1727.

29. Stoumbos VD, Klein ML. Syphilitic retinitis in a patient with acquired-immunodeficiency syndrome-related complex [letter to the editor]. *Am J Ophthalmol.* 1987;2:103.

30. Joyce PW, Haye KR, Ellis ME. Syphilitic retinitis in a homosexual man with concurrent HIV infection: case report. *Genitoruin Med.* 1989;65:244.

31. Levy JH, Liss RA, Maguire AM. Neurosyphilis and ocular syphilis in patients with concurrent human immunodeficiency virus infection. *Retina.* 1989;9:175.

32. Zambrano W, Perez GM, Smith JL. Acute syphilitic blindness in AIDS. *J Clin Neuro Ophthalmol.* 1987;7:1.

33. Tomsak RL, Lystad LD, Katirji MB, Brassel TC. Rapid response of syphilitic optic neuritis to posterior sub-Tenon's steroid injection. *J Clin Neuro Ophthalmol.* 1992;12:6.

34. Zaidman GW. Neurosyphilis and retrobulbar neuritis in a patient with AIDS. *Ann Ophthalmol.* 1986;18:260.

35. Halperin LS. Neuroretinitis due to seronegative syphilis associated with human immunodeficiency virus. *J Clin Neuro Ophthalmol.* 1992;12:171.

36. Smith JL, Byrne SF, Cambron CR. Syphiloma/gumma of the optic nerve and human immunodeficiency virus seropositivity. *J Clin Neuro Ophthalmol.* 1990;10:175.

37. Hart G. Syphilis tests in diagnostic and therapeutic decision making. *Ann Intern Med.* 1986;104:368.

38. Johnson PDR, Graves SR, Stewart L, et al. Specific syphilis serological tests may become negative in HIV infection. *AIDS.* 1991;5:419.

39. Haas JS, Bolan G, Larsen SA, et al. Sensitivity of treponemal tests for detecting prior

treated syphilis during human immuno-deficiency virus infection. *J Infect Dis.* 1990; 162:862.

40. Recommendations for diagnosing and treating syphilis in HIV-infected patients. *MMWR.* 1988;37:600.

41. Gadde J, Spence M, Wheeler B, Adkinson NF Jr. Clinical experience with penicillin skin testing in a large inner-city STD clinic. *JAMA.* 1993;270:2456.

42. Dowell ME, Ross PG, Musher DM, et al. Response of latent syphilis or neurosyphilis to ceftriaxone therapy in persons infected with human immunodeficiency virus. *Am J Med.* 1992;93:481.

43. Duncan WC. Failure of erythromycin to cure secondary syphilis in a patient infected with the human immunodeficiency virus. *Arch Dermatol.* 1989;125:82.

44. Belin MW, Balth AL, Hay PB. Secondary syphilitic uveitis. *Am J Ophthalmol.* 1981;92:210.

45. Levy JH, Liss RA, Maguire AM. Neurosyphilis and ocular syphilis in patients with concurrent human immunodeficiency virus infection. *Retina.* 1989;9:175.

46. Klauder JV, Dublin GJ. Syphilitic uveitis. *Arch Ophthalmol.* 1946;35:384.

47. Carter JB, Hamill HJ, Matoba AY. Bilateral syphilitic optic neuritis in a patient with a positive test for HIV. *Arch Ophthalmol.* 1987;105:1485.

48. Steere AC, Malawista SE, Snydman DR, et al. Lyme arthritis: an epidemic of oligoarticular arthritis in children and adults in three Connecticut communities. *Arthritis Rheum.* 1977;20:7.

49. Steere AC. *Borrelia burgdorferi* (Lyme disease, Lyme borreliosis). In: Mandell GL, Douglas RG Jr, Bennett JE, eds. *Infectious Diseases.* 3rd ed. New York: Churchill Livingstone; 1990.

50. Oliver JH Jr, Owsley MR, Hutcheson HJ, et al. Conspecificity of the ticks *Ixodes scapularis* and *I. dammini* (Acari: Ixodidae). *J Med Entomol.* 1993;30:54.

51. Spach DH, Liles WC, Campbell GL, et al. Tick-borne diseases in the United States. *N Engl J Med.* 1993;329:936.

52. Lyme disease—United States, 1991–1992. *MMWR.* 1993;42:345.

53. Kornmehl EW, Lesser RL, Jaros P, et al. Bilateral keratitis in Lyme disease. *Ophthalmology.* 1989;96:1194.

54. Baum J, Barza M, Weinstein P, et al. Bilateral keratitis as a manifestation of Lyme disease. *Am J Ophthalmol.* 1988;105:75.

55. Steere AC, Duray PH, Kauffmann DJH, Wormser GP. Unilateral blindness caused by infection with Lyme disease spirochete, *Borrelia burgdorferi. Ann Intern Med.* 1985; 103:382.

56. Bertuch AW, Rocco E, Schwartz EG. Lyme disease: ocular manifestations. *Ann Ophthalmol.* 1988;20:376.

57. Winward KE, Smith JL, Culbertson WW, Paris-Hamelin AP. Ocular Lyme borreliosis. *Am J Ophthalmol.* 1989;108:651.

58. Lang GE, Schonherr U, Naumann GOH. Retinal vasculitis with proliferative retinopathy in a patient with evidence of *Borrelia burgdorferi* infection [letter to the editor]. *Arch Ophthalmol.* 1991;109:243.

59. Lightman DA, Brod RD. Branch retinal artery occlusion associated with Lyme disease. *Arch Ophthalmol.* 1991;109:1198.

60. Jacobson DM, Frens DB. Pseudotumor cerebri syndrome associated with Lyme disease [letter to the editor]. *Am J Ophthalmol.* 1989;107:81.

61. Bialasiewicz AA, Ruprecht KW, Naumann GOH, Blenk H. Bilateral diffuse choroiditis and exudative retinal detachments with evidence of Lyme disease [letter to the editor]. *Am J Ophthalmol.* 1988;105:419.

62. Duffy J. Lyme disease. *Infect Dis Clin North Am.* 1987;1:511.

63. Pachner AR, Steere AC. The triad of neurologic manifestations of Lyme disease: meningitis, cranial neuritis, and radiculoneuritis. *Neurology.* 1985;35:47.

64. Flach AJ, Lavoie PE. Episcleritis, conjunctivitis, and keratitis as ocular manifestations of Lyme disease. *Ophthalmology.* 1990;97:973.

65. Mombaerts IM, Maudgal PC, Knockaert DC. Bilateral follicular conjunctivitis as a manifestation of Lyme disease. *Am J Ophthalmol.* 1991;112:96.

66. Dattwyler RJ, Volkman DJ, Luft BJ, et al. Seronegative Lyme disease: dissocation of specific T- and B-lymphocyte responses to *Borrelia burgdorferi. N Engl J Med.* 1988;319:1441.

67. Aaberg TM. The expanding ophthalmologic spectrum of Lyme disease. *Am J Ophthalmol.* 1989;107:77.

68. Rosenbaum JT, Rahn DW. Prevalence of

Lyme disease among patients with uveitis. *Am J Ophthalmol.* 1991;112:462.

69. Treatment of Lyme disease. *Med Lett Drugs Ther.* 1988;30:65.

70. Steere AC, Pachner AR, Malawista SE. Neurologic abnormalities of Lyme disease: successful treatment with high-dose intravenous penicillin. *Ann Intern Med.* 1983;99:767.

71. Farrar WE. Leptospira species (leptospirosis). In: Mandell GL, Douglas RG Jr, Bennett JE, eds. *Infectious Diseases.* 3rd ed. New York: Churchill Livingstone; 1990.

72. Alexander A, Baer A, Fair JR, et al. Leptospiral uveitis: report of bacteriologically verified case. *Arch Ophthalmol.* 1952;48:292.

73. Barkay S, Garzozi H. Leptospirosis and uveitis. *Ann Ophthalmol.* 1984;16:164.

74. Daley CL, Small PM, Schecter GF, et al. An outbreak of tuberculosis with accelerated progression among persons infected with the human immunodeficiency virus. *N Engl J Med.* 1992;326:231.

75. Des Prez RM, Heim CR. Mycobacterial diseases. In: Mandell GL, Douglas RG Jr, Bennett JE, eds. *Infectious Diseases.* 3rd ed. New York: Churchill Livingstone; 1990.

76. Frieden TR, Sterling T, Pablos-Mendez A, et al. The emergence of drug-resistant tuberculosis in New York City. *N Engl J Med.* 1993;328:521.

77. Tuberculosis morbidity in the United States: final data, 1990. *MMWR CDC Surveill Summ.* 1991;40:23.

78. Woods AC. *Endogenous Inflammations of the Uveal Tract.* Baltimore: Williams & Wilkins; 1961.

79. Schlaegel TF, O'Connor GR. Metastatic nonsuppurative uveitis. *Int Ophthalmol Clin.* 1977;17:87.

80. Donahue HC. Ophthalmologic experience in a tuberculosis sanatorium. *Am J Ophthalmol.* 1967;64:742.

81. Rosen PH, Spalton DJ, Graham EM. Intraocular tuberculosis. *Eye.* 1990;4:486.

82. Nussenblatt RB, Palestine AG. Bacterial and fungal diseases. In: *Uveitis: Fundamentals and Clinical Practice.* Chicago: Year Book Medical Publishers; 1989.

83. Gur S, Silverstone BZ, Zylberman R, Berson D. Chorioretinitis and extrapulmonary tuberculosis. *Ann Ophthalmol.* 1987;19:112.

84. Mansour AM, Haymond R. Choroidal tuberculomas without evidence of extra-

ocular tuberculosis. *Graefe's Arch Clin Exp Ophthalmol.* 1990;228:382.

85. Cangemi FE, Friedman AH, Josephberg R. Tuberculoma of the choroid. *Ophthalmology.* 1980;87:252.

86. Jabbour NM, Faris B, Trempe CL. A case of pulmonary tuberculosis presenting with a choroidal tuberculoma. *Ophthalmology.* 1985;92:834.

87. Lyon CE, Grimson BS, Peiffer RL, Merritt JC. Clinicopathological correlation of a solitary choroidal tuberculoma. *Ophthalmology.* 1985;92:845.

88. Khalil M, Lindley S, Matouk E. Tuberculosis of the orbit. *Ophthalmology.* 1985;92:1624.

89. Yon Kim J, Carroll CP, Opremcak EM. Antibiotic-resistant tuberculous choroidits [letter to the editor]. *Am J Ophthalmol.* 1993;115:259.

90. Snider DE Jr, Cohn DL, Davidson PT, et al. Standard therapy for tuberculosis, 1985. *Chest.* 1985;87:117S.

91. Iseman MD. Treatment of multidrug-resistant tuberculosis. *N Engl J Med.* 1993;329:784.

92. British Thoracic Society. A controlled trial for 6 months' chemotherapy in pulmonary tuberculosis: results during the 36 months after the end of chemotherapy and beyond. *Br J Dis Chest.* 1984;78:330.

93. Snider DE Jr, Zierski M, Graczyk J, et al. Short-course tuberculosis chemotherapy studies conducted in Poland during the past decade. *Eur J Respir Dis.* 1986;68:12.

94. Rosenbaum JT, Wernick R. The utility of routine screening of patients with uveitis for systemic lupus erythematosus or tuberculosis. A Bayesian analysis. *Arch Ophthalmol.* 1990;108:1291.

95. Abrams J, Schlaegel TF Jr. The role of the isoniazid therapeutic test in tuberculous uveitis. *Am J Ophthalmol.* 1982;94:511.

96. Wacker WB, Donoso LA, Kalsow CM, et al. Experimental allergic uveitis: isolation, characterization and localization of a soluble uveitis-pathogenic antigen from bovine retinal. *J Immunol.* 1977;119:1949.

97. Nussenblatt RB, Kuwabara T, de Monasterio FM, et al. S-antigen uveitis in primates: a new model for human disease. *Arch Ophthalmol.* 1981;99:1090.

98. Bullock WE. *Mycobacterium leprae* (leprosy). In: Mandell GL, Douglas RG Jr, Bennett JE,

eds. *Infectious Diseases*. 3rd ed. New York: Churchill Livingstone; 1990.

99. Binford C, Meyers W, Walsh G. Leprosy. *JAMA*. 1982;247:2283.

100. Brandt F, Malla O. Ocular findings in leprous patients. *Albrecht von Grafes Arch Klin Exp Ophthalmol*. 1981;217:27.

101. Slem G. Clinical studies of ocular leprosy. *Am J Ophthalmol*. 1971;71:431.

102. Allen JH, Byers JL. The pathology of ocular leprosy. I. Cornea. *Arch Ophthalmol*. 1960; 64:216.

103. Spaide R, Nattis R, Lipka A, D'Amico R. Ocular findings in leprosy in the United States. *Am J Ophthalmol*. 1985;100:411.

104. Allen JH. Pathology of ocular leprosy. II. Miliary lepromas of the iris. *Am J Ophthalmol*. 1966;61:987.

105. WHO Study Group. Chemotherapy of leprosy for control programmes. *WHO Tech Rep Ser*. 1982;675.

106. Hastings RC, Jacobson RR. Activity of ansamycin against *Mycobacterium leprae* in mice [letter]. *Lancet*. 1983;2:1079.

107. Hastings RC, Richard VR, Jacobson RR. Ansamycin activity against rifampicin-resistant *Mycobacterium leprae* [letter]. *Lancet*. 1984;1:1130.

108. Mikolich DJ, Boyce JM. *Brucella* species. In: Mandell GL, Douglas RG Jr, Bennett JE, eds. *Infectious Diseases*. 3rd ed. New York: Churchill Livingstone; 1990.

109. Woods AC. *Endogenous Uveitis*. Baltimore, Williams & Wilkins; 1956.

110. Rolando I, Carbone A, Haro D, et al. Retinal detachment in chronic brucellosis. *Am J Ophthalmol*. 1985;99:733.

111. Dobbins WO III. Whipple's disease. In: Mandell GL, Douglas RG Jr, Bennett JE, eds. *Principles and Practice of Infectious Diseases*. 3rd ed. New York: Churchill Livingstone; 1990.

112. Dobbins WO III, Kawanishi H. Bacillary characteristics in Whipple's disease; an electron microscopic study. *Gastroenterology*. 1981;80:1468.

113. Fleming JL, Wiesner RH, Shorter RG. Whipple's disease: clinical, biochemical, and histopathologic features and assessment of treatment in 29 patients. *Mayo Clin Proc*. 1988;63:539.

114. Maizel H, Ruffin JM, Dobbins WO III. Whipple's disease. A review of 19 patients from one hospital and a review of the literature since 1950. *Medicine (Balt)*. 1970;49: 175.

115. Disdier P, Harle J-R, Vidal-Morris D, et al. Chemosis associated with Whipple's disease. *N Engl J Med*. 1991;112:217.

116. Fout RL, Rao NA, Issarescu S, McEntee WJ. Ocular involvement in Whipple's disease. Light and electron microscopic observations. *Arch Ophthalmol*. 1978;96:1431.

117. Avila MP, Jalkh AE, Feldman E, et al. Manifestations of Whipple's disease in the posterior segment of the eye. *Arch Ophthalmol*. 1984;102:384.

118. Durant WJ, Flood T, Goldberg MF, et al. Vitrectomy and Whipple's disease. *Arch Ophthalmol*. 1984;102:848.

10
Fungal Diseases

Histoplasmosis

The ocular histoplasmosis syndrome (OHS) or presumed ocular histoplasmosis syndrome (POHS) is a multifocal chorioretinitis epidemiologically linked to *Histoplasma capsulatum*.

Etiology

H. capsulatum is a dimorphic fungus with both yeast and filamentous forms.[1] Human disease is caused by the yeast form.

Epidemiology

Histoplasmosis has worldwide distribution and is endemic in the midwestern United States. Ocular signs of histoplasmosis are found in 2% to 13% of persons within an endemic region.[2,3] It is particularly prevalent along the Ohio and Mississippi River valleys, where 80% of adults have positive skin tests for histoplasmin.[4] Bird droppings in soil (including chickens and pigeons) provide an environment for fungal growth in these regions.

Histoplasmosis affects both males and females equally. Although the initial infection is thought to occur sometime during childhood, ocular manifestations do not occur until the age of 20 to 50 years, with an average age of 41 years.[4] Human leukocyte antigen HLA-B7 has been associated with the development of disciform macular lesions and HLA-Dr22 with peripheral histoplasmosis spots.[5,6] The disease is bilateral in 60% of patients and is less common in dark-skinned races.[7]

Pathogenesis

Primary infection occurs after inhalation of fungal spores in the lungs.[1] Macrophages carry the organism to the liver, spleen, and choroid. A granulomatous reaction with epithelioid cells, Langhans' cells, and lymphocytic infiltration occurs around the sites of infection. The immune response is able to eradicate the organism, but a persistent lymphocytic infiltration can remain around undigested cell wall components and chitin.[1,8]

Focal areas of choroiditis in the macula result in retinal pigment epithelium (RPE) proliferation and subretinal neovascularization membrane (SRNVM) formation.[9,10] Originating from the choroid, these vessels lack tight junctions and can leak fluid, lipid, and blood into the subretinal space. Chronic exudation and hemorrhage result in formation of a fibrovascular scar. Peripheral "histo spots" and peripapillary scarring may exhibit lymphocytic infiltration when active. Inactive lesions show scarring and a fibrous reaction. Organisms are not seen within the areas of choroiditis.[10,11]

Clinical Presentation

Primary infection with histoplasmosis is usually subclinical. Systemic manifestations when present are usually mild and may be flu-like.[1] Immunosuppressed patients may develop severe disease, with cavitary lung lesions and miliary dissemination throughout the body.[1,12] *H. capsulatum* has been identified in the eyes of these patients.[12]

Ocular manifestations of histoplasmosis have a characteristic pattern.[10,11] The eye is quiet without anterior uveitis or vitritis. The presence of active inflammatory cells in the vitreous should suggest other conditions. Macular disciform scar, peripapillary pigment changes, and peripheral "histo spots" make up the diagnostic triad of ocular histoplasmosis[9,11,13] (Fig. 10.1). Macular lesions may begin with a small focus of choroiditis.[7] The development of SRNVMs with serous exudation, hemorrhage, and lipid formation will cause metamorphopsia.[14] Healing occurs with subretinal disciform scar formation.[4,8,15] Peripapillary pigment changes represent prior episodes of juxtapapillary choroiditis.[9,10] Neovascularization and juxtapapillary hemorrhage may occur in the area. Atrophic "histo spots" are typically pigmented in the center and are discrete.[13] About 5% of patients develop linear arrangements of these "punched out" chorioretinal scars called linear equatorial streaks.[16] Massive intraocular hemorrhage has rarely been observed in ocular histoplasmosis.[17,18]

Diagnosis

Ocular histoplasmosis is a clinical diagnosis.[4,19] A healthy patient with a quiet eye and the triad of peripapillary pigment scarring, histo spots, and macular lesions establishes the diagnosis.

Fluorescein angiography may help demonstrate areas of active choroiditis and subretinal neovascular membrane formation. Areas of active choroiditis block early in the study and stain late. Choroidal neovascular membranes have an early hyperfluorescence followed by further leakage of fluorescein dye into the retina.

Chest radiograph may show calcified pulmonary nodules indicative of old granulomatous disease.[1] A 1:1000 histoplasmin skin test is positive in 90% of patients; however, skin testing has been associated with worsening of the clinical course. Skin testing is rarely needed for the diagnosis and should be performed with caution in these patients.

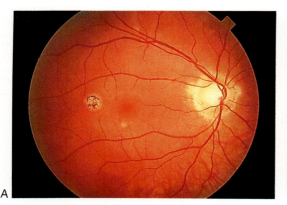 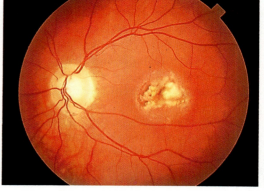

Figure 10.1. Infectious uveitis—histoplasmosis. The triad of ocular histoplasmosis includes peripapillary pigment changes (**A**), atrophic peripheral "histo spots," and disciform macular scar (**B**).

Differential Diagnosis

Subretinal neovascular membrane formation and disciform macular scars may occur in patients with angioid streaks and high myopia and in age-related macular degeneration. Peripheral "histo spots" and the peripapillary choroiditis are not typically found in these other conditions. Multifocal choroiditis can be seen in sarcoidosis, tuberculosis, and idiopathic multifocal choroiditis and panuveitis syndrome. These disorders will typically be characterized by significant vitritis.

Treatment

It is important to discern inactive scars from active choroiditis and choroidal neovascularization. Areas of active choroiditis may be treated with oral or regional corticosteroids in an attempt to prevent subsequent choroidal neovascularization. Sub-Tenon's triamcinolone, 40 mg, or a pulse of high-dose oral corticosteroid can reduce the severity of choroiditis in most patients. Antifungal agents do not play a role in the ocular histoplasmosis syndrome.[20]

Subretinal neovascular membranes with an edge between 200 and 2500 μm from the center of the foveal avascular zone (FAZ) are called extrafoveal. When these SRNVMs are located between 1 and 200 μm from the center of the FAZ, they are considered juxtafoveal. Subfoveal SRNVMs are lesions within 1 μm of the center of the FAZ. Juxtafoveal SRNVMs and extrafoveal lesions should be treated with focal laser photocoagulation. The multicenter Macular Photocoagulation Study Group demonstrated a visually significant benefit from such therapy.[21,22] A six-line loss of vision occurred in 50% of untreated patients compared with 22% of laser-treated patients over a 24-month period.[21] The neovascular membrane is typically outlined with 100-μm spots for 0.1 second. The power is determined by the intensity of the tissue reaction. The desired burn is an intense whitish yellow lesion (Fig. 10.2). The margins of the membrane are then filled in with contiguous 200-μm laser spots for 0.2 seconds. The center is then overlapped by 200- to 500-μm burns for 0.5 seconds.

The treatment of subfoveal lesions is more challenging. Observation, administration of sub-Tenon's triamcinolone, and oral corticosteroids have all been used to improve the visual prognosis for these lesions. Recent advances in vitreoretinal

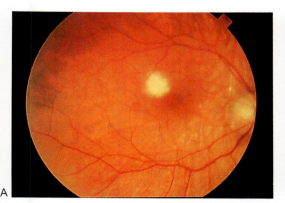
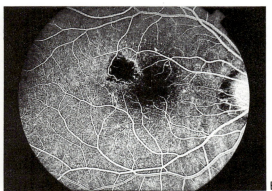

Figure 10.2. Laser photocoagulation—histoplasmosis. Extrafoveal subretinal neovascular membrane immediately after focal laser photocoagulation. **A:** The burn is intense, and **B,** fluorescein angiography performed 3 weeks later shows no evidence of recurrence.

surgical techniques have allowed these membranes to be removed via submacular surgery.[15] Postoperative visual acuity has improved in many patients; however, recurrent neovascularization is common (30%–50%).[23]

Prognosis

Histoplasmosis is often a bilateral disease and can result in legal blindness from loss of macular function. Fortunately, peripheral vision is not affected. Laser therapy has greatly improved the visual prognosis for patients with juxtafoveal and extrafoveal neovascular membranes. The best prognosis is for patients with extrafoveal lesions.

The presence of subfoveal lesions carries a worse prognosis: 85% of patients with subfoveal SRNVMs have worse than 20/40 acuity and 75% have less than 20/200 vision; however, 15% of such patients will retain 20/40 or better vision without therapy.[24] Future treatments should consider such a natural history.

Candidiasis

Candidiasis is an opportunistic fungal infection that can cause focal areas of chorioretinitis, vitritis, and endophthalmitis.

Etiology

Candida albicans and other *Candida* species are a dimorphic fungus with both yeast and filamentous forms.[25]

Epidemiology

Candida is normally present on the skin and mucous membranes and is considered part of the normal flora in human beings.[25] It can cause disease with breach of the skin and with relative immunosuppression. Indwelling catheters, intravenous (IV) drug abuse, chronic antibiotic use, immunosup-

pressive therapy, and poorly controlled diabetes are predisposing risk factors for infection.[26–29]

Pathogenesis

Once *Candida* gains access to the bloodstream, it can disseminate to all parts of the body.[27,29,30] As a result of the high blood flow to the choroid, up to 30% of patients with candidemia have eye findings. Mononuclear cell infiltration occurs at the metastatic sites of infection.

Clinical Presentation

Fever, chills, and malaise are common constitutional complaints with candidemia.[25] In the eye, the infection most often begins in the choroid and subsequently produces multifocal, fluffy white areas of chorioretinitis.[31] As the fungus grows, the lesions expand and can break through the retina into the vitreous cavity, causing a vitritis. Vitreous "puffballs" are characteristic and can

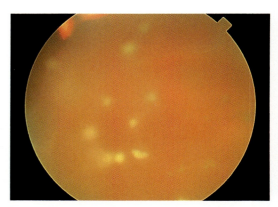

Figure 10.3. Infectious uveitis—*Candida*. *Candida* endophthalmitis masquerading as idiopathic intermediate uveitis. The patient was an IV drug abuser. "Puffballs" can be seen in the vitreous cavity. The vitritis was medically unresponsive and a diagnostic vitrectomy was performed. Cultures grew *Candida*, and the patient was treated with intraocular and IV amphotericin.

be a useful diagnostic sign of endogenous fungal endophthalmitis (Fig. 10.3).

Diagnosis

The diagnosis is made with a high degree of clinical suspicion. Multifocal chorioretinitis and vitritis in a patient with a history of indwelling catheters, IV drug abuse, immunosuppression, or antibiotic use should suggest *Candida* endophthalmitis. Blood cultures or cultures from the removed catheters can confirm the diagnosis.[25,31] A diagnostic vitrectomy may be required in patients without an obvious source to establish the diagnosis.[30,32,33]

Differential Diagnosis

Toxoplasmosis may cause a focal area of fluffy chorioretinitis and an overlying vitritis. These patients are otherwise healthy and the lesion is typically adjacent to an older, pigmented retinochoroidal scar. Endogenous bacterial endophthalmitis can have a similar picture but is usually more fulminant and can be associated with ocular pain, hypopyon, and chemosis.

Treatment

Intravenous amphotericin B is the treatment of choice (0.5–1 mg/kg/per day).[26,27,30–32] A total amphotericin B dose should range between 0.5 and 1.5 g.[25,28] Other antifungal agents can be used in certain settings, including flucytosine, myconazole, and rifampin.[22] Cases of severe fungal endophthalmitis should be treated with vitrectomy and intraocular amphotericin (5 μg/0.1 ml).[32]

Prognosis

The prognosis is often determined by the severity of the underlying systemic illness and predisposing factors. If the systemic immunosuppression cannot be reversed, then recurrent or persistent infection is likely. Visual prognosis depends on the location of the metastatic lesion. Macular lesions carry a poorer visual prognosis than extramacular sites of infection. Intravenous and intraocular antifungal agents and adjunctive vitrectomy can sterilize most cases of *Candida endophthalmitis.*[27–32]

Coccidiomycosis

Coccidiomycosis, also called San Joaquin or valley fever, is an infectious fungal disease that can cause a chorioretinitis.

Etiology

Coccidioides is a dimorphic fungus with yeast and filamentous forms.[33] The filamentous form has characteristic hypha called arthroconidia when in host tissues. The fungal spores form spherules with multiple internal endospores.

Epidemiology

Coccidioides is endemic in the Western hemisphere and is most prevalent along the coastal areas from California to Argentina.[33]

Pathogenesis

Inhalation of spores results in a focal pulmonary infection. The endospores are carried by macrophages to other sites throughout the body.[30] Polymorphonuclear neutrophils, monocytes, and macrophages are recruited and produce a suppurative inflammation that evolves to a granulomatous reaction. Epithelioid cells and caseating necrosis can occur.

Clinical Presentation

Less than 1% of those infected are symptomatic. Fever, malaise, cough, night sweats, and chest pain can be symptoms of an acute infection and pneumonitis.[33]

Ocular involvement may occur with disseminated disease. A multifocal chorioretinitis similar to histoplasmosis may be seen.[3-37] Lesions are "punched out" when inactive, but appear yellowish white when active. They are small, 0.1 to 0.25 disc diameters, and can occur throughout the fundus. Patients may develop a granulomatous iritis with posterior synechiae during the course of the disease.[38,39] In severe cases, the infection may result in an endogenous fungal endophthalmitis.[40]

Diagnosis

Patients with active, multifocal chorioretinal lesions, with or without intraocular inflammation, who live in an endemic area should be suspected of coccidiomycosis.[33] Active pulmonary disease may show a pneumonitis and characteristic "coin lesions" on chest radiograph. Skin testing with coccidioidin (1:10,000) or spherulin (1:1,000) will be positive. Within 4 weeks of infection, precipitating (90%) and complement-fixing (10%) antibodies can be detected. Vitreous biopsy can be performed in cases of suspected fungal endophthalmitis.[40]

Differential Diagnosis

Candidiasis may cause a similar fungal endophthalmitis but occurs in immunocompromised patients or those with risk factors such as indwelling catheters. Histoplasmosis can cause multifocal chorioretinal scars similar to coccidiomycosis but rarely causes an acute systemic illness and is not associated with active intraocular inflammation.

Treatment

Intravenous amphotericin (1 mg/kg/per day) is the treatment of choice.[33,41] A total dose of 0.5 to 1.5 g can be given. Intraocular amphotericin (5 μg/0.1 ml) can be used at the time of vitrectomy in cases of suspected fungal endophthalmitis. Miconazole is an alternative antifungal agent used in the treatment of this disease.[33,41]

Prognosis

Visual prognosis depends on the location of the chorioretinal lesions and on prompt diagnosis in cases of fungal endophthalmitis. Vitrectomy combined with IV and intraocular amphotericin can sterilize the eye in most cases.[41]

Sporotrichosis

Sporotrichosis is a disseminated fungal disease caused by *Sporothrix schenckii*.[42]

Etiology

S. schenckii is a dimorphic, cigar-shaped fungus found in soil. The yeast form is found within host tissues.[42]

Epidemiology

Disease occurs after injury with plant material and thorns. Ocular involvement is rare in sporotrichosis.

Pathogenesis

Skin or eyelid infections can develop after a perforating injury contaminated by soil.[42] Hematogenous spread results in metastatic foci of infection. A necrotizing granulomatous reaction occurs at the site of infection.[42,43]

Clinical Presentation

Sporotrichosis most often affects the lung, bones, and eye.[42] In the eye, disseminated infection can result in a necrotizing, granulomatous retinochoroiditis.[43,44] The anterior segment may have granulomatous iridocyclitis with posterior synechiae.[44-46] Subretinal fluid can develop with severe chorioretinitis. In one case, the organism was cultured from the subretinal fluid.[45] An endogenous fungal endophthalmitis may occur in advanced cases.[45]

Diagnosis

Culture of the involved site will document the presence of the fungus.[43] Cultures from the aqueous humor or vitreous can also establish the diagnosis when endophthalmitis is suspected.

Differential Diagnosis

Other forms of fungal endophthalmitis may present in a similar fashion. Microbiologic techniques and cultures will determine the etiologic agent in cases of suspected fungal endophthalmitis.

Treatment

Skin lesions can be treated with saturated solution of potassium iodide (SSKI) and with IV amphotericin.[42] Intraocular involvement requires systemic amphotericin (0.5 mg/kg/per day) for a total dose of 2 to 2.5 g and, in cases of active endophthalmitis, vitrectomy and intraocular amphotericin (5 µg/0.1 ml).

Prognosis

Visual prognosis depends on the site of metastatic infection and on prompt diagnosis and treatment.

Cryptococcosis

Cryptococcal infection is an opportunistic fungal infection that can cause a chorioretinitis and endophthalmitis.

Etiology

Cryptococcus neoformans is an encapsulated yeast-like fungus.[47]

Epidemiology

C. neoformans is endemic in pigeons and other birds.[47] Bird droppings contaminate the soil with the fungus and fungal spores.

Pathogenesis

Most patients with cryptococcal infections are immunocompromised.[47-51] Cryptococcal disease can be found in up to 9% of persons with acquired immunodeficiency syndrome (AIDS). Primary pulmonary infection results in hematogenous dissemination to other organs. The central nervous system (CNS) and eye are commonly involved.

Clinical Presentation

Headache and other CNS complaints may be present with cryptococcal encephalitis and meningitis. Ocular examination may reveal papilledema from elevated intracranial pressure.[48-51] The other cranial nerves (abducens) may be affected.[50] Metastatic infection of the choroid can result in a multifocal chorioretinitis.[50,51] These lesions are often in a peripapillary location (Fig. 10.4).

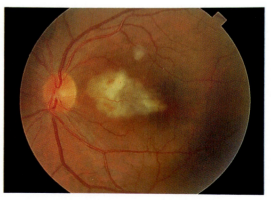

Figure 10.4. Infectious uveitis—*Cryptococcus*. Fungal retinitis in an immunocompromised patient with cryptococcal meningitis.

Patients may have a chronic iridocyclitis but minimal vitritis. A few patients have been reported with severe panuveitis.

Diagnosis

Immunocompromised patients with CNS complaints and focal chorioretinitis should undergo cerebral spinal fluid (CSF) analysis.[47] India ink staining will demonstrate the encapsulated fungi. Cultures from the CSF confirm the diagnosis. Diagnostic vitrectomy may be indicated in patients with panuveitis and CNS complaints to help establish the diagnosis.

Differential Diagnosis

Multifocal chorioretinitis and CNS complaints in an immunocompromised patient may be caused by toxoplasmosis, candidiasis, tuberculosis, and syphilis. Laboratory testing, chest radiograph, and skin testing can help differentiate these diseases from cryptococcal infection.

Treatment

Intravenous amphotericin B (0.5 mg/kg per day) should be given. Intravitreal amphotericin (5 µg/0.1 ml) can be given if vitrectomy is performed in the setting of suspected fungal endophthalmitis. Amphotericin B can be combined with flucytosine and may result in higher cure rates.[42] It is interesting to note that although cyclosporin A therapy results in systemic immunosuppression, as a natural antibiotic it has antifungal activity against *C. neoformans*.[52] Patients on this drug may be less susceptible to infection because of this antibiotic activity.

Prognosis

The disease may be fatal if not diagnosed early. Antifungal agents are required in CNS and ocular disease to minimize morbidity. The underlying and predisposing systemic immunosuppression should be addressed to improve the long-term prognosis.

References

1. Lloyd JE, des Prez RM, Goodwin RA Jr. Histoplasma capsulatum. In: Mandell GL, Douglas RG Jr, Bennett JE, eds. *Principles and Practice of Infectious Diseases*. 3rd ed. New York: Churchill Livingstone; 1990.
2. Asbury T. The status of presumed ocular histoplasmosis: including a report of a survey. *Trans Am Ophthalmol Soc*. 1966;64:371.
3. Davidorf FH, Anderson JD. Ocular lesions in the Earth Day 1970 histoplasmosis epidemic. *Int Ophthalmol Clin*. 1975;15:51.
4. Schlaegel TF Jr. *Ocular Histoplasmosis*. New York: Grune & Stratton; 1977.
5. Godfrey WA, Sabates R, Cross DE. Association of presumed ocular histoplasmosis with HLA-B7. *Am J Ophthalmol*. 1978;85:854.
6. Braley RE, Meredith TA, Aaberg TM, et al. The prevalence of HLA-B7 in presumed ocular histoplasmosis. *Am J Ophthalmol*. 1978;85:859.
7. Gass JDM, Wilkinson CP. Follow-up study of presumed ocular histoplasmosis. *Trans Am Acad Ophthalmol Otolaryngol*. 1972;76:672.
8. Nussenblatt RB, Palestine AG. Ocular histoplasmosis. In: David K. Marshall, ed. *Uveitis: Fundamentals and Clinical Practice*. Chicago: Year Book Medical Publishers; 1989.
9. Khalil MK. Histopathology of presumed ocular histoplasmosis. *Am J Ophthalmol*. 1982;94:369.
10. Makley TA Jr, Craig EL, Long JW. Histopathology of presumed ocular histoplasmosis. *Palestra Oftalmologica Panamericana*. 1977;1:72.
11. Walma D, Schlaegel TJ Jr. Presumed histoplasmic choroiditis. *Am J Ophthalmol*. 1964;57:107.
12. Scholz R, Green WR, Kutys R, et al. *Histoplasma capsulatum* in the eye. *Ophthalmology*. 1984;91:1100.
13. Smith RE, Ganley JP, Knox DL. Presumed ocular histoplasmosis. II. Patterns of peripheral and peripapillary scarring in persons with nonmacular disease. *Arch Ophthalmol*. 1972;87:251.

14. Ryan SR Jr. De novo subretinal neovascularization in the histoplasmosis syndrome. *Arch Ophthalmol.* 1976;94:321.
15. Thomas MA, Grand MG, Williams DF, et al. Surgical management of subfoveal choroidal neovascularization. *Ophthalmology.* 1992;99:952.
16. Fountain JA, Schlaegel TF Jr. Linear streaks of the equator in the presumed ocular histoplasmosis syndrome. *Arch Ophthalmol.* 1981;99:244.
17. Kranias G. Vitreous hemorrhage secondary to presumed ocular histoplasmosis syndrome. *Ann Ophthalmol.* 1985;17:295.
18. Makley TA Jr, Davidorf FH, Chambers RB, et al. Massive intraocular hemorrhage in the ocular histoplasmosis syndrome. *Contemp Ophthalmic Forum.* 1987;5:55.
19. Woods AC, Wahlen HE. The probable role of benign histoplasmosis in the etiology of granulomatous uveitis. *Am J Ophthalmol.* 1960;49:205.
20. Makley TA, Long JW, Suit T. Therapy of chorioretinitis presumed to be caused by histoplasmosis. *Int Ophthalmol Clin.* 1975;15:181.
21. Macular Photocoagulation Study Group. Argon laser photocoagulation for histoplasmosis. Results of a randomized clinical trial. *Arch Ophthalmol.* 1983;101:1347.
22. Macular Photocoagulation Study Group. Krypton laser photocoagulation for neovascular lesions of ocular histoplasmosis. Results of a randomized clinical trial. *Arch Ophthalmol.* 1987;105:1499.
23. Thomas MA, Kaplan HJ. Surgical removal of subfoveal neovascularization in the presumed ocular histoplasmosis syndrome. *Am J Ophthalmol.* 1991;111:1.
24. Olk RJ, Burgess DB, McCormick PA. Subfoveal and juxtafoveal subretinal neovascularization in the presumed ocular histoplasmosis syndrome. *Ophthalmology.* 1984;91:1592.
25. Edwards JE Jr. Candida species. In: Mandell GL, Douglas RG Jr, Bennett JE, eds. *Principles and Practice of Infectious Diseases.* 3rd ed. New York: Churchill Livingstone; 1990.
26. Stern WH, Tamura E, Jacobs RA. Epidemic postsurgical *Candida parapsilosis* endophthalmitis. *Ophthalmology.* 1985;92:1701.
27. Griffin JR, Pettit TH, Fishman LS, Foos RY. Blood-borne *Candida* endophthalmitis. *Arch Ophthalmol.* 1973;89:450.
28. Joshi N, Hamory BH. Endophthalmitis caused by non-*Albicans* species of *Candida. Rev Infect Dis.* 1991;13:281.
29. Elliott JH, O'Day DM, Gutow GS, et al. Mycotic endophthalmitis in drug abusers. *Am J Ophthalmol.* 1979;88:66.
30. McDonnell PJ, McDonnell JM, Brown RH, Green WR. Ocular involvement in patients with fungal infections. *Ophthalmology.* 1985;92:706.
31. Kinyoun JL. Treatment of *Candida* endophthalmitis. *Retina.* 1982;2:215.
32. Axelrod AJ, Peyman GA. Intravitreal amphotericin B treatment of experimental fungal endophthalmitis. *Am J Ophthalmol.* 1973;76:584.
33. Stevens DA. *Coccidiodes immitis.* In: Mandell GL, Douglas RG Jr, Bennett JE, eds. *Principles and Practice of Infectious Diseases.* 3rd ed. New York: Churchill Livingstone; 1990.
34. Levitt JM. Ocular manifestations of coccidioidomycosis. *Am J Ophthalmol.* 1948;31:1626.
35. Alexander PB, Goodley EL. Disseminated coccidioidomycosis with intraocular involvement. *Am J Ophthalmol.* 1967;64:283.
36. Zakka KA, Foos RY, Brown WJ. Intraocular coccidioidomycosis. *Surv Ophthalmol.* 1978;22:313.
37. Boyden BS, Yee DS. Bilateral coccidioidal choroiditis: a clinicopathologic case report. *Trans Am Acad Ophthalmol Otolaryngol.* 1971;76:1006.
38. Brown WC, Kellenberger RE, Hudson KE: Granulomatous uveitis associated with disseminated coccidioidomycosis. *Am J Ophthalmol.* 1958;45:102.
39. Bell R, Font RL. Granulomatous anterior uveitis caused by *Coccidioides immitis. Am J Ophthalmol.* 1972;74:93.
40. Hagele AJ, Evans PH, Larwood TR. Primary endophthalmic coccidioidomycosis. Report of a case of exogenous primary coccidioidomycosis of the eye diagnosed prior to enucleation. In: Ajello L, ed. *Coccidioidomycosis.* Tucson: University of Arizona Press; 1967:37–39.
41. Blumenkranz MS, Stevens DA. Therapy of endogenous fungal endophthalmitis. Miconazole or amphotericin B for coccidioidal and candidal infection. *Arch Ophthalmol.* 1980;98:1216.
42. Bennett JE. *Sporothrix schenckii.* In: Mandell

GL, Douglas RG Jr, Bennett JE, eds. *Principles and Practice of Infectious Diseases*. 3rd ed. New York: Churchill Livingstone; 1990.

43. Font RL, Jakobiec FA. Granulomatous necrotizing retinochoroiditis caused by *Sporotrichum schenckii*. *Arch Ophthalmol*. 1976;94:1513.

44. Gordon D. Ocular sporotrichosis. *Arch Ophthalmol*. 1947;37:56.

45. Cassady J, Foerster H. *Sporotrichum schenckii* endophthalmitis. *Arch Ophthalmol*. 1971;85:71.

46. Levy J. Intraocular sporotrichosis: report of a case. *Arch Ophthalmol*. 1971;85:574.

47. Diamond RD. *Cryptococcus neoformans*. *Principles and Practice of Infectious Diseases*. 3rd ed. New York: Churchill Livingstone; 1990.

48. Jabs DA, Green WR, Fox R, et al. Ocular manifestations of acquired immune deficiency syndrome. *Ophthalmology*. 1989;96:1092.

49. Pepose JS, Holland GN, Nestor MS, et al. Acquired immune deficiency syndrome. *Ophthalmology*. 1985;92:472.

50. Kestelyn P, Taelman H, Bogaerts J, et al. Ophthalmic manifestations of infections with *Cryptococcus* neoformans in patients with the acquired immunodeficiency syndrome. *Am J Ophthalmol*. 1993;116:721.

51. Morinelli EN, Dugel PU, Riffenburgh R, Rao NA. Infectious multifocal choroiditis in patients with acquired immune deficiency syndrome. *Ophthalmology*. 1993;100:1014.

52. Mody CH, Toews GB, Lipscomb MF. Cyclosporin A inhibits the growth of *Cryptococcus neoformans* in a murine mode. *Infect Immunol*. 1988;56:7.

11
Protozoal Diseases

Toxoplasmosis

Toxoplasmosis is a protozoal infectious disease that can cause a necrotizing retinochoroiditis.

Etiology

Toxoplasma gondii is an obligate intracellular parasitic protozoan.[1] It has three common forms: the oocyst or soil form (10–12 μm), the trophozoite or active infectious form (4–8 μm), and the tissue cyst or latent form (10–200 μm). Tissue cysts contain hundreds of *Toxoplasma* organisms.

Epidemiology

Toxoplasmosis is a zoonosis, with the cat being the natural host.[1] The cat excretes oocysts, which are ingested by other domestic animals. Human beings become infected by ingesting the cysts in undercooked meats and by fecal-oral routes: 10% of mutton, 10% of beef, and 25% of pork contain oocysts of toxoplasmosis.[1,2] On serologic testing, 3% to 70% of adults are positive for *Toxoplasma* organisms.

Once ingested, the oocyst produces trophozoites in the gastrointestinal (GI) tract. The trophozoites travel in the lymph and bloodstream with resultant central nervous system (CNS) and ocular infection. Trophozoites may also travel via the placental route to a fetus during pregnancy. In the United States, 2 to 6/1000 women acquire the disease during pregnancy.[2] Maternal infection during pregnancy results in a 40% transmission rate to the child.[2] Indeed, most cases of ocular toxoplasmosis are thought to be congenital. Only 1% occur as a result of a de novo acquired infection. Worldwide, toxoplasmosis is the most common cause of posterior uveitis.[3]

Pathogenesis

Toxoplasmosis is disseminated throughout the body by infected macrophages and lymphocytes.[1] The cells lodge in retinal capillaries and produce a focal necrotizing retinal infection.[3-5] The contiguous choroid and vitreous are secondarily involved. An acquired cell-mediated immune response is thought to destroy the replicating trophozoites.[1] Local B-cell production of antibody may induce tissue cyst formation. Latent tissue cysts spontaneously lyse throughout life, producing recurrent infections. Hypersensitivity reaction to *Toxoplasma* antigens do not appear to play a role in triggering recurrences of retinochoroiditis in animal models of ocular toxoplasmosis.[6]

Clinical Presentation

Most cases of acquired toxoplasmosis are either subclinical or present with a mild flu-like illness.[1] Retinochoroiditis is rare in acquired toxoplasmosis. In an outbreak of toxoplasmosis in 1977 in Atlanta, Georgia, only 1% of 37 acutely infected persons developed ocular lesions.[9] A more severe meningoencephalitic form of acquired toxoplasmosis may result in retinal infection in 16% of patients.[1]

Congenital toxoplasmosis has an active, severe form that may result in miscarriage, hydrocephalus, seizures, and calcification of the choroid plexus in the brain.[1] A less fulminant, inactive form of congenital toxoplasmosis results in latent infection and the characteristic ocular disease.[7,8]

Congenital ocular toxoplasmosis is usually bilateral[3,4,10] (Fig. 11.1). Siblings of patients with ocular toxoplasmosis typically do not have eye findings.[9-12] This supports the existence of a transplacental route of infection with a low risk for maternal transmission to subsequent children. Inactive pigmented scars often can be seen in the peripheral retina or posterior pole of both eyes of affected individuals. Clusters of toxoplasmosis scars or "satellite" lesions represent previous episodes of disease activation. Recurrent toxoplasmosis retinitis is typically unilateral.

Patients with ocular toxoplasmosis will complain of floaters and blurred vision with a reactivation.[3,4,11-13] The anterior segment can have a granulomatous iridocyclitis with heavy "mutton fat" keratic precipitates. Secondary cataract, posterior synechiae, and glaucoma may be present. The vitreous often has marked cellular infiltration, flare, and opacification. Granulomatous precipitates can form on the posterior vitreous face (see Fig. 2.21). In severe cases, the retinochoroidal lesion is obscured by the vitritis and appears only as a "headlight in the fog."

Fundus examination reveals a fluffy, whitish yellow focus of retinitis (see Fig. 2.24). Characteristically, the active lesion is located adjacent to an older pigmented, "mother" scar. Retinal vasculitis, phlebitis, and optic neuritis are commonly seen.[14-16] Severe papillitis may occur alone or associated with vitritis and adjacent retinitis.[15] A stellate neuroretinitis can occur in younger patients.[16] Retinal detachment, vitreous scarring, and epiretinal membrane formation are sequelae of severe inflammation.

A variation of ocular toxoplasmosis is punctate outer retinal toxoplasmosis (PORT).[17-20] This condition is characterized by multifocal areas of retinitis localized to the outer layers of the retina, typically within the posterior pole (Fig. 11.2). Vitritis is often mild. Lesions may be adjacent to an older pigmented scar. It is possible that the patient does not recognize

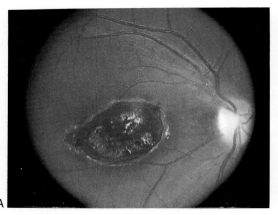
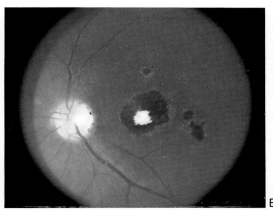

A   B

Figure 11.1. Infectious uveitis—congenital ocular toxoplasmosis. A, B: Inactive chorioretinal scars in the maculae of a patient with congenital toxoplasmosis.

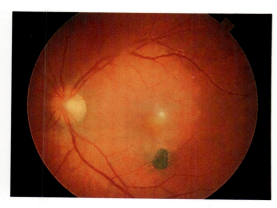

Figure 11.2. Infectious uveitis—punctate outer retinal toxoplasmosis. PORT in a patient with decreasing visual acuity and floaters. The lesions may be multiple and may be associated with an older hyperpigmented scar.

peripheral PORT until they coalesce and form a larger area of full-thickness retinitis.

Toxoplasmosis in immunocompromised patients and persons with acquired immunodeficiency syndrome (AIDS) may be atypical. De novo lesions not associated with older pigmented scars, multiple active lesions, and massive retinal necrosis have been described in these patients.[21–26] A brushfire form of retinitis resembling cytomegalovirus (CMV) retinitis has been described.[27] The advancing edge of the retinitis is creamy and not associated with significant hemorrhage. Unlike CMV retinitis, a significant vitritis is often noted in patients. Toxoplasmosis also can cause a form of infectious optic neuritis in AIDS.[28]

Diagnosis

Children born with an active congenital toxoplasmosis will have cerebral calcifications, seizures, bilateral retinochoroiditis (85%), and a positive immunoglobulin M (IgM) titer for toxoplasmosis.[1] Patients with latent congenital toxoplasmosis may be asymptomatic and can be diagnosed by the presence of characteristic ophthal-

moscopic lesions.[3,4] Serologic testing via enzyme-linked immunoadsorbent assay (ELISA) for IgG and IgM have largely replaced the indirect fluorescent antibody (IFA) and dye tests. A threefold rise in IgG titer or positive IgM titer is serologic evidence for an acquired infection.[1] Because *T. gondii* is an obligate intracellular organism and the retinal lesions are relatively small, antibody titers have low correlation to disease activity. Any positive titer, even undiluted or 1:1, in the setting of characteristic fundus lesions supports the clinical diagnosis.[3–9,11–13,29,30]

Fluorescein angiography may be helpful and will desmonstrate diffuse retinal vasculitis and chorioretinal anastomotic vessels.[31] Active areas of retinitis block early and become hyperfluorescent late in the study.

Toxoplasmosis can be identified in ocular tissues through histologic staining and the demonstration of tissue cysts. Polymerase chain reaction has been used to detect the organism in paraffin-embedded ocular sections.[32]

Differential Diagnosis

Tuberculosis, syphilis, *Candida*, and CMV may all cause a focal infectious retinitis. History, physical examination, characteristic satellite retinal lesions, and laboratory testing can help establish the correct diagnosis.

Treatment

It is not necessary to treat all cases of active retinal toxoplasmosis.[3,4,33,34] Small, peripheral lesions with minimal vitritis can be observed. Healing occurs over 1 to 3 months. Active lesions that threaten the optic nerve and macula and peripheral retinitis associated with severe vitreous reaction should be treated with antiprotozoal therapy. In a recent survey of the members of the American Uveitis Society, the most common agents used in the United States are pyrimethamine, sulfadiazine, clindamycin, sulfisoxazole, tetracycline, and minocycline.[34]

An alternative treatment protocol is the use of the fixed combination antibiotic trimethoprim-sulfamethoxazole twice a day. This agent has proved effective both in vitro and in vivo against *T. gondii*.[35–37] Trimethoprim-sulfamethoxazole can be delivered on a twice-a-day regimen and has fewer serious side effects. Table 11.1 lists several common regimens available for the treatment of ocular toxoplasmosis.[38,39]

Oral prednisone, 40 to 80 mg, can be added to antibiotic therapy after the patient has been on antibiotics for 24 to 48 hours. Regional corticosteroids should not be used because of their profound local immunosuppressive effect. When used alone without antiprotozoal agents, corticosteroids can cause a protozoal-mediated acute retinal necrosis similar to the acute retinal necrosis syndrome (ARN/BARN).[40]

Other adjunctive treatments have been used, including focal laser photocoagulation, cryoablation, and injection of sub-Tenon's clindamycin (50 mg in 1 ml).[34,41–45] In chronically immunosuppressed patients,

Table 11.1. Antiprotozoal therapy for ocular toxoplasmosis.

Regimen #1
Pyrimethamine (Daraprim)
  Load: 50 mg p.o. b.i.d. for first day
  Maintenance: 25 mg p.o. q.d. or b.i.d. for 2–8 weeks
Sulfadiazine
  Load: 1 g p.o. q.i.d. for first day
  Maintenance: 500 mg p.o. q.i.d. for 2–8 weeks with
    fluids
Folinic acid (Leucovorin): 3–5 mg p.o. three times a
  week; monitor CBC and platelet count weekly

Regimen #2
Clindamycin (Cleocin): 300 mg p.o. t.i.d. or q.i.d. for 3–
  4 weeks
Sulfadiazine 500 mg p.o. q.i.d.

Regimen #3
Trimethoprim (160 mg)/sulfamethoxazole (800 mg)
  (Bactrim DS or Septra) one p.o. b.i.d. for 2–6 weeks
Add clindamycin 300 mg p.o. q.i.d. (for zone I lesions)

---

prolonged maintenance antiprotozoal therapy may be required.[28]

One recent study demonstrated no reduction in duration of disease with several antibiotic therapeutic regimens compared to observation alone.[46] The size of the lesion was significantly reduced with therapy, however, and is an important consideration when treating lesions that threaten the macula or optic nerve.

Prognosis

Untreated, toxoplasmosis resolves within 3 weeks to 6 months. With treatment, resolution can be observed within 2 to 6 weeks. Recurrent disease is common, with an average of three attacks over a lifetime. Sequelae of the severe inflammation include retinal detachment and epiretinal membrane formation and vitreous opacification.[46] Retinal detachment repair during active disease can be challenging and may be associated with excessive postoperative scarring and proliferative vitreoretinopathy. Vitrectomy can improve vision in patients with media opacification or periretinal fibrosis.[47] Medically unresponsive glaucoma and cataract are also common complications of toxoplasmosis.

Amoebiasis

Amoebiasis is a protozoal infection caused by species of pathogenic amoeba.

Etiology

Several species of amoeba are pathogenic in human beings. *Naegleria fowleri, Entamoeba histolytica, Entamoeba coli,* and *Acanthamoeba* species have all been reported to cause human disease.[48,49] The free-living trophozoites can form cysts (10–20 μm) that are resistant to disinfectants and antibiotics. Heat sterilization kills these protozoal cysts.

Epidemiology

Amoeba have worldwide distribution, with 10% of the world population infected.[48-50] Their cysts are present in soil, dust, and water. Infection rates have been higher among homosexuals (31.7%) than heterosexuals (1.2%).[51]

Pathogenesis

Amoeba and their cysts can be inhaled or can gain access to the host via contaminated water through breaks in the skin or mucous membranes.[48,49] *N. fowleri* can enter the nose and directly penetrate the cribriform plate. Contaminated contact lenses can carry the amoeba to the cornea and result in amoebic keratitis. Polymorphonuclear (PMN) infiltration and tissue necrosis occur at the site of infection.

Clinical Presentation

Amoebic dysentery, liver abscess, encephalitis, and granulomatous amoebic encephalomeningitis are systemic manifestations of disseminated amoebic infection.[48-50]

The most common eye involvement is a chronic amoebic keratitis and sclerokeratitis.[52-54] The keratitis is indolent and may have a characteristic ring-like stromal infiltrate.[55] The keratitis can be associated with a nongranulomatous iridocyclitis, keratitic precipitates (KP), and hypopyon. A multifocal choroiditis and chorioretinitis have rarely been reported with *E. histolytica* and *Acanthamoeba* infection.[56,57]

Diagnosis

Systemic symptoms and signs of diarrhea, abdominal pain, or CNS symptoms may suggest an extraocular source for amoebic disease.[48,49] Patients who wear contact lenses and develop a medically unresponsive chronic keratitis should undergo culture or corneal biopsy to establish the diagnosis.[52-54] Trichrome stains will demonstrate the organism with a prominent karyosome (red) against the green cytoplasm of the amoeba. Amoeba can be grown in agar on a lawn of *Escherichia coli* bacteria.[49]

Differential Diagnosis

Keratouveitis can be seen in herpetic diseases and syphilis. Other forms of bacterial keratitis may resemble amoebic keratitis. Corneal scraping and culture can differentiate these diseases.

Treatment

Although no drug is specific for the treatment of amoebiasis, several agents have been used to treat the disease. Emetine, amphotericin B, miconazole, propamidine isothionate, ketoconazole, neomycin, polymyxin, and tobramycin have all been used in treating systemic and corneal disease.[57-60] Surgical debridement via drainage of an abscess or penetrating keratoplasty often is necessary to effect a cure.[60-62]

Prognosis

The prognosis is often poor. Effective, nontoxic antiprotozoal agents for amoeba are not available. Tissue cysts can resist antibiotic therapy and disease recurrence is common.

Trypanosomiasis

Trypanosomiasis or "sleeping sickness" is a protozoal infection caused by *Trypanosoma* species.

Etiology

T. gambiense and *T. rhodesiense* are flagellated protozoal parasites that may have ocular manifestations.[63]

Epidemiology

The tsetse fly is the vector for human sleeping sickness.[63] The disease is limited to river basin areas of Africa, the breeding areas of tsetse flies. Travel may increase the geographic distribution of patients with this disease.

Pathogenesis

Infected tsetse flies inoculate the bite wound with saliva containing the trophozoites.[63,64] In the blood or lymphatics, the trophozoites undergo extracellular binary division and result in the development of fever and malaise. The organism disseminates to the brain and other organ systems. Once in the brain and left untreated, the disease progresses to coma and death.

Clinical Presentation

Patients with sleeping sickness present with fever and CNS complaints. Later in the disease course, the patient becomes debilitated and lapses into coma.[63,64]

In the eye, the trophozoites can invade the vessel walls and cause an iridocyclitis, keratitis, retinal vasculitis, and hemorrhagic retinitis.[65–67] Ocular findings may be a result of infection or a response to protozoal antigens.

Diagnosis

Patients with a history of exposure to endemic areas in Africa and who have fever, CNS complaints, and uveitis or a hemorrhagic retinal vasculitis should undergo Wright or Giemsa staining procedures to look for parasites in the blood.

Differential Diagnosis

Behçet's disease, sarcoidosis, syphilis, systemic lupus erythematosus, and other forms of vasculitis can all be associated with systemic disease and hemorrhagic retinal vasculitis.

Treatment

Suramin, melarsoprol, and pentamidine have been used to treat trypanosomal disease.[63,64]

Prognosis

CNS involvement can result in coma and death.

Giardiasis

Giardiasis is a protozoal infection that can cause GI disease. It has been associated with several forms of uveitis, retinal vasculitis, and chorioretinitis.

Etiology

Giardia lamblia is a flagellated, binucleate protozoan with both free-living (trophozoite) and cystic forms.[68,69]

Epidemiology

Giardia is found in contaminated water worldwide. Wild animals such as deer, horse, beaver, and rabbit carry the organism. In the United States, 3.9% of stool specimens from asymptomatic subjects are positive for the *Giardia*.

Pathogenesis

Drinking contaminated water results in GI infection.[68,69] The trophozoites replicate in the small intestine and encyst in the lower bowel. It is not known whether the organism actually travels outside the bowel to the eye or whether the associated ocular and systemic manifestations are secondary to an allergic event.

Clinical Presentation

Systemic symptoms include diarrhea, bloating, anorexia, and constipation.[68,69] Cramping, weight loss, belching, and gas are other common complaints. Headache, skin rash, and seizures have also been reported with *Giardia* infection.

Patients with giardiasis can develop a nongranulomatous iridocyclitis and vitritis.[70–73] Hemorrhagic retinal vasculitis and retinal vascular sheathing have been observed associated with giardiasis.[74] Cases of peripheral choroiditis, exudative retinal detachment, and retinal edema have been reported as well.[71]

Diagnosis

Giardiasis can be diagnosed via stool specimen for ova and parasite.[68,69] A peripheral eosinophilia can be noted in 9% of patients.

Differential Diagnosis

Gastrointestinal complaints and uveitis can occur in inflammatory bowel syndrome (IBD), amoebiasis, and Whipple's disease. Patients with IBD experience episodic bloody diarrhea and an acute, alternating, nongranulomatous iridocyclitis. Patients with Whipple's disease develop arthritis associated with the chronic diarrhea. Jejunal biopsy is often performed in both Whipple's disease and giardiasis to confirm the diagnosis.

Treatment

Quinacrine (Atabrine), 50 to 100 mg, three times a day and metronidazole (Flagyl), 250 mg, orally three times a day for 10 days can be used to treat giardiasis.[68,69] Cure rates are high and approximate 90% to 95%.[75]

Prognosis

The systemic and visual prognosis is good with proper therapy.

Pneumocystosis

Pneumocystosis is an opportunistic protozoal infection that can cause a pneumonitis and multifocal subretinal infiltrate in immunocompromised hosts.

Etiology

Pneumocystis carinii has characteristics of protozoa, bacteria, and fungi.[76] It is currently classified as protozoa.

Epidemiology

P. carinii is a communicable, air-borne disease and is the most common cause of pneumocystic pneumonia (PCP) in immunocompromised patients; 60% to 90% of persons with AIDS patients develop PCP.[76] *Pneumocystis* choroiditis is rare. All reported ocular cases have been in patients with advanced AIDS.

Pathogenesis

The organism is inhaled and in immunocompromised hosts can cause focal pneumonitis. Primary pulmonary infection is hematogenous dissemination in the body and to the eye. In the eye, multifocal areas of infection occur in the choroid.[77–80] Inflammation is minimal in the areas of choroidal necrosis. Many cystic *P. carinii* organisms can be seen in these areas.

Clinical Presentation

Systemic manifestations of PCP include fever, cough, and shortness of breath. Chest radiograph may reveal infiltrates or cavitary lung lesions. *Pneumocystis* organisms, when metastatic to the choroid, result in multifocal, subretinal, yellowish white infiltrates. There is little associated vitritis. The lesions are large (300–3000 μm) and are typically located in the posterior pole.[77]

Diagnosis

Pneumocystis pneumonia should be suspected in any immunocompromised patient with pulmonary complaints. Chest radiographs and sputum analysis help establish the diagnosis.[76] Bronchoalveolar lavage via bronchoscopy can increase diagnostic accuracy. Ocular findings are very characteristic, and diagnosis can be made on clinical grounds.

Differential Diagnosis

Tuberculosis, syphilis, and toxoplasmosis may all have atypical clinical courses in AIDS and may cause a multifocal choroiditis.

Treatment

Intravenous pentamidine and oral trimethoprim sulfamethoxazole are the antibiotics of choice for *P. carinii* choroiditis.[76–80]

Prognosis

The development of *Pneumocystis* pneumonia is one of the most common opportunistic infections diagnostic of AIDS and is fatal without treatment. Long-term antibiotic therapy is required to control the infection in immunocompromised patients. Visual prognosis is poor as the choroiditis occurs in the later stages of AIDS.[79,81]

References

1. McCabe RE, Remington JS. *Toxoplasma gondii.* In: Mandell GL, Douglas RG Jr, Bennett JE, eds. *Principles and Practice of Infectious Diseases.* 3rd ed. New York: Churchill Livingstone; 1990.
2. Dubey JP. A review of toxoplasmosis in pigs. *Vet Parasitol.* 1986;19:181.
3. Smith RE, Nozik RA. Toxoplasmic retinochoroiditis. In: *Uveitis. A Clinical Approach to Diagnosis and Management.* 2nd ed. Baltimore: Williams & Wilkins; 1989.
4. Nussenblatt RB, Palestine AG. Ocular toxoplasmosis. In: David K. Marshall, ed. *Uveitis. Fundamentals and Clinical Practice.* Chicago: Year Book Medical Publishers; 1989.
5. O'Connor GR. The influence of hypersensitivity on the pathogenesis of ocular toxoplasmosis. *Trans Am Ophthalmol Soc.* 1970; 68:501.
6. Newman PE, Ghosheh R, Tabbara KF, et al. The role of hypersensitivity reactions to Toxoplasma antigens in experimental ocular toxoplasmosis in nonhuman primates. *Am J Ophthalmol.* 1982;94:159.
7. Langer H. Repeated congenital infection with toxoplasma gondii. *Obstet Gynecol.* 1963;21:318.
8. Aronson SB. Annual review. The uvea. *Arch Ophthalmol.* 1969;81:736.
9. Akstein RB, Wilson LA, Teutsch SM. Acquired toxoplasmosis. *Ophthalmology.* 1982; 89:1299.
10. Perkins ES. Ocular toxoplasmosis. *Br J Ophthalmol.* 1973;57:1.
11. Jacobs L, Cook MK, Wilder HC. Serologic data on adults with histologically diagnosed toxoplasmic chorioretinitis. *Trans Am Acad Ophthalmol Otolaryngol.* 1954;58:193.
12. Ashbell PA, Vermund SH, Hofeldt AJ. Presumed toxoplasmic retinochoroiditis in four siblings. *Am J Ophthalmol.* 1982;94:656.
13. Hogan MJ, Kimura SJ, O'Connor GR. Ocular toxoplasmosis. *Arch Ophthalmol.* 1964;72:592.
14. Morgan CM, Gragoudas ES. Branch retinal artery occlusion associated with recurrent toxoplasmic retinochoroiditis. *Arch Ophthalmol.* 1987;105:130.
15. Folk JC, Lobes LA. Presumed toxoplasmic papillitis. *Ophthalmology.* 1984;91:64.
16. Fish RH, Hoskins JC, Kline LB. Toxoplasmosis neuroretinitis. *Ophthalmology.* 1993;100: 1177.
17. Friedmann CT, Knox DL. Variations in recurrent active toxoplasmic retinochoroiditis. *Arch Ophthalmol.* 1969;81:481.
18. Doft BH, Gass DM. Punctate outer retinal toxoplasmosis. *Arch Ophthalmol.* 1985;103: 1332.
19. Matthews JD, Weiter JJ. Outer retinal toxoplasmosis. *Ophthalmology.* 1988;95:941.
20. Doft BH, Gass JD. Outer retinal layer toxoplasmosis. *Graefes Arch Clin Exp Ophthalmol.* 1986;224:78.
21. Yeo JH, Jakobiec FA, Iwamoto T, et al. Opportunistic toxoplasmic retinochoroiditis

following chemotherapy for systemic lymphoma. *Ophthalmology.* 1983;90:885.

22. Parke EW II, Font RL. Diffuse toxoplasmic retinochoroiditis in a patient with AIDS. *Arch Ophthalmol.* 1986;104:571.

23. Heinemann M-H, Gold JM, Maisel J. Bilateral toxoplasma retinochoroiditis in a patient with acquired immune deficiency syndrome. *Retina.* 1986;6:224.

24. Holland GN, Engstrom RE Jr, Glasgow BJ, et al. Ocular toxoplasmosis in patients with the acquired immunodeficiency syndrome. *Am J Ophthalmol.* 1988;106:653.

25. Cochereau-Massin I, LeHoang P, Lauteri-Frau M, et al. Ocular toxoplasmosis in human immunodeficiency virus-infected patients. *Am J Ophthalmol.* 1992;114:130.

26. Moorthy RS, Smith RE, Rao NA. Progressive ocular toxoplasmosis in patients with acquired immunodeficiency syndrome. *Am J Ophthalmol.* 1993;115:742.

27. Elkins BS, Holland GN, Opremcak EM, et al. Ocular toxoplasmosis misdiagnosed as cytomegalovirus retinopathy in immunocompromised patients. *Ophthalmology.* In press.

28. Grossniklaus HE, Specht CS, Allaire G, Leavitt JA. *Toxoplasma gondii* retinochoroiditis and optic neuritis in acquired immune deficiency syndrome. *Ophthalmology.* 1990; 97:1342.

29. Cursons RTM. DIG-ELISA for the serologic diagnosis of toxoplasmosis. *Am J Clin Pathol.* 1982;77:459.

30. Weiss MJ, Velazquez N, Hofeldt AJ. Serologic tests in the diagnosis of presumed toxoplasmic retinochoroiditis. *Am J Ophthalmol.* 1990;109:407.

31. Hausmann N, Richard G. Acquired ocular toxoplasmosis. A fluorescein angiography study. *Ophthalmology.* 1991;98:1647.

32. Brezin AP, Egwuagu CE, Burnier M Jr, et al. Identification of *Toxoplasma gondii* in paraffin-embedded sections by the polymerase chain reaction. *Am J Ophthalmol.* 1990;110: 559.

33. Fajardo RV, Furgiuele FP, Leopold IH. Treatment of toxoplasmosis uveitis. *Arch Ophthalmol.* 1962;67:50.

34. Enstrom RE, Holland GN, Nussenblatt RB, Jabs DA. Current practices in the management of ocular toxoplasmosis. *Am J Ophthalmol.* 1991;111:601.

35. Seah SKK. Chemotherapy in experimental toxoplasmosis: comparison of the efficacy of trimethoprim-sulfur and pyrimethamine-sulfur combinations. *J Trop Med Hyg.* 1975; 78:150.

36. Nguyen BT, Stadtsbaeder S. Comparative effects of cotrimoxazole (trimethoprim-sulphamethoxazole), pyrimethamine-sulphadiazine and spiramycin during a virulent infection with *Toxoplasma gondii* (Beverley strain) in mice. *Br J Pharmacol.* 1983;79:923.

37. Grossman PL, Krahenbuhl JL, Remington JS. In vivo and in vitro effects of trimethoprim and sulfamethoxazole on *Toxoplasma* infection. In: Siegenthaler W, Luthy R, eds. *Current chemotherapy. Proceedings of the Tenth International Congress of Chemotherapy.* Washington, DC: American Society of Microbiology; 1978:135.

38. Opremcak EM, Scales DK, Sharpe MR. Trimethoprim-sulfamethoxazole therapy for ocular toxoplasmosis. *Ophthalmology.* 1992;99: 920.

39. Rothova A, Buitenhuis HJ, Meenken C, et al. Therapy of ocular toxoplasmosis. *Int Ophthalmol.* 1989;13:415.

40. Sabates R, Pruett RC, Brockhurst RJ. Fulminary ocular toxoplasmosis. *Am J Ophthalmol.* 1981;92:497.

41. Rollins DF, Tabbara KJ, Ghosheh R, Nozik RA. Minocycline in experimental ocular toxoplasmosis in the rabbit. *Am J Ophthalmol.* 1982;93:361.

42. Lakhanpal V, Schocket SS, Nirankari VS. Clindamycin in the treatment of toxoplasmic retinochoroiditis. *Am J Ophthalmol.* 1983;95:605.

43. Dobbie JG. Cryotherapy in the management of toxoplasma retinochoroiditis. *Trans Am Acad Ophthalmol Otolaryngol.* 1968;72:364.

44. Tabbara KF, Dy-Liacco J, Nozik RA, et al. Clindamycin in chronic toxoplasmosis. *Arch Ophthalmol.* 1979;97:542.

45. Ghartey KN, Brockhurt RJ. Photocoagulation of active toxoplasmic retinochoroiditis. *Am J Ophthalmol.* 1980;89:858.

46. Rothova A, Meenken C, Buitenhuis HJ, et al. Therapy for ocular toxoplasmosis. *Am J Ophthalmol.* 1993;115:517.

47. Fitzgerald CR. Pars plana vitrectomy for vitreous opacity secondary to presumed toxoplasmosis. *Arch Ophthalmol.* 1980;98:321.

48. Ravdin JI, Petri WA Jr. *Entamoeba histolytica* (amebiasis). In: Mandell GL, Douglas RG Jr,

Bennett JE, eds. *Principles and Practice of Infectious Diseases*. 3rd ed. New York: Churchill Livingstone; 1990.

49. Petri WA Jr, Ravdin JI. Free-living amoebae. In: Mandell GL, Douglas RG Jr, Bennett JE, eds. *Principles and Practice of Infectious Diseases*. 3rd ed. New York: Churchill Livingstone; 1990.

50. Kean BH, Sun T, Ellsworth RM, eds. Entamebiasis. In: *Color Atlas/Text of Ophthalmic Parasitology*. New York: Igaku-Shoin; 1991.

51. Kean BH, William DC, Luminais SK. Epidemic of amebiasis and giardiasis in a biased population. *Br J Vener Dis*. 1979;55:375.

52. Mannis MJ, Tamaru R, Roth AM, et al. *Acanthamoeba* sclerokeratitis. Determining diagnostic criteria. *Arch Ophthalmol*. 1986;104:1313.

53. Cohen EJ, Buchannan HW, Laughrea PA, et al. Diagnosis and management of *Acanthamoeba* keratitis. *Am J Ophthalmol*. 1985;100:389.

54. Moore MB, McCulley JP, Luckenbach M, et al. *Acanthamoeba* keratitis associated with soft contact lenses. *Am J Ophthalmol*. 1985;100:396.

55. Theodore FH, Jakobiec FA, Juechter KB, et al. The diagnostic value of a ring infiltrate in acanthamoebic keratitis. *Ophthalmology*. 1985;92:1471.

56. Johns KJ, O'Day DM, Feman SS. Chorioretinitis in the contralateral eye of a patient with *Acanthamoeba* keratitis. *Ophthalmology*. 1988; 95:635.

57. Kean BH. The treatment of amebiasis. A recurrent agony. *JAMA*. 1976;235:501.

58. Watt G, Padre LP, Adapon B, et al. Nonresolution of an amebic liver abscess after parasitologic cure. *Am J Trop Med Hyg*. 1986; 35:501.

59. Larkin DFP, Kilvington S, Dart JKG. Treatment of *Acanthamoeba* keratitis with polyhexamethylene biguanide. *Ophthalmology*. 1992;99:185.

60. Cohen EJ, Parlato CJ, Arentsen JJ, et al. Medical and surgical treatment of *Acanthamoeba* keratitis. *Am J Ophthalmol*. 1987;103:615.

61. Meisler DM, Ludwig IH, Rutherford I, et al. Susceptibility of *Acanthamoeba* to cryotherapeutic method. *Arch Ophthalmol*. 1986;104:130.

62. Blackman HJ, Rao NA, Lemp MA, Visvesvara GS. *Acanthamoeba* keratitis successfully treated with penetrating keratoplasty: suggested immunogenic mechanisms of action. *Cornea*. 1984;3:125.

63. Kirchhoff LV. Agents of African trypanosomiasis (sleeping sickness). In: Mandell GL, Douglas RG Jr, Bennett JE, eds. *Principles and Practice of Infectious Diseases*. 3rd ed. New York: Churchill Livingstone; 1990.

64. African trypanosomiasis. In: BH Kean, MD, Tseih Sun, MD, Robert M Ellsworth, MD, eds. *Color Atlas/Text of Ophthalmic Parasitology*. New York: Igaku-Shoin; 1991.

65. Rodger FC. *Eye Disease in the Tropics*. Edinburgh: Churchill Livingstone; 1981:83.

66. Mortelmans J, Neetans A. Ocular lesions in experimental *Trypanosoma brucei* infection in cats. *Acta Zool Pathol Antverpiensia*. 1975;62:149.

67. Buissonniere RF, de Boissieu D, Tell G, et al. Uveomeningitis revealing a West African trypanosomiasis in a 12 year old girl. *Arch Fr Pediatr*. 1989;46:517.

68. Hill DR. *Giardia lamblia*. In: Mandell GL, Douglas RG Jr, Bennett JE, eds. *Principles and Practice of Infectious Diseases*. 3rd ed. New York: Churchill Livingstone; 1990.

69. Kean BH, Tsieh S, Ellsworth RM. Giardiasis. In: *Color Atlas/Text of Ophthalmic Parasitology*. New York: Igaku-Shoin; 1991.

70. Barraquer I. Sur la coincidence de la lambliase et de certaines lesions du fond de l'oeil. *Bull Soc Pathol Exot (Paris)*. 1938;31:55.

71. Carroll M, Anast BP, Birth CL. Giardiasis and uveitis. *Arch Ophthalmol*. 1961;65:775.

72. Sucs FE, Zanen A. Ocular manifestations secondary to giardiasis. *Bull Soc Belge Ophthalmol*. 1986;219:63.

73. Anderson ML, Griffith DG. Intestinal giardiasis associated with ocular inflammation. *J Clin Gastroenterol*. 1985;7:169.

74. Knox DL, King J Jr. Retinal arteritis, iridocyclitis, and giardiasis. *Ophthalmology*. 1982;89:1303.

75. Davidson RA. Issues in clinical parasitology: the treatment of giardiasis. *Am J Gastroenterol*. 1984;79:256.

76. Walzer PD. *Pneumocystis carinii*. In: Mandell GL, Douglas RG Jr, Bennett JE, eds. *Principles and Practice of Infectious Diseases*. 3rd ed. New York: Churchill Livingstone; 1990.

77. Shami MJ, Freeman W, Friedberg D, et al. A multicenter study of *Pneumocystis* choroidopathy. *Am J Ophthalmol.* 1991;112:15.

78. Pneumocystosis. In: Kean BH, Sun Tsieh, Ellsworth RM, eds. *Color Atlas/Text of Ophthalmic Parasitology.* New York: Igaku-Shoin; 1991.

79. Dugel PU, Rao NA, Forster DJ, et al. *Pneumocystis carinii* choroiditis after long-term aerosolized pentamidine therapy. *Am J Ophthalmol.* 1990;110:113.

80. Foster RE, Lowder CY, Meisler DM, et al. Presumed *Pneumocystis carinii* choroiditis. *Ophthalmology.* 1991;98:1360.

81. Freeman WR, Gross JG, Labelle J, et al. *Pneumocystis carinii* choroidopathy. A new clinical entity. *Arch Ophthalmol.* 1989;107:863.

12
Helminthic Diseases

Toxocariasis

Toxocariasis is a nematode disease that may cause systemic disease or local ocular disease.

Etiology

Toxocara canis and *T. cati* are common roundworm parasites of dogs and cats. Humans are not a natural host for the worm, which is unable to complete its life cycle in human infection. *Toxocara* larvae are 357 to 445 μm long and 18 to 21 μm in diameter.[1] *T. canis* is most often the cause of toxocariasis.

Epidemiology

Toxocara has worldwide distribution; most reported cases are in the United States.[2] Between 33% and 100% of dogs have evidence for *Toxocara* infection; 10% of humans have serologic evidence for exposure to *Toxocara*.[3,4]

Pathogenesis

In adult dogs, infection is acquired by ingesting ova or larval stages of the worm.[5] Ova are considered first-stage larvae and can be found in soil and feces. Second-stage larvae hatch and gain access to the bloodstream and are found in infected tissues. A third-stage larva can be found in

lungs and saliva of dogs. These larvae are swallowed to enter the fourth larval stage in the intestine and feces of puppies. In humans, ova (first-stage larvae) are ingested from soil and undercooked foods. Third-stage larvae are acquired by handling infected puppies. The ova hatch in the intestine and bore through the intestinal mucosa. In the bloodstream, the larvae get trapped in the small capillaries and bore into surrounding tissues.[1,5] In the retina, the dead larva incites an intense eosinophilic abscess. Later, granuloma formation and scarring surround the organism.

Clinical Presentation

T. canis can cause a systemic illness called visceral larval migrans (VLM), which is not associated with ocular disease. VLM can occur in children 2 to 3 years of age and presents with fever, hepatosplenomegaly, cough, and a pruritic skin rash.[1,6,7] A peripheral eosinophilia and leukocytosis is found on laboratory testing.

Ocular toxocariasis or ocular larval migrans (OLM) has three classic, clinical presentations.[3,4,8,9] In young children (2–9 years), parents note a leukocoria. The eye is typically white and quiet with reduced visual acuity. Ocular examination reveals a panuveitis or "endophthalmitis" associated with hypopyon, posterior synechiae, and cataract. Traction retinal detachment may also be present.

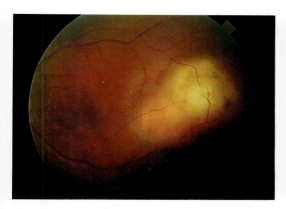

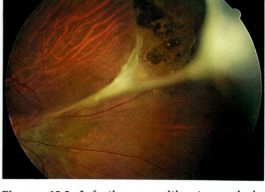

Figure 12.1. Infectious uveitis—toxocariasis. An inflammatory granuloma in the posterior pole of a patient with ocular toxocariasis.

Figure 12.2. Infectious uveitis—toxocariasis. Peripheral retinal granuloma with a falciform retinal fold in an asymptomatic patient. The inflammatory granuloma was noted on routine dilated fundus examination.

A second form of toxocariasis occurs in older children between 4 and 14 years.[3,4,8,10] These children and young adults have poor visual acuity in one eye. An inflammatory granuloma can be seen in the posterior pole on fundus examination (Fig. 12.1). The lesions often have a dark center representing the dead larva. The overlying vitreous may have inflammatory cells. With active inflammation, the adjacent retina may be edematous, with a localized serous/exudative detachment.

The third form of toxocariasis occurs in children and young adults between the ages of 6 and 40 years.[3,4,8,10,11] Patients may be asymptomatic, and on routine examination a peripheral retinal granuloma is noted, which may involve the pars plana and ciliary body (Fig. 12.2). A traction falciform fold can be noted extending from the optic disc toward the mass. Vision may be affected if the retinal traction involves the macula.

Diagnosis

The clinical picture is often characteristic. Enzyme-linked immunoadsorbent assay (ELISA) testing for *Toxocara* antibodies can support the diagnosis. The antigen load is small in ocular toxocariasis, and the antibody titer is often low.[1] Any titer, even a 1:2, is significant in the proper clinical setting.[1,8,11,12] Aqueous or vitreous biopsy may be necessary in younger children in whom retinoblastoma or true endophthalmitis is suspected.[8] Eosinophils are noted on cytologic examination. Ultrasound will not demonstrate calcification and can help differentiate *Toxocara* granuloma from retinoblastoma.[1,5]

Differential Diagnosis

Retinoblastoma may cause a leukocoria and an "endophthalmitis"-like picture with a pseudohypopyon. Family history, the presence of multiple retinal lesions, and calcification can help differentiate the two diseases. Vitreous biopsy demonstrates tumor cells. Leukocoria can be seen in Coats' disease, retinopathy of prematurity, familial exudative vitreoretinopathy, and persistent hyperplastic vitreous. Retinal granuloma formation may also occur in ascariasis, tuberculosis, sarcoidosis, and syphilis. In contrast, retinal toxoplasmosis causes a necrotizing lesion without granuloma formation.

Treatment

Puppies should be treated with piperazine as soon as they are weaned to prevent disease transmission. Inactive *Toxocara* granulomas require no therapy. When they are associated with vitritis, retinal edema, or exudative retinal detachment, periocular corticosteroids are the treatment of choice.[8,10] Oral prednisone can also be effective in controlling the secondary inflammation. Anthelminthic agents do not play a role in ocular toxocariasis, as the larva incites inflammation and granuloma formation only after its death.[8] Vitreoretinal surgery can be performed in the presence of severe endophthalmitis to clear the media and control the inflammation.[13,14]

Prognosis

Visual prognosis is poor with the panuveitis form and with macular granuloma. Peripheral lesions are often unnoticed and have the best potential for vision.

Ascariasis

Ascariasis is a helminthic disease caused by the nematode *Ascaris lumbricoides*.

Etiology

A. lumbricoides is a free-living roundworm found in soil.[1] The worm is 150 to 350 mm long.

Epidemiology

A. lumbricoides has worldwide distribution. Approximately 25% of the world's population is infected.[15]

Pathogenesis

Infection occurs via fecal-oral routes or via ingestion of contaminated soil.[1] The larvae hatch in the intestine and enter the bloodstream.[15] They travel to the lungs and complete their life cycle by being swallowed and passed through the intestines.

Clinical Presentation

The migrating worms can cause wheezing when in the lungs. Itching and intestinal obstruction can occur.[1] In the eye, the larvae have been proposed to cause a clinical picture similar to that of *Toxocara*, with the development of inflammatory granuloma.[16–18] In Africa, atypical bilateral Mooren's corneal ulcers are associated with severe ascariasis.[19]

Diagnosis

Peripheral eosinophilia can be found on testing. Ova and parasites should be sought in stool samples.[1,15]

Differential Diagnosis

Toxocariasis, sarcoidosis, tuberculosis, and syphilis can cause a peripheral retinal granuloma formation.

Treatment

Pyrantel pamoate can be used to kill the nematodes. Associated intraocular inflammation can be controlled with periocular or oral corticosteroids.

Prognosis

As with ocular toxocariasis, visual prognosis depends on the location of the granuloma.

Onchocerciasis

Onchocerciasis is a microfilarial disease that causes "river blindness."

Etiology

Onchocerca volvulus is a thread-like, nematode that causes human disease. The adult female worm is 230 to 500 mm long, and the male is 16 to 42 mm long.[20] Microfilariae are 220 to 360 μm long and 5 to 9 μm in diameter. The adult female worm can produce up to one million microfilariae per year and can live within host tissues for 8 to 12 years.[20] As many as 200 million microfilariae can be present in an individual infected patient.[20]

Epidemiology

O. volvulus has worldwide distribution. Human disease is concentrated, however, in tropical Africa, Central and South America, and the Arabian Peninsula.[20] It is estimated that 40 million people are infected with *O. volvulus* and 2 million of those are blind from the ocular complication.[21,22] In endemic areas, 40% of patients develop eye disease.

Pathogenesis

The female black fly (Simulium) transmits the disease. The fly acquires the microfilariae by sucking blood from an infected host. The disease is transmitted during the next blood meal. Once in humans, adult worms mature slowly in the subcutaneous tissues, producing millions of microfilariae. These areas (called onchocercoma) develop subcutaneous, encapsulated fibrous nodules that contain clusters of worms. The worms die over a 2- to 12-year lifespan. An inflammatory response may occur with the death of the worms.

Clinical Presentation

The systemic manifestations include an itching dermatitis and subcutaneous nodules containing microfilaria or mature worms.[21-24] Lymphatic obstruction can result in elephantiasis.[21,23,25] The microfilaria gain access to the eye and cause several forms of inflammation. In the cornea, punctate keratitis with "snowflake opacities" occurs around dead microfilariae.[26,27] A

severe stromal keratitis occurs with further invasion of the cornea by living microfilaria.[26-28] In the anterior chamber, the free-swimming worms cause a nongranulomatous iridocyclitis, posterior synechiae, cataract, and glaucoma. Bilateral patchy chorioretinitis, retinal scarring, and optic atrophy occur late in the disease process[26-28] and account for a large degree of visual impairment.

Diagnosis

Biopsy of the skin nodules (onchocercoma) demonstrates the parasite. Ocular paracentesis can also demonstrate the presence of microfilariae within the aqueous.

Differential Diagnosis

Keratitis and iridocyclitis, with or without chorioretinitis and optic atrophy, can be seen in patients with syphilis. Syphilis does not have the characteristic subcutaneous nodules.

Treatment

Prevention of disease transmission in endemic areas is critical to control the disease worldwide. The Onchocerciasis Control Programme, begun in 1974, focused on spraying larvacide on Simulium breeding sites.[29] This effort has reduced disease transmission to zero over a 10-year period. Surgical removal of the skin nodule can reduce the worm load. Nodulectomy may even improve visual prognosis.[1,30,31] Diethylcarbamazine (Hetrazan) (0.5–6 mg/kg in three divided doses) can kill most of the microfilariae, but not the adult worms.[32] Suramin (17 mg/kg IV each week for 6 weeks) can kill both microfilaria and adult worms; however, this drug is nephrotoxic.[33] Single-dose Ivermectin (150 μg/kg) is microfilariacidal and can help clear the body and the cornea of the microfilariae.[34] Most anthelminthic therapies are associated with severe systemic reactions (Mazzotti reaction) when a massive parasite killing occurs. Topical corticosteroids can control this often severe inflammation.

Prognosis

Many of the ocular cicatricial changes are permanent. In certain endemic areas, 40% of the adult population is blind from ocular complications of *O. volvulus* infection.

Loiasis

Loiasis is a microfilarial parasitic disease that can affect humans.

Etiology

Loa loa eye worms are long (70 mm) nematodes.[35] They are 350 to 430 μm in diameter.

Epidemiology

Loiasis is endemic in West and Central Africa. The prevalence rate is 50% to 90% in some regions.[36] The disease is transmitted by Chrysops, a mango fly.[35] Microfilariae are ingested by the fly during biting. An infected fly can transmit the disease by inoculating the larvae in a new host.

Pathogenesis

Once in the tissues, the microfilariae develop into an adult worm over 4 to 7 years. Migration of the worm causes cutaneous swelling from antigen or mechanical reactions.[36]

Clinical Presentation

Repeated bouts of hot, erythematous areas of skin swelling (calabar swelling) is the most common symptom.[37] The worm can migrate through the tissues of the eye including the conjunctiva, anterior chamber, vitreous, or subretinal spaces.[38,39] The worm may also cause a secondary uveitis

and a retinopathy.[40–42] Vascular obstruction, intraretinal hemorrhage, and exudation have been noted with invasion of the retinal vessels.

Diagnosis

The diagnosis is made on clinical grounds by directly observing the motile worm in the eye.

Differential Diagnosis

The observation of a migrating *Loa loa worm* is pathognomonic.

Treatment

The worm can be surgically removed from the eye.[39] Diethylcarbamazine can kill both adult worms and microfilariae.[35] Rapid death of a large load of worms can produce a Jarisch-Herxheimer–like reaction with fever, chills, and coma.[36]

Prognosis

The visual prognosis is good with therapy and removal of the worm from the eye.

Cysticercosis

Cysticercosis is caused by the encysted tapeworm larva, *Taenia solium*.

Etiology

T. solium, or tapeworm, is a long, ellipsoid cestode.[43] The adult worm has a scolex and 800 to 900 proglottids. The worm can reach a length of 2 to 3 meters and may live in the intestine for up to 25 years.[43,44] The larva of *T. solium* is called *Cysticercus cellulosae* and contains a protoscolex.

Epidemiology

The worm has worldwide distribution and humans are the definitive host. Transmission occurs via fecal-oral routes and consumption of undercooked meats.

Pathogenesis

Once the worm is ingested, it attaches with its scolex to the GI tract and releases larvae, which can travel throughout the body or encyst and be excreted in the feces.[43] Larval cysts can reach sizes greater than 1 cm in diameter. Tissue inflammation occurs with the death of the larva.

Clinical Presentation

Many patients with tapeworm are entirely asymptomatic.[45] Mild GI complaints include diarrhea, anorexia, and constipation.[44,46] Subcutaneous lesions (24%) may occur with migration of the larva in systemic cysticercosis.[47] The larvae can cause multiple cystic lesions in the brain and elevated intracranial pressure in 60% to 90% of patients with clinical disease.[48]

The larva may gain access to the eye and form cysts in the vitreous or subretinal space in 13% to 46% of patients.[49–51] The living parasite with protoscolex can be seen undulating in these spaces.[43] With the death of the tapeworm, a severe panuveitis can occur, which can be bilateral[49] (Fig.

12.3A). Less common is orbital, subconjunctival, and anterior chamber involvement.[43]

Diagnosis

Ocular cysticercosis can be diagnosed on clinical grounds. Biomicroscopy and ophthalmoscopy can demonstrate the encysted larva. Ultrasound can demonstrate the hard protoscolex within the cysts[52] (Fig. 12.3B). Computed tomography (CT) or magnetic resonance imaging (MRI) of the brain reveals multiple cystic lesions when the CNS is involved.[48] Serologic tests are available but not specific for *T. solium*.[48] Eosinophilia may be noted on paracentesis or in vitrectomy specimens.

Differential Diagnosis

The clinical observation of the encysted larva with a protoscolex is distinctive.

Treatment

Surgical removal of the intraocular cysts can prevent the severe inflammation that occurs with the death of the worm.[49,50] Praziquantel (50 mg/kg/per day) can kill the tapeworm and can be used for neurocysticercosis, but may be associated with worsening of the ocular disease.[53,54]

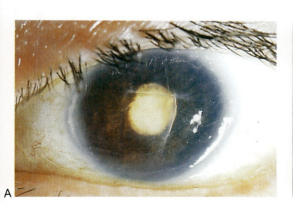 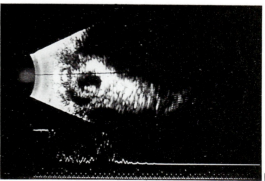

Figure 12.3. Infectious uveitis—cysticercosis. A: A hypotonus left eye in a patient with severe, bilateral diffuse uveitis. **B:** The ultrasound demonstrates the presence of a cystic lesion with a calcified protoscolex.

Prognosis

Untreated, the disease has a poor visual prognosis as a result of the severe inflammatory response.

Diffuse Unilateral Subacute Neuroretinitis

Diffuse unilateral subacute neuroretinitis (DUSN), also called "unilateral wipe-out syndrome," is caused by a motile nematode.

Etiology

The nematode responsible for DUSN has not been specifically identified. A raccoon ascarid, Baylisascaris, has been postulated to be responsible for DUSN in several cases.[1,55–59]

Epidemiology

More than 100 cases of DUSN have been described in the literature. The average age of patients is 14 years, with a range of 11 to 65 years. Males are affected slightly more often than females (1.5:1). The Midwest and southeastern United States appear to be the "endemic" regions for DUSN. The responsible worm appears to be larger (1500–2000 μm) in the Midwest than the worm seen in the Southeast (400–1200 μm).[60,61] Recently, DUSN documented to be due to Baylisascaris has been reported in California.[59]

Pathogenesis

DUSN appears to be caused by an immunologic or toxic reaction to the worm and worm by-products. Death of the worm appears to cause little intraocular inflammation. A small focal granuloma may be seen in some cases, but is not typical.

Clinical Presentation

DUSN is a biphasic disease.[60,61] Patients will experience a unilateral, insidious decrease in visual acuity. Early in the course of the disease, the fundus develops multiple, postequatorial, evanescent crops of grayish white dots (400–1500 μm). There is often an associated nongranulomatous vitritis, retinal vasculitis, and papillitis. Careful ophthalmoscopy, contact lens examination, and fundus photography reveal a motile nematode in the retina.

The second phase of the disease occurs with a toxic "wipe-out" of the retinal pigment epithelium (RPE), retina, and optic nerve[60,61] (Fig. 12.4). Afferent pupillary defect, massive RPE disruption (sparing the macula), sheathed/narrowed vessels, and optic atrophy develop. A small, whitish subretinal granuloma may form around the worm.

Diagnosis

The diagnosis can be made clinically.[60,61] Finding a motile subretinal worm confirms

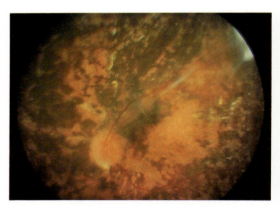

Figure 12.4. Infectious uveitis—DUSN. Fundus photograph of a patient with "unilateral wipe-out" and widespread disruption of the RPE in untreated DUSN. A small, subretinal granuloma was noted surrounding the worm in the superotemporal retina.

the diagnosis. Fluorescein angiogram reveals disc edema and early blockage, with late staining in the lesions. Electrophysiologic testing reveals a decreased electroretinogram (ERG). Laboratory testing is unremarkable. Increased lactate dehydrogenase (LDH) and serum glutamic-oxaloacetic transaminase (SGOT) have been reported. *T. canis* titers are negative.[61]

Differential Diagnosis

Multiple evanescent white dot syndrome (MEWDS), acute multifocal placoid pigment epitheliopathy, and toxocariasis can cause a similar fundus picture. The presence of a motile nematode assists in the diagnosis.[61,62]

Treatment

Laser photocoagulation of the worm results in death of the worm and minimal post-laser inflammation. Such treatment can prevent the severe "wipe-out" and is the treatment of choice.[60,62] Oral thiabendazole (22 mg/kg) for 2 to 4 days has caused death of the worm in the fundus in four cases.[63]

Prognosis

The prognosis is poor without early treatment because of optic atrophy and "unilateral wipe-out."

References

1. Kean BH, Sun T, Ellsworth RM. Toxocariasis, ascariasis, and baylisascariasis. In: *Color Atlas/Text of Ophthalmic Parasitology.* New York: Igaku-Shoin; 1991:105.
2. Glickman LT, Schantz PM. epidemiology and pathogenesis of zoonotic toxocariasis. *Epidemiol Rev.* 1981;3:230.
3. Woodruff AW. Toxocariasis. *Br Med J.* 1970; 3:663.
4. Mok CH. Visceral larva migrans. *Clin Pediatr.* 1968;7:565.
5. Molk R. Ocular toxocariasis: a review of the literature. *Ann Ophthalmol.* 1983;15:216.
6. Neafie RC, Connor DH. Visceral larva migrans. In: Binford CH, Connor DH, eds. *Pathology of Tropical and Extraordinary Diseases.* Washington DC: Armed Forces Institute of Pathology; 1976:433.
7. Arean VM, Crandall CA. Toxocariasis. In: Marcial-Rojas RA, ed. *Pathology of Protozoal and Helminthic Diseases.* Baltimore: Williams & Wilkins; 1971:808.
8. Ocular toxocariasis. In: Smith RE, Nozik RA, eds. *Uveitis: A Clinical Approach to Diagnosis and Management.* 2nd ed. Baltimore: Williams & Wilkins; 1989:135.
9. *Toxocara canis* infection. In: Nussenblatt RB, Palestine AG, eds. *Uveitis: Fundamentals and Clinical Practice.* Chicago: Year Book Medical Publishers; 1989:355.
10. Shields JA. Ocular toxocariasis. A review. *Surv Ophthalmol.* 1984;28:361.
11. Wilder H. Nematode endophthalmitis. *Trans Am Acad Ophthalmol Otolaryngol.* 1950;55:99.
12. Kieler RA. *Toxocara canis* endophthalmitis with low ELISA titer. *Ann Ophthalmol.* 1983; 15:447.
13. Wilkinson CP, Welch RB. Intraocular *Toxocara. Am J Ophthalmol.* 1971;71:9221.
14. Hagler WS, Pollard ZF, Jarrett WH, et al. Results of surgery for ocular *Toxocara canis. Ophthalmology.* 1981;88:1081.
15. Pawlowski ZS. Ascariasis. *Clin Gastroenterol.* 1978;7:157.
16. Price AJ Jr, Wadsworth JAC. An intraretinal worm. *Arch Ophthalmol.* 1970;83:768.
17. Parsons HE. Nematode chorioretinitis: report of a case with photographs of a viable worm. *Arch Ophthalmol.* 1953;47:799.
18. Calhoun FP. Intraocular invasion by the larva of the *Ascaris. Arch Ophthalmol.* 1937; 18:963.
19. Majekodunmi AA. Ecology of Mooren's ulcer in Nigeria. *Doc Ophthalmol.* 1980;49:211.
20. Kean BH, Sun T, Ellsworth RM. Onchocerciasis. In: *Color Atlas/Text of Ophthalmic Parasitology.* New York: Igaku-Shoin; 1991.
21. Connor DH, Neafie RC. Onchocerciasis. In: Binford CH, Connor DH, eds. *Pathology of Tropical and Extraordinary Diseases.* Washington DC: Armed Forces Institute of Pathology; 1976:360.

22. WHO. *WHO Expert Committee on Onchocerciasis: Third Report, Techn Report Ser No 752.* Geneva: World Health Organization; 1987.

23. Gibson DW, Heggie C, Connor DH. Clinical and pathologic aspects of onchocerciasis. *Pathol Annu.* 1980;15(pt 2):195.

24. Connor DH. Onchocerciasis. *N Engl J Med.* 1978;298:379.

25. Gibson DW, Connor DH. Onchocercal lymphadenitis: clinicopathologic study of 34 patients. *Trans Roy Soc Trop Med Hyg.* 1978; 72:137.

26. Anderson J, Fuglsang H. Ocular onchocerciasis. *Trop Dis Bull.* 1977;74:257.

27. Paul EV, Zimmerman LE. Some observations on the ocular pathology of onchocerciasis. *Hum Pathol.* 1970;1:581.

28. Anderson J, Font RL. Ocular onchocerciasis. In: Binford CH, Connor DH, eds. *Pathology of Tropical and Extraordinary Diseases.* Washington DC: Armed Forces Institute of Pathology; 1976:373.

29. WHO. *Ten Years of Onchocerciasis Control in West Africa: Review of the Work of the Onchocerciasis Control Programme in the Volta River Basin Area From 1974 to 1984.* Geneva: World Health Organization; 1985.

30. Zea-Flores G. *Nodulectomy and Its Effects on Guatemalan Onchocerciasis.* Geneva: World Health Organization; 1986.

31. Guderian RH, Proafio RS, Beck B, et al. The reduction in microfilariae loads in the skin and eye after nodulectomy in Ecuadorian onchocerciasis. *Trop Med Parasitol.* 1987;38: 275.

32. Drugs for parasitic infections. *Med Lett.* 1988;30:15.

33. Rolland A, Rougemont A, Thylefors B. *Suramin in the Treatment of Onchocerciasis.* Geneva: World Health Organization; 1986.

34. Soboslay PT, Newland HS, White AT, et al. Ivermectin effect on microfilariae of *Onchocerca volvulus* after a single oral dose in humans. *Trop Med Parasitol.* 1987;38:8.

35. Kean BH, Sun T, Ellsworth RM. Loiasis. In: *Color Atlas/Text of Ophthalmic Parasitology.* New York: Igaku-Shoin; 1991.

36. Hawking F. The distribution of human filariasis throughout the world. Part III. *Africa Trop Dis Bull.* 1977;74:650.

37. Negesse Y, Lanoie LO, Neafie RC, et al. Loiasis: "calabar" swellings and involvement of deep organs. *Am J Trop Med Hyg.* 1985;34: 537.

38. Lee BYP, McMillan R. *Loa loa*: ocular filariasis in an African student in Missouri. *Ann Ophthalmol.* 1984;16:456.

39. Gendelman D, Blumberg R, Sadun A. Ocular *Loa loa* with cryoprobe extraction of subconjunctival worm. *Ophthalmology.* 1984;91: 300.

40. Choyce DP. Uveitis in tropical ophthalmology. *Trans Ophthalmology Soc UK.* 1976;96: 145.

41. Toussaint D, Danis P. Retinopathy in generalized *Loa-loa* filariasis. A clinicopathological study. *Arch Ophthalmol.* 1965;74:470.

42. Price DH, Hopps HC. Loiasis (the eye worm, loa worm). In: Marcial-Rojas RA, ed. *Pathology of Protozoal and Helminthic Diseases.* Baltimore: Williams & Wilkins, 1971:917.

43. Kean BH, Sun T, Ellsworth RM. Cysticercosis. In: *Color Atlas/Text of Ophthalmic Parasitology.* New York: Igaku-Shoin; 1991.

44. Beaver PC, Jung RC, Cupp EW. *Clinical Parasitology.* 9th ed. Philadelphia: Lea & Febiger; 1984:512.

45. Pawlowski Z, Schultz MD. Taeniasis and cysticercosis (*Taenia saginata*). *Adv Parasitol.* 1972;10:269.

46. Castillo M. Intestinal taeniasis. In: Marcial-Rojas RA, ed. *Pathology of Protozoal and Helminthic Diseases.* Baltimore: Williams & Wilkins; 1971:618.

47. Marquez-Monter H. Cysticercosis. In: Marcial-Rojas RA, ed. *Pathology of Protozoal and Helminthic Diseases.* Baltimore: Williams & Wilkins; 1971:592.

48. McCormick GF, Zee CA, Heiden J. Cysticercosis cerebri: review of 127 cases. *Arch Neurol (Chicago).* 1982;39:534.

49. Topilow HW, Yimoyines DI, Freeman HM, et al. Bilateral multifocal intraocular cysticercosis. *Ophthalmology.* 1981;88:1166.

50. Kruger-Leite E, Jalkh AE, Quiroz H, et al. Intraocular cysticercosis. *Am J Ophthalmol.* 1985;99:252.

51. Messner KH, Kaminerer MD. Intraocular cysticercosis. *Arch Ophthalmol.* 1979;97:1103.

52. Guillory SL, Zinn KM. Intravitreal *Cysticercus cellulosae*: ultrasonographic and fluorescein angiographic features. *Bull NY Acad Med.* 1980;56:655.

53. Pearson RD, Guerrant RL. Praziquantel: a

major advance in anthelminthic therapy. *Ann Intern Med.* 1983;99:193.

54. Santos R, Chavarria M, Aquirre AE. Failure of medical treatment in two cases of intraocular cysticercosis. *Am J Ophthalmol.* 1984;97:249.

55. Kazacos KR, Vestre WA, Kazacos EA, et al. Diffuse unilateral subacute neuroretinitis syndrome: a probable cause. *Arch Ophthalmol.* 1984;102:967.

56. Kazacos KR, Raymond LA, Kazacos EA, et al. The raccoon ascarid: a probable cause of human ocular larva migrans. *Ophthalmology.* 1985;92:1735.

57. Kazacos KR, Boyce WM. *Baylisascaris* larva migrans. *J Am Med Vet Assoc.* 1989;195:894.

58. Kazacos KR, Vestre WA, Kazacos EA. Raccoon ascarid larvae (*Baylisascaris procyonis*) as a cause of ocular larva migrans. *Invest Ophthalmol Vis Sci.* 1984;25:1177.

59. Goldberg MA, Kazacos KR, Boyce WM, et al. Diffuse unilateral subacute neuroretinitis. *Ophthalmology.* 1993;100:1695.

60. Gass JDM, Scelfo R. Diffuse unilateral subacute neuroretinitis. *J Roy Soc Med.* 1978;71:95.

61. Gass JDM, Braunstein RA. Further observations concerning the diffuse unilateral subacute neuroretinitis syndrome. *Arch Ophthalmol.* 1983;101:1689.

62. Raymond LA, Gutierrez Y, Strong LE, et al. Living retinal nematode destroyed by photocoagulation. *Ophthalmology.* 1978;85:944.

63. Gass JDM, Callanan DG, Bowman B. Oral therapy in diffuse unilateral subacute neuroretinitis. *Arch Ophthalmol.* 1992;110:675.

13
Insect Disease

Ophthalmomyiasis

Ophthalmomyiasis is an ocular disorder caused by the maggot of the botfly.

Etiology

The larval stage of the insect botfly (of the order Diptera) is responsible for ophthalmomyiasis. Certain botflies are obligatory parasites and require living tissue to develop. Other larvae are facultative or accidental ocular parasites.[1-3]

Epidemiology

The sheep nasal botfly (*Oestrus ovis*) is the most common cause of external ophthalmomyiasis.[4-6] Ophthalmomyiasis interna is thought to be due to cattle botfly maggots.[7-9] Orbital disease is secondary to maggots from the Calliphoridae family.[3,10,11] The eye can be involved in 5% of cases of myiasis.[1]

Pathogenesis

The fly eggs are laid in the mucous membrane of the nose and conjunctival cul-de-sac. The maggot bores through the conjunctiva and can gain access internally by penetrating the cornea/sclera. There is minimal inflammation while the maggot is alive. Inflammation occurs with the death of the organism.

Clinical Presentation

In external disease, maggots will be noted in the conjunctival cul-de-sac. Eyelid twitching and motion will be noted.[1] In internal ophthalmomyiasis, patients may be asymptomatic or complain of a unilateral decrease in visual acuity.[12,13] On examination a single motile maggot may be found in the anterior chamber, vitreous cavity, or subretinal space. When it is in the subretinal space, the maggot leaves behind trails or "railroad tracks" throughout the fundus.[13] There may be a mild inflammation in the anterior chamber and vitreous.[7,8]

Diagnosis

The diagnosis can be made on clinical grounds by observing the motile larva.

Differential Diagnosis

The clinical picture is pathognomonic.

Treatment

The treatment of choice is surgical removal of the maggot from the conjunctiva, vitreous, or subretinal spaces.[1] Corticosteroids can be used to treat intraocular inflammation. Photocoagulation can treat subretinal larvae but may result in severe post-laser inflammation.[14]

Prognosis

The prognosis is variable.

References

1. Kean BH, Sun T, Ellsworth RM. Ophthalmomyiasis. In: Kean BH, Sun T, Ellsworth RM, eds. *Color Atlas/Text of Ophthalmic Parasitology*. New York: Igaku-Shoin; 1991:105.
2. Beaver PC, Jung RC, Cupp EW. *Clinical Parasitology*. 9th ed. Philadelphia: Lea & Febiger; 1984:680.
3. Kersten RC, Showkrey NM, Tabbara KF. Orbital myiasis. *Ophthalmology*. 1986;93:1228.
4. Cameron JA, Shoukrey NM, Al-Garni AA. Conjunctival ophthalmomyiasis caused by the sheep nasal botfly *(Oestrus ovis)*. *Am J Ophthalmol*. 1991;112:331.
5. Harvey JT. Sheep botfly: ophthalmomyiasis externa. *Can J Ophthalmol*. 1986;21:92.
6. Reingold WJ, Robin JB, Leipa D, et al. *Oestrus ovis* ophthalmomyiasis externa. *Am J Ophthalmol*. 1984;97:7.
7. Mason GI. Bilateral ophthalmomyiasis interna. *Am J Ophthalmol*. 1981;91:65.
8. Edwards K, Meredith TA, Hagler WS, et al. Ophthalmomyiasis. *Am J Ophthalmol*. 1984;97:605.
9. Vine A, Schatz H. Bilateral posterior interior ophthalmomyiasis. *Ann Ophthalmol*. 1981;13:1041.
10. Mathur SP, Makhija JM. Invasion of the orbit by maggots. *Br J Ophthalmol*. 1967;51:406.
11. Wood TR, Slight JR. Bilateral orbital myiasis. Report of a case. *Arch Ophthalmol*. 1970;84:692.
12. Anderson WB. Ophthalmomyiasis interna: case report and review of the literature. *Trans Am Acad Ophthalmol Otolaryngol*. 1934;39:218.
13. Gass JDM, Lewis RA. Subretinal tracks in ophthalmomyiasis. *Arch Ophthalmol*. 1976;94:1500.
14. Forman AR, Cruess AF, Benson WE. Ophthalmomyiasis treated by argon-laser photocoagulation. *Retina*. 1984;4:163.

14
Animal Disease

Although animals are not considered infections, ocular inflammatory diseases caused by animal hairs are presented in this section. In a broad sense, caterpillar and tarantula hair–associated ocular inflammation is a result of an external macroorganism "infection."

Ophthalmia Nodosa

Ophthalmia nodosa is a term used to describe the harmful effects of insect cilia, animal hairs, and vegetable filaments on the eye.[1-4]

Etiology

Tarantula and caterpillar hairs are capable of embedding within the skin, sclera, cornea, and vitreous.[1-4] The hairs are barbed and can migrate through ocular tissues.

Epidemiology

Tarantula are sold as pets throughout the United States. Rose-haired tarantulas from Texas are popular varieties because of their more even, docile temperament.

Pathogenesis

Tarantulas broadcast barbed hairs by the rhythmic beating of the hind legs against their abdomen as a defense mechanism.[2-4] These hairs can embed and migrate through tissues, causing skin irritation and ophthalmia nodosa.

Clinical Presentation

The ocular surface can receive the barbed hairs from the abdomen of a tarantula.[2-4] In the sclera they cause nodular episcleritis and scleritis. In the cornea they cause a multifocal keratitis. On biomicroscopy, the hairs can be noted at various levels of the cornea. When they migrate through the cornea or sclera, they can be seen on the endothelium, in the lens, and within the vitreous. They often develop granulomatous and characteristically oval or linear precipitates around the hairs (Fig. 14.1A). Oval "snowballs" and "snowmen" can be noted in the vitreous. A multifocal punctate chorioretinitis can be noted at the entrance site in the pars plana and retina anterior to the equator (Fig. 14.1B).

Diagnosis

The diagnosis can be made by noting the fine clear hairs in the cornea and the distinctive oval keratitic precipitates (KP) and vitreous snowmen.[2-4] A history of exposure to a tarantula supports the clinical diagnosis.

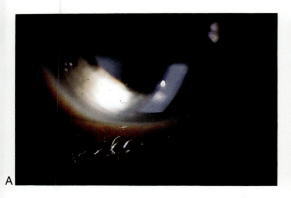

A

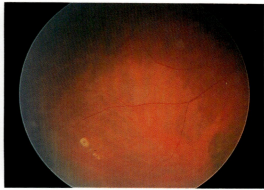

B

Figure 14.1. Ophthalmia nodosa. A: Oval granulomatous KPs surround tarantula hairs entering the anterior chamber. Three KPs can be seen on the nasal cornea, and a large KP can be noted in an area with overlying focal keratitis. The patient presented with a nodular scleritis. **B:** Dilated fundus examination demonstrated multifocal chorioretinal scars with hyperpigmented centers. Vitreous "snowmen" could be seen surrounding the hairs in the inferior vitreous base.

Differential Diagnosis

Filaments from vegetable matter can cause ophthalmia nodosa.

Treatment

Treatment begins with the recommendation that the patient avoid the offending animal. Tarantula hairs can be removed when they protrude from the eyelid or the cornea. Deeper hairs can be left alone and observed. The keratitis, KP, and vitreous inflammation can be treated with topical corticosteroids. Vitrectomy could be considered for hairs poised and approaching the macula to prevent macular lesions.

Prognosis

Prognosis is good and greater care in handling these animals, including eye protection, should be emphasized.

References

1. Stulting RD, Hooper RJ, Cavanagh HD. Ocular injury caused by tarantula hairs. *Am J Ophthalmol.* 1983;96:118.
2. Dean RC. Ophthalmia nodosa: a case report. *Ann Ophthalmol.* 1982;14:1177.
3. Hered RW, Spaulding AG, Sanitato JJ, Wander AH. Ophthalmia nodosa caused by tarantula hairs. *Ophthalmology.* 1988;95:166.
4. Rutzen AR, Weiss JS, Kachadoorian H. Tarantula hair ophthalmia nodosa. *Am J Ophthalmol.* 1992;116:381.

Ocular Inflammation Associated with Immunologic Disease

15
Type I Hypersensitivity

Most of the disorders that have a type I hypersensitivity reaction as the predominant pathophysiologic mechanism are inflammatory diseases of the ocular surface. The choroid has a population of mast cells; however, their role in uveitis and retinal edema is not well defined.[1]

Hay Fever

Hay fever is a recurrent seasonal rhinitis and conjunctivitis.

Etiology

Air-borne allergens including tree and grass pollens and molds are the source of hay fever.[2]

Epidemiology

This seasonal disease is more common in temperate zones with abundant plant life. Desert and extremely cold climates do not support appropriate vegetation.

Pathogenesis

The allergen is inhaled and comes in contact with the mucous membranes of the eyes and upper respiratory tract. The resident mast cells of the mucosa have been primed with allergen-specific immunoglobulin E (IgE) on their surface.[2–5] With cross-linking of the surface IgE, these cells degranulate, releasing vasoactive amines including histamine, heparin, slow-reacting substance, and prostaglandins. These mediators cause itching, increased vascular permeability, and swelling.

Clinical Presentation

Rhinitis, mild itching, and sneezing are hallmarks of hay fever.[2,4] Clinical findings may be minimal. An acute, watery, mild papillary conjunctivitis and chemosis may be noted on biomicroscopic examination. The cornea is clear characteristically.

Diagnosis

Family history is often positive for hay fever.[2] The seasonal nature of the symptoms helps establish the diagnosis. Mucosal scraping can demonstrate eosinophils if the hay fever is chronic or severe.

Differential Diagnosis

Vernal and atopic keratoconjunctivitis can have similar clinical features. Chemical irritants may produce similar complaints but without significant itching.

Treatment

Efforts should be made to eliminate the allergen from the environment.[2,4] Topical vasoconstrictors can produce ocular comfort. Topical and oral antihistamines can help alleviate some of the symptoms. Topical corticosteroids are effective in controlling the disease, but have a high risk for abuse, and secondary complications of cataract and glaucoma can occur. Disodium cromoglycate (2%) is a safe, effective therapy for allergic ocular surface diseases.[6,7] This agent is a mast-cell membrane stabilizing drug and has been shown to help allergic rhinitis and asthma.[8,9] Lodoxamide (0.1%) is another mast-cell membrane stabilizing agent that has been shown to be effective in treating allergic keratoconjunctivitis.[10]

Prognosis

The visual prognosis is good.

Atopic Keratoconjunctivitis

Atopic keratoconjunctivitis (AKC) is a year-round allergic disease that involves the conjunctiva and cornea.

Etiology

The cause of AKC is not known.[2,11–13] The perennial allergens involved with atopy may be dust, mold spores, dander, cosmetics, and certain pollens.

Epidemiology

AKC is a year-round disorder that affects men more than women, with an age range of 29 to 47 years. Seventy percent of patients have a history of asthma, eczema, or concurrent hay fever; 5% to 10% of the population have atopic dermatitis.[2] The disease can last years but typically resolves by the age of 50 years.

Pathogenesis

Although there appears to be a predominant type I hypersensitivity reaction, other immune events may participate in the response.[2,12,14,15] Basophils, eosinophils, mast cells, and lymphocytes are all present in the tissues. A type IV delayed hypersensitivity may play a mediating role.

Clinical Presentation

Atopic dermatitis is usually present. The skin is often wrinkled and thickened.[11,12] When the eyelids are involved, the skin becomes indurated and may develop secondary staphylococcal infection. The tear film often has a thick, whitish discharge.[2,11,12] The conjunctiva is pale and superficial vessels are dilated. Limbal Trantas' dots and concretions are commonly found. The cornea may have superficial punctate keratitis, a fine pannus formation, subepithelial scarring, and ulcer formation. An anterior subcapsular cataract can develop in long-standing disease.[13]

Diagnosis

The history of perennial ocular symptoms and atopic dermatitis establishes the diagnosis. A family history of atopic disease is helpful. Patients may have elevated serum IgE and an eosinophilia.[12]

Differential Diagnosis

Hay fever is seasonal and mild and is not associated with conjunctival scarring or corneal involvement. Vernal keratoconjunctivitis is a seasonal disorder and does not involve the skin.

Treatment

Efforts to eliminate allergens from the environment can be helpful. Systemic antihistamine and topical vasoconstrictors can alleviate some of the symptoms. Oral terfenadine (60–120 mg two times a day) or astemizole (10 mg a day) have been used, with alleviation of ocular and systemic symptoms. Topical corticosteroids can be used in severe situations but may be abused. Cromolyn (2%–4%) and lodoxamide (0.1%) can stabilize mast cell degeneration and are effective topical agents in atopic disease.[10] Plasmapheresis has been used to control severe cases of atopic disease.[16]

Prognosis

The disease can last years. Corneal scaring can impair vision in patients with severe AKC.

Vernal Keratoconjunctivitis

Vernal keratoconjunctivitis (VKC) is a recurrent, seasonal allergic disorder.

Etiology

The exact etiology of VKC is not known.[2,17] Spring pollens are the primary allergen that cause VKC.[18]

Epidemiology

VKC has worldwide distribution and is more common in warmer climates. Patients with VKC often have a family history of atopic disease. The disease occurs most commonly in boys (2:1) and may last for 10 years.[2] Eighty percent of patients are younger than 14 years.[2]

Pathogenesis

VKC appears to have components of both type I and type IV hypersensitivity.[2,17] A basophilic cutaneous hypersensitivity reaction is found with eosinophils, basophils, mast cells, lymphocytes, and plasma cells.[19] The tears have increased IgE levels.[18]

Clinical Presentation

Itching is the hallmark of VKC.[2,17] Symptoms are severe and seasonal, occurring in

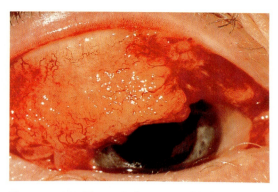

Figure 15.1. Type I hypersensitivity—vernal keratoconjunctivitis. Giant papillary conjunctivitis in a patient with active VKC.

the spring. The tears have a whitish ropy discharge. Giant papillary conjunctivitis is noted on the palpebral conjunctiva (Fig. 15.1). Trantas' dots are noted at the limbus. Occasionally, a "shield" ulcer occurs on the cornea.

Diagnosis

VKC is a clinical diagnosis.[2,17] Family history, severe seasonal itching, and the characteristic papillary conjunctivitis in young males establishes the diagnosis. Conjunctival scraping reveals eosinophils.

Differential Diagnosis

Hay fever and AKC may have similar presentations. Hay fever is seasonal but has mild itching and no corneal involvement.

Treatment

Efforts to eliminate allergens from the environment can be helpful. Patients often improve in cooler climates.[2] Cromolyn sodium and lodoxamide (0.1%) can prevent mast-cell degranulation and can help the symptoms of VKC.[10,20] In severe cases, brief courses of topical corticosteroids can be used with caution.[17] Topical steroids can be overused and increase the chances for cataract and glaucoma. Systemic antihistamines may help control some of the symptoms of VKC. Topical cyclosporine (2%) has been used in these patients, with improvement in the severity of ocular symptoms.[21]

Prognosis

VKC may last 10 years but typically "burns out" with age.

References

1. de Kozak Y, Sainte-Laudy J, Benveniste J, Faure J-P. Evidence for immediate hypersensitivity phenomena in experimental autoimmune uveoretinitis. *Eur J Immunol*. 1981;11: 612.
2. Allansmith MR, Abelson MB. Ocular allergies. In: Smolin G, Thoft RA, eds. *The Cornea: Scientific Foundations and Clinical Practice*. 2nd ed. Boston: Little, Brown; 1987.
3. Gell PGH, Coombs RRA, eds. *Clinical Aspects of Immunology*. Oxford: Blackwell; 1968.
4. Hogan MJ. Atopic keratoconjunctivitis. *Am J Ophthalmol*. 1953;36:937.
5. Blumenthal M, Casale T, Dockhorn R, et al. Efficacy and safety of nedocromil sodium ophthalmic solution in the treatment of seasonal allergic conjunctivitis. *Am J Ophthalmol*. 1992;113:56.
6. Friday GA, Biglan AW, Hiles DA, et al. Treatment of ragweed allergic conjunctivitis with cromolyn sodium 4% ophthalmic solution. *Am J Ophthalmol*. 1983;95:169.
7. Cox J. Disodium cromoglycate (FPL670) (Intal): a specific inhibitor of reaginic antigen-antibody mechanisms. *Nature*. 1967;216: 1329.
8. Bernstein IL, Siegel SC, Blanden ML, et al. A controlled study of cromolyn sodium sponsored by the drug committee of the American Academy of Allergy. *J Allergy Clin Immunol*. 1972;50:235.
9. Handleman NI, Friday GA, Schwartz HJ, et al. Cromolyn sodium nasal solution in the prophylactic treatment of pollen induced seasonal allergic rhinitis. *J Allergy Clin Immunol*. 1977;59:237.
10. Caldwell DR, Verin P, Hartwich-Young R, et al. Efficacy and safety of lodoxamide 0.1% vs cromolyn sodium 4% in patients with vernal keratoconjunctivitis. *Am J Ophthalmol*. 1992; 113:632.
11. Hogan MJ. Atopic keratoconjunctivitis. *Am J Ophthalmol*. 1953;50:937.
12. Foster CS, Calonge M. Atopic keratoconjunctivitis. *Ophthalmology*. 1990;97:992.
13. Beethan WP. Atopic cataract. *Arch Ophthalmol*. 1940;24:21.
14. Braude LS, Chandler JW. Atopic corneal disease. *Int Ophthalmol Clin*. 1984;24:145.
15. Rich LF, Hanifin JM. Ocular complications of atopic dermatitis and other eczemas. *Int Ophthalmol Clin*. 1985;25:61.
16. Aswad MI, Tauber J, Baum J. Plasmapheresis treatment in patients with severe atopic keratoconjunctivitis. *Ophthalmology*. 1988;95: 444.
17. Foster CS. Vernal keratoconjunctivitis. *Perspect Ophthalmol*. 1980;4:35.
18. Ballow M, Donshik PC, Mendelson L, et al. IgG specific antibodies to rye grass and ragweed pollen antigens in the tear secretions of patients with vernal conjunctivitis. *Am J Ophthalmol*. 1983;95:161.
19. Trocmé SD, Kephart GM, Bourne WM, et al. Eosinophil granule major basic protein deposition in corneal ulcers associated with vernal keratoconjunctivitis. *Am J Ophthalmol*. 1993;115:640.
20. Foster CS, Duncan J. Randomized clinical trial of topically administered cromolyn sodium for vernal keratoconjunctivitis. *Am J Ophthalmol*. 1980;90:175.
21. Bleik JH, Tabbara KF. Topical cyclosporine in vernal keratoconjunctivitis. *Ophthalmology*. 1991;98:1679.

16
Type II Hypersensitivity

In autoimmune diseases with a type II hypersensitivity mechanism, autoantibodies are directed against cell-associated antigens. Subsequent activation of complement and recruitment of leukocytes result in local tissue inflammation.

Cicatricial Pemphigoid

Cicatricial pemphigoid (CP) or ocular cicatricial pemphigoid (OCP) is a systemic autoimmune disorder that affects the mucous membranes of the body, including the eye.[1-4]

Etiology

The etiology is unknown. Immunologically active autoantibodies can be found in the basement membranes associated with mucosal epithelium.[1-4] Several antiglaucoma drugs (epinephrine, pilocarpine, and echothiophate) have been associated with OCP.[5,6]

Epidemiology

Human leukocyte antigen HLA-B12 has been found in 45% of patients with OCP.[7] Women are affected more than men by an approximate 2:1 ratio.[8,9] The disease is uncommon in persons under the age of 30 years, with an average age of 68 years.[8]

Pathogenesis

In CP, autoantibodies are directed against the basement membranes of conjunctival, buccal, nasal, esophageal, rectal, and vaginal mucosal membranes.[1-9] These antibodies can be of any class (IgG, IgM, IgD, IgA, IgE) and are immunologically active. Activation of complement and the local deposition of immunoreactants (C3, C4, fibrinogen) result in the recruitment of polymorphonuclear neutrophils (PMN) and lymphocytes. Subepithelial bullae formation and subsequent scarring occur. There is a reduction of goblet cells and metaplasia of the mucosal epithelium, with parakeratosis and keratinization of the membranes.

In contrast to bullous pemphigoid, only 10% of patients have circulating antibasement membrane antibodies, and circulating antiepithelial antibodies are rare, suggesting local or regional antibody production.[4]

Clinical Presentation

The eye is involved in 70% of patients with CP. Nonscarring cutaneous lesions and bullae formation can be found in 25% of patients with ocular CP.

CP has several ocular staging systems.[2-4,8,9] It is important in any system to account for nonimmunologic, secondary, or reactive inflammation. Sicca, trichiasis, en-

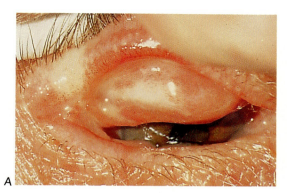
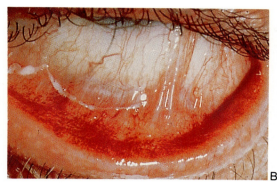

Figure 16.1. Type II hypersensitivity—cicatricial pemphigoid. A: An area of subepithelial fibrosis and conjunctival hyperemia in a patient with CP. **B:** Symblepharon formation can be noted in another patient with active CP.

tropion, keratinization of the lid margin, and secondary bacterial blepharitis may all cause ocular irritation and redness unrelated to an active immunologic disease. These factors should be addressed to minimize complications of OCP and to help ascertain true disease activity.

Ocular findings in stage I OCP include papillary conjunctivitis and linear subepithelial fibrosis[1,3] (Fig. 16.1A). This fibrosis can be observed most readily on the upper palpebral conjunctiva. A mucoid discharge and punctate staining of the epithelium can be seen with rose Bengal staining at this stage of the disease. Stage II OCP is characterized by progressive subepithelial scarring with conjunctival foreshortening, which can be best appreciated in the cul-de-sac areas. In stage III OCP, patients begin to develop symblepharon formation, often with entropion and progressive trichiasis (Fig. 16.1B). Corneal neovascularization may be prominent. Stage IV, or end-stage disease, is characterized by keratinization of the cornea and ankyloblepharon.

Diagnosis

The diagnosis can be made on clinical grounds.[1] Blood testing is not helpful. Some patients may have a positive antinuclear antibody (ANA) test and an increase

in circulation immune complexes. Conjunctival biopsy confirms the diagnosis and should be considered before instituting systemic chemotherapy.[1–4,10] Linear deposition of immunoglobulin, C3, C4, fibrinogen, and properdin factor B in the lamina lucida of the conjunctiva basement membrane can be found in 67% to 100% of patients. Immunohistologic studies should include assays to detect all classes of immunoglobulin including IgG, IgM, IgA, IgD, and IgE.

Differential Diagnosis

Chemical or thermal burns, Stevens-Johnson syndrome, Sjögren's syndrome, and trachoma may all have conjunctival scarring, corneal findings, and sicca.[1] Stevens-Johnson syndrome is characterized by an acute, explosive onset with marked systemic involvement.[11] Conjunctival biopsy in these patients does not demonstrate basement membrane deposition of antibodies at the basement membrane.

Treatment

The secondary sequela of OCP, including the sicca, trichiasis, entropion, and blepharitis, needs to be continually addressed. Artificial tears and ointments are helpful.[1,2]

Lash removal or ablation may be required for recurrent trichiasis. Entropion repair may be needed.[1]

The active, immunologic disease should be controlled by systemic immunosuppressive therapy. Palpebral and bulbar conjunctival hyperemia can be used to measure disease activity and is graded on a scale of 1 to 4. Oral dapsone (75–150 mg/day) can control the disease in many patients.[8,12] Pulses of oral prednisone or low-dose oral corticosteroids often are needed to gain initial control. Patients should be screened for G-6-PD (glucose-6-phosphate dehydrogenase) deficiency before initiating dapsone therapy and minimize hematologic complications.

Patients who fail to respond to dapsone or are intolerant to its side effects are candidates for second-generation immunosuppressive agents. Cyclophosphamide, azathioprine, and cyclosporin have all been used.[3,8,13–16] Cyclophosphamide has been used with the greatest success as reported in the literature. Under the direction of a chemotherapist, 1 to 2 mg/kg per day of cyclophosphamide should be administered initially. Response to therapy should include both elimination of conjunctival inflammation and halting conjunctival shrinkage. Careful follow-up for complications associated with these drugs is required because of the potential side effects including leukopenia, cystitis, and pulmonary fibrosis. One third of patients achieve remission without need for immunosuppression.[13] Relapses may occur in 22% of patients.[13]

Prognosis

CP has a variable clinical course. Management of the ocular complications is often the most challenging aspect of CP. Untreated patients may progress to blindness from severe ocular surface disease. With therapy, the active immunologic disease can often be halted with better visual prognosis. Advances in keratoprosthesis may allow some visual rehabilitation for end-stage disease.

Lens-Induced Uveitis

Lens-induced uveitis has also been called phacoantigenic uveitis, phacoallergic uveitis, and phacoanaphylactic endophthalmitis.[17,18]

Etiology

The lens has several autoantigens including alpha, beta, and gamma crystallins.[19] These antigens are normally enveloped within the basement membrane of the lens within the eye. The blood–eye barrier, unique anterior chamber–associated immune events, embryologic development of the immune system and lens give these antigens relative immunologic "privilege."[17] These "sequestered" lens proteins can be the target of an autoimmune response. Denatured lens proteins occurring with advanced cataracts may be less able to promote a true lens-induced uveitis.[20,21]

Epidemiology

Surgical or nonsurgical injury to the lens capsule exposes the lens proteins to the ocular immunologic milieu, which may lead to an autoimmune response.[17] Patients who have experienced trauma or who have undergone complicated cataract surgery may develop a true lens-induced uveitis. Sympathetic ophthalmia may also develop after ocular trauma, and 20% of these patients have histologic evidence for lens-induced uveitis.[22]

Pathogenesis

Much of the literature supports a primary role for autoantibodies in the generation of lens-induced uveitis.[17–19,23–25] When these autoantibodies are directed against lens epithelial cells, a type II hypersensitivity mechanism appears responsible for the inflammation. In animal models, lens-induced uveitis can be transferred by hyperimmune serum.[2] Antibodies directed against soluble lens proteins would support a type III hypersensitivity component as well. Other investigators have demonstrated a cell-mediated immune response in lens-induced uveitis.[23,26–28] Skin testing, lymphocyte proliferation assays, and limiting dilution assays demonstrate that T cells may be capable of responding to the autologous lens antigens. There is no evidence for a type I "phacoanaphylactic reaction."

Skin microorganisms such as *Propionibacterium acnes* may participate in the development of lens-induced uveitis by providing an exogenous "adjuvant" effect.[29–32] Microbial cultures are negative in true lens-induced uveitis and microorganisms are not seen on pathologic specimens. A zonal granulomatous reaction is noted around the lens fragments on histologic examination.[17,18] PMNs, macrophages, giant cells, and lymphocytes surround the lens material and lens basement membrane.

Clinical Presentation

Patients with lens-induced uveitis are typically healthy, with mild to severe unilateral anterior uveitis.[1,2,33–38] Early in the course, the disease may be nongranulomatous; as the disease becomes more chronic, the inflammation often becomes granulomatous. Lens-induced uveitis can begin within weeks of the injury. Mutton fat (KP), posterior synechiae, and glaucoma are common (see Figs. 2.3 and 2.10). There is relative sparing of the posterior segment. The choroid can be thickened in severe cases and in a recent pathologic review, 76% of cases had histologic evidence for choroidal inflammation.[2,39] Lens-induced uveitis has been described in eyes after phacoemulsification and with lens dislocation.[35–38]

Diagnosis

Diagnosis of patients with lens-induced uveitis can be challenging.[17,18] A history of insult to the lens occurring with a unilat-

eral, granulomatous anterior uveitis suggests the diagnosis. Aqueous and vitreous aspirate yield negative cultures and demonstrate amorphous lens material surrounded by macrophages, PMN, and lymphocytes.[17,18] Skin testing, lymphocyte proliferation studies, and assays to determine the presence of circulating antilens antibodies have limited availability. Ultrasound may reveal retained lens fragments and choroidal thickening in the involved eye.

Differential Diagnosis

The differential diagnosis includes traumatic uveitis, chronic anaerobic endophthalmitis, fungal endophthalmitis, sympathetic ophthalmia, and phacolytic glaucoma.[17,18] Traumatic inflammation resolves spontaneously and is not typically granulomatous. Chronic anaerobic endophthalmitis from *Propionibacterium* species can closely resemble lens-induced uveitis. Both produce a chronic, smoldering anterior uveitis after surgical or nonsurgical trauma. Often, diagnostic aqueous and vitreous biopsy and cultures are required to differentiate these two conditions. Sympathetic ophthalmia is a bilateral disease that commonly involves the posterior uveal tract. Phacolytic glaucoma is associated with elevated intraocular pressures and macrophages containing lens material.

Treatment

Although corticosteroids can moderate the uveitis, lens-induced uveitis is often chronic. Surgical removal of all lens antigen and capsule is usually required.[31,35] Vitrectomy techniques are often helpful in removing all lens material from these eyes. Perioperative control of the uveitis may require intraocular dexamethasone (400 μg/0.1 ml), sub-Tenon's triamcinolone (40 mg/1 ml), and oral prednisone (1 mg/kg per day). The ocular fluids should undergo culture (aerobic, anaerobic, and fungal) and cytologic study to help confirm the diagnosis. If a chronic anaerobic endophthalmitis is suspected, intraocular antibiotics can be given at the time of surgery (vancomycin, 1 mg/0.1 ml).

Prognosis

Untreated, the clinical course may be prolonged. With removal of lens material and appropriate anti-inflammatory therapy, intraocular inflammation typically resolves. Chronic cystoid macular edema may compromise final visual acuity.

References

1. Fujikawa LS, Nussenblatt RB. The cornea and dermatologic disorders. In Smolin G, Thoft RA, eds. *The Cornea*. 2nd ed. Boston: Little, Brown; 1987:367.
2. Mondino BJ, Brown SI. Ocular cicatricial pemphigoid. *Ophthalmology*. 1981;88:95.
3. Foster CS, Wilson LA, Ekins MB. Immunosuppressive therapy for progressive ocular cicatricial pemphigoid. *Ophthalmology*. 1982;89:340.
4. Mondino BJ. Cicatricial pemphigoid and erythema multiforme. *Ophthalmology*. 1990;97:939.
5. Hirst LW, Werblin T, Novak M. Drug-induced cicatrizing conjunctivitis simulating ocular pemphigoid. *Cornea*. 1982;1:121.
6. Hirst LW, Werblin T, Novak M, et al. Drug-induced cicatrizing conjunctivitis simulating ocular pemphigoid. *Cornea*. 1982;1:121.
7. Mondino BJ, Brown SI, Rabin BS. HLA antigens in ocular cicatricial pemphigoid. *Arch Ophthalmol*. 1979;97:479.
8. Foster CS. Cicatricial pemphigoid. *Trans Am Ophthalmol Soc*. 1986;84:95.
9. Mondino BJ, Brown SI. Ocular cicatricial pemphigoid. *Ophthalmology*. 1981;88:95.
10. Mondino BJ, Ross AN, Rabin BS, Brown SI. Autoimmune phenomena in ocular cicatricial pemphigoid. *Am J Ophthalmol*. 1977;83:443.
11. Chan LS, Soong HK, Foster CS, et al. Ocular cicatricial pemphigoid occurring as a sequela of Stevens-Johnson syndrome. *JAMA*. 1991;266:1543.
12. Rogers RS, Seehafer JR, Perry HO. Treatment of cicatricial (benign mucous membrane) pemphigoid with dapsone. *J Am Acad Dermatol*. 1982;6:215.
13. Neumann R, Tauber J, Foster CS. Remission and recurrence after withdrawal of therapy for ocular cicatricial pemphigoid. *Ophthalmology*. 1991;98:858.
14. Mondino BJ, Brown SI. Immunosuppressive therapy in ocular cicatricial pemphigoid. *Am J Ophthalmol*. 1983;96:453.
15. Dave VK, Vickers CFH. Azathioprine in the treatment of mucocutaneous pemphigoid. *Br J Dermatol*. 1974;90:183.
16. Brody HJ, Pirozzi DJ. Benign mucous membrane pemphigoid: response to therapy with cyclophosphamide. *Arch Dermatol*. 1977;113:1598.
17. Müller-Hermelink HK, Daus W. Recent topics in the pathology of uveitis. In: Kraus-Mackiw E, O'Connor RG, eds. *Uveitis: Pathophysiology and Therapy*. 2nd rev. ed. New York: Thieme Medical Publishers; 1986:155.
18. Thach AB, Marak GE Jr, McLean IW, Green WR. Phacoanaphylactic endophthalmitis: a clinicopathologic review. *Int Ophthalmol*. 1991;15:271.
19. Sandberg HO, Closs O. The humoral immune response to alpha, beta and gamma crystallins of the human lens. *Scand J Immunol*. 1979;10:549.
20. Fisher RF. The changes with age in the biophysical properties of the capsule of the human crystalline lens in relation to cataract. *Interdiscipl Topics Gerontol*. 1978;13:131.
21. Maraini G, Mangili R. Differences in proteins and in the water balance of the lens in nuclear and cortical types of senile cataract. In: *The Human Lens in Relation to Cataract*. Ciba Foundation Symposium 19. Amsterdam: Elsevier; 1973:79.
22. Allen JC. Sympathetic uveitis and phacoanaphylaxis. *Am J Ophthalmol*. 1967;63:281.
23. Gery I, Nussenblatt R, BenEzra D. Dissociation between humoral and cellular immune response to lens antigens. *Invest Ophthalmol Vis Sci*. 1981;20:32.
24. Nissen SH, Andersen P, Andersen HMK. Antibodies to lens antigens in cataract and after cataract surgery. *Br J Ophthalmol*. 1981;65:63.
25. Deschenes J, Baines M, Anteka A. Investigation of antilens antibodies in uveitis and cat-

aract. In: *ARVO Abstracts*. St. Louis: Mosby–Year Book; 1989:83.

26. Simpson W, Wild G, Figg K, Milford-Ward A. Human T-cell mediated response to homologous lens antigen. *Exp Eye Res*. 1989;48: 49.

27. Marak GE, Rao NA. Lens protein binding lymphocytes. *Ophthalmic Res*. 1983;15:6.

28. Hammer H, Olah M. Cellular hypersensitivity to lenticular protein in lens-induced uveitis. *Albrecht Von Graefes Arch Klin Exp Ophthalmol*. 1974;192:339.

29. Roussel TJ, Culbertson WW, Jaffee NS. Chronic postoperative endophthalmitis associated with *Propionibacterium acne*. *Arch Ophthalmol*. 1987;105:1119.

30. Meisler DM, Palestine AG, Vastine DW, et al. Chronic *Propionibacterium* endophthalmitis after extracapsular cataract extraction and intraocular lens implantation. *Am J Ophthalmol*. 1986;102:733.

31. Cusumano A, Busin M, Spitznas M. Is chronic intraocular inflammation after lens implantation of bacterial origin? *Ophthalmology*. 1991;98:1703.

32. Smith RE. Inflammation after cataract surgery. *Am J Ophthalmol*. 1986;102:788.

33. Wirostko E, Spalter HF. Lens-induced uveitis. *Arch Ophthalmol*. 1967;78:1.

34. Allen JC, de Venecia GB. Lens-induced uveitis in the opposite untraumatized eye. *Ann Ophthalmol*. 1970; **[vol 6]**:19.

35. Wohl L, Lucier AC, Kline OR Jr, Galman BD. Pseudophakic phacoanaphylactic endophthalmitis. *Ophthalmic Surg*. 1986;17:234.

36. Smith RE, Weiner P. Unusual presentation of phacoanaphylaxis following phacoemulsification. *Ophthalmic Surg*. 1976;7:65.

37. Belfort R Jr, Nussenblatt RB, Lottemberg C, et al. Spontaneous lens subluxation in uveitis. *Am J Ophthalmol*. 1990;110:714.

38. Croxatto JO, Lombardi A, Malbran ES. Inflamed eye in Marfan's syndrome with posteriorly luxated lens. *Ophthalmologica*. 1986; 193:23.

39. Hodes BL, Stern G. Phacoanaphylactic endophthalmitis: echographic diagnosis of phacoanaphylactic endophthalmitis. *Ophthalmic Surg*. 1976;7:60.

17
Type III Hypersensitivity

This section describes collagen vascular diseases with evidence for a type III hypersensitivity component. Other immunologic events and mechanisms may be participating in the pathogenesis of this group of diseases as well. These disorders are typically multisystemic with protean manifestations affecting the joints, muscles, bursae, and tendons. Ocular inflammation is common and is often considered a major diagnostic criterion for establishing a clinical diagnosis in several of these disorders (Table 17.1).[1]

To appreciate the significance of ocular involvement in the rheumatic diseases, one must first have an accurate understanding of connective tissue. Connective tissue and structures are the matrix that support individual cells, tissues, and organs. This ground substance is produced by specialized connective tissue cells that secrete various fibers (collagen, reticulin, and elastin) as well as a group of mucopolysaccharides called proteoglycans.[2] Hyaluronic acid, chondroitin sulfate, dermatan sulfate, keratan sulfate, and heparin sulfate comprise the common polysaccharides found in the connective tissue proteoglycans.[3]

Collagen fibers can be subdivided further by their polypeptide structure into six types (collagen types I–VI).[4] Each tissue and organ maintains a distinct connective tissue environment by varying these individual components, thereby affecting optimal structure and function. In rheumatologic diseases, inflammation of these supportive structures and milieu results in tissue and organ dysfunction.

The eye, perhaps more than any other organ, maintains a unique connective tissue environment. In the cornea, keratocytes secrete both type II and type IV collagen, as well as chondroitin and keratan sulfate.[2,5] This connective tissue combination results in strong tissue that becomes transparent as a result of unique lamellar fiber orientation and active endothelial cell dehydration. Hyalocytes in the vitreous produce hyaluronic acid and type II collagen, which forms a clear gel that allows transmission of light and provides support for the globe and retina.[2,6] The retina and choroid possess connective tissue and a complex vascular system comprised of type III and type IV collagen.[1] These circulations are critical for retinal function and general nutrition of the eye. Each of these ocular tissues performs critical functions in the visual system and is exquisitely sensitive to inflammation.

Separate connective tissues and structures within the eye can become inflamed in the various rheumatic diseases. Wegener's granulomatosis, rheumatoid arthritis, and polyarteritis nodosa can affect the cornea and produce peripheral ulcerative keratopathy. Reiter's syndrome is defined by the triad of urethritis, arthritis, and inflammation of the conjunctiva and iris. Juvenile rheumatoid arthritis (JRA) commonly pro-

Table 17.1. Collagen vascular diseases with ocular involvement.

Diffuse connective tissue diseases
Rheumatoid arthritis
Juvenile rheumatoid arthritis
Systemic lupus erythematosus
Progressive systemic sclerosis
Polymyositis/dermatomyositis
Necrotizing vasculitis and other vasculopathies
   Polyarteritis nodosa group
      Classic polyarteritis nodosa
      Churg-Strauss syndrome
      Cogan's syndrome
   Wegener's granulomatosis
   Temporal arteritis
   Behçet's disease
Sjögren's syndrome
Relapsing polychondritis

Arthritis associated with spondylitis (HLA–B27–associated)
Ankylosing spondylitis
Reiter's syndrome
Psoriatic arthritis
Arthritis associated with chronic inflammatory bowel
   disease (Crohn's disease, ulcerative colitis)

Miscellaneous
Erythema multiforme

duces a chronic iridocyclitis. Ankylosing spondylitis, Reiter's syndrome, psoriatic arthritis, and the chronic inflammatory bowel diseases produce an acute inflammation of the iris and ciliary body. It is important, therefore, to evaluate all patients who present with ocular inflammation or uveitis for symptoms and signs of an underlying connective tissue disease.

Rheumatic diseases often present in the eye before the onset of significant systemic involvement. The eye may even be the primary target of several diseases such as Behçet's disease, Reiter's syndrome, and ankylosing spondylitis. The importance of performing a careful review of systems and physical examination cannot be underestimated. Particular attention should be paid to the skin, joints, central nervous system (CNS), lungs, gastrointestinal (GI) tract, and kidneys. Involvement of these systems can help the ophthalmologist determine that an underlying collagen vascu-

lar disease is the etiology for the ocular inflammation. For example, iritis in a patient complaining of large-joint arthritis could represent JRA, systemic lupus erythematosus (SLE), Wegener's granulomatosis, or Behçet's disease. Oral ulcers, malaise, skin rash, and uveitis may be found in SLE, Behçet's disease, and sarcoidosis. Genital/urethral pain and uveitis may represent Behçet's disease, polyarteritis nodosa, or Reiter's syndrome.

Laboratory evaluation and consultation with an internist/rheumatologist can help confirm the presence of a collagen vascular disease and result in diagnosis and the initiation of proper systemic therapy. Local ocular therapy in rheumatic disorders without attention to the underlying systemic process universally results in suboptimal control of the ocular inflammation and risks potentially life-threatening complications of uncontrolled systemic disease.

Ankylosing Spondylitis

Ankylosing spondylitis (AS), or Marie-Strümpell disease, is a systemic collagen vascular disease associated with spondylitis, arthritis, and uveitis.[7]

Etiology

The etiology of AS is unknown. It has a strong association with human leukocyte antigen HLA-B27; 90% to 100% percent of AS patients have this tissue type, which is present in approximately 5% to 14% of Americans.[7–10] The disease has been associated with *Klebsiella* and chlamydial infections.[11]

Epidemiology

Clinical disease typically occurs in young men between the ages of 20 and 30 years.[7] About 1% of the male population is affected and 20% of those with HLA-B27 haplotype develop AS.[7,12] The disease is often silent in women and can be under-diagnosed. Women have less spinal involvement and more peripheral disease.[13] Several studies have associated HLA-B27 haplotype with the development of idiopathic, acute, anterior uveitis (50–100%) alone.[14–16]

Pathogenesis

Ankylosing spondylitis causes a bilateral, chronic symmetric arthritis in the lumbosacral spine and sacroiliac joint. The primary site of inflammation is at the insertion of ligaments and capsules into bone (enthesopathy). This accounts for the clinical presentation, including inflammation of the Achilles tendon and vertebra. In the eye it causes a unilateral, alternating, acute, nongranulomatous inflammation.

Clinical Presentation

Patients with AS may complain of low back pain and stiffness, which worsens with inactivity and is frequently troublesome at night.[7,12,13] The onset is insidious. It is not unusual for young patients to deny or minimize the nature and extent of the low back pain. About half of patients are relatively asymptomatic (50%). Extraspinal involvement includes Achilles tendonitis and plantar fasciitis.

Patients with AS develop sudden onset of ocular pain, redness, and photophobia.[7,17] Vision is typically good. On biomicroscopic examination, a limbal hyperemia, fine keratic precipitates (KP), posterior synechiae, and a prominent cellular reaction with marked flare and fibrin can be seen. The cellular response can be severe enough to cause hypopyon. The disease is typically unilateral but is recurrent and can be alternating.[18] Secondary glaucoma and cataract are not uncommon. The posterior segment is not typically involved. Cystoid macular edema (CME) can occur with prolonged or severe cases of anterior uveitis. The macular edema responds to therapies that address the anterior uveitis.

Diagnosis

The presence of a recurrent, alternating, nongranulomatous, acute iridocyclitis in a young man with lower back pain is suggestive of the diagnosis; however, women should not be overlooked. Sacroiliac and lumbar spine films may verify the diagnosis. A bilateral and symmetric sclerosis or fusion can be noted. HLA typing can be performed for B27 tissue antigen.[7,17] Bone scanning or magnetic resonance imaging (MRI) may assist in the diagnosis if plain films are normal.

Differential Diagnosis

Reiter's syndrome, Crohn's disease, and psoriatic arthritis are other HLA-B27–associated collagen vascular diseases that can have recurrent, acute, nongranulomatous iridocyclitis and sacroiliitis. Some patients have features of several of these HLA-B27–associated diseases simultaneously.

Treatment

Rheumatologic consultation should be advised to assist with care for the potentially crippling arthritis.[7] Physical therapy, extension exercises and nonsteroidal anti-inflammatory drugs (NSAIDs) can help prevent complications of this disease. Indomethacin may be particularly efficacious.[7]

Iridocyclitis can be severe and may last several weeks (4–12 weeks). At the first sign of inflammation, the patient should initiate aggressive topical corticosteroid treatment. One drop every hour, or in severe cases 3 drops an hour, should be started at the onset. Homatropine (5%) or scopolamine (0.25%) should be prescribed for ciliary spasm and to break posterior synechiae. If treatment is delayed, it can become difficult to achieve control with drops alone. Periocular injection of triamcinolone (40 mg/1 ml) can be given in resistant cases. Oral prednisone can be used for severe attacks.[17]

Patients who experience frequent recurrent attacks should receive a maintenance course of NSAIDs (indomethacin, 75 mg SR PO BID) to slow the frequency of the attacks.[18] In some patients, the ocular inflammation becomes chronic. Weekly, low-dose methotrexate (5–15 mg/week in divided doses) can help moderate disease progression. In severe cases, pars plana lensectomy and vitrectomy can be performed in eyes with recurrent inflammation, cataract, vitreous opacification, and medically unresponsive CME.[19]

Prognosis

The prognosis is generally good for this form of acute uveitis. Unlike some chronic forms of uveitis, the symptoms are severe enough to bring the patient into therapy. Attacks are relatively short and can usually be controlled. In recalcitrant cases, cataract, glaucoma, and macular edema may limit visual acuity. Spinal complications can be minimized with proper medical attention.

Behçet's Disease

Behçet's disease is a systemic necrotizing vasculitis with protean manifestations. It was first described by a Turkish physician in 1937.[20]

Etiology

The etiology is unknown but is thought to have a strong autoimmune component. Several HLA associations have been established in other countries, but have not proved useful in the United States.[20–22] HLA-B5, HLA-B51 (ocular), HLA-B12 (oral and skin), and HLA-B27 (joint) have all been associated with certain forms of Behçet's disease. English walnuts appear to stimulate lymphocytes in patients with Behçet's disease and have been anecdotically associated with disease recurrences.[23]

Epidemiology

Behçet's disease has worldwide distribution, but is much more common in the Orient and Middle East.[24] In Japan, Behçet's disease has accounted for as much as 20% of all cases of uveitis. In the United States, the disease is found equally in men and women and affects the 20- to 40-year-old age group.[25,26]

Pathogenesis

Behçet's vasculitis involves small to medium-sized vessels. A perivascular infiltrate with polymorphonuclear neutrophils and mononuclear cells can be found around the veins and arteries.[20,25] This infiltrate is often associated with vessel thrombosis, tissue hemorrhage, and necrosis. Immunoreactants, including immune complexes C3 and C4, and immunoglobulin deposition may be found in the vessel walls.[20,25,26]

Clinical Presentation

A 6- to 10-year prodrome with recurrent or chronic malaise, fever, and sore throat may be present.[27] The classic triad of recurrent aphthous oral ulcers (100%), genital ulcers (84%), and uveitis (66%) establishes the clinical diagnosis (Fig. 17.1). The oral ulcers are painful, may occur in clusters of two to five lesions, and may precede other findings for years. They can occur anywhere within the mouth and gums. The borders are regular and not "heaped up." Genital lesions may be asymptomatic or quite evident. With healing a scar may remain in the area of prior ulceration. Cutaneous vasculitis and erythema nodosum (66%) are also considered major criteria. Arthritis (66%) and meningoencephalitis (22%) are also common.[20,25–28] The gastrointestinal (GI), renal, pulmonary, and cardiovascular systems may be involved and are considered "minor" findings in this syndrome.

The eye may be the first and/or pre-

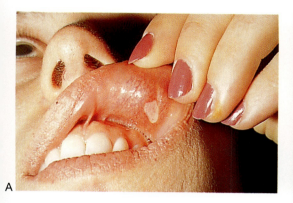
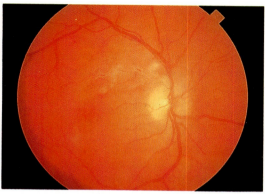

Figure 17.1. Type III hypersensitivity—Behçet's disease. A: Aphthous oral ulcer in a patient with Behçet's disease. B: Fundus photograph of the same patient showing vitritis, occlusive retinal arteriolitis with intraretinal hemorrhage, and cotton-wool spots. The optic disc is edematous.

dominant organ involved in Behçet's disease.[25–28] More characteristically, uveitis follows the other systemic findings by 1 to 3 years. Systemic and ocular symptoms typically wax and wane. Patients often present with an acute loss of vision associated with a bilateral (80%) uveitis.[25] The ocular inflammation may be severe and relapsing. A nongranulomatous iridocyclitis with hypopyon, posterior synechiae, and hyphema are common (see Fig. 2.18). On fundus examination, there may be a severe vitritis, disc edema, and attenuation of the arterioles.[26] A serious finding in Behçet's disease is the presence of an occlusive retinal vasculitis with surrounding intraretinal hemorrhage and retinal edema (Fig. 17.1B). CME, cataract, glaucoma, and retinal detachment can occur as a secondary complication of the uveitis and retinal vasculitis.[26]

Diagnosis

The diagnosis is based on clinical findings. There are several systems for the clinical diagnosis of Behçet's. The Japanese system divides Behçet's disease into complete, incomplete, suspect, and possible Behçet's disease[29] (Table 17.2).

Table 17.2. Diagnostic criteria for Behçet's disease: Japanese system.

Complete: Four major symptoms (oral ulcers, uveitis, genital ulcers, skin lesions)
Incomplete: Three major symptoms or uveitis with one major symptom
Suspect: Two nonocular major symptoms
Possible: One major symptom

The complete form consists of oral ulcers, genital ulcers, uveitis, and nonulcerative skin lesions. The presence of other minor findings such as erythema nodosa and phlebitis associated with the multisystemic involvement can assist in the diagnosis. Laboratory testing may help by demonstrating an elevated erythrocyte sedimentation rate (ESR), C-reactive protein, immune complexes, and a positive antinuclear antibody (ANA) test.

HLA typing can also be helpful in diagnosing incomplete forms of Behçet's disease. Properdin factor B, serum lysozyme, and alpha-1 acid glycoprotein are also elevated in Behçet's disease.[30] Pathergy and dermatographism, although much extolled, have not proved to be sensitive tests for Behçet's disease in the United States. Fluorescein angiography can be used to help document the ischemic retinal vasculitis and follow response to therapy.[28] CME and disc edema often result from the chronic inflammation. Choroidal vessels may be involved and demonstrate delayed filling or localized choroidal infarction.

Differential Diagnosis

Reiter's syndrome can be associated with acute anterior uveitis, oral ulcers, sacroiliitis and arthritis, and urethritis. The uveitis is recurrent and unilateral and is not associated with retinal vasculitis. Patients with sarcoidosis can develop oral ulcers, large joint arthralgias, and chronic uveitis with retinal vasculitis. Sarcoidosis is associated with hilar adenopathy, systemic anergy, and elevated serum angiotensin-converting enzyme (ACE) and lysozyme levels.

Treatment

Treatment of Behçet's disease is characteristically challenging.[20,26-28] Patients may experience multiple relapses and the disease may persist for many years. Explosive exacerbations may develop after periods of relative inactivity or remission. Mild forms may be controlled initially with prednisone and colchicine (0.6 mg orally, twice a day).[31] In most cases, Behçet's disease requires more aggressive immunosuppressive therapy. Periocular and oral corticosteroids can assist in controlling severe, acute episodes of ocular inflammation. Dapsone, 50 to 100 mg a day, and thalidomide have also been used to treat manifestations of Behçet's disease.

Chlorambucil (0.1–0.15 mg/kg per day) or cyclophosphamide (1–2 mg/kg per day) has been the mainstay of therapy.[32] Cyclophosphamide may be associated with fewer and more predictable systemic side effects and has been used to treat Behçet's disease in the United States.[26,33] Cyclosporine-A (4 mg/kg per day) also has recently proved effective in controlling this disease and has

become the treatment of choice at some centers.[32–37] Therapy may be required for several years. Careful monitoring for side effects and complications of immunosuppressive therapy is required.

Prognosis

Even with treatment, up to 74% of patients lose useful visual acuity secondary to retinal vasculitis (see Fig. 2.29). Early treatment with immunosuppressive agents may improve the visual prognosis.[38] When the CNS is involved, Behçet's disease can be fatal in up to 40% of patients.

Chürg-Strauss Syndrome

See under polyarteritis nodosa group of necrotizing vasculopathies (p. 213).

Cogan's Syndrome

See under polyarteritis nodosa group of necrotizing vasculopathies (p. 214).

Dermatomyositis and Polymyositis

Dermatomyositis and polymyositis (DM-PM) are a group of autoimmune diseases that cause an inflammatory, diffuse myopathy and dermatitis.[39]

Etiology

The etiology, as for other collagen vascular diseases, is unknown. An autoimmune mechanism is suspected. DM-PM can be associated with other collagen vascular diseases and malignancies, including rheumatoid arthritis, systemic lupus erythematosus, polyarteritis nodosa, and viral infections.[39]

Epidemiology

This rare disease (5 cases/1 million population) can affect both children and adults.[39]

Pathogenesis

These diseases may be mediated by microvascular damage from immune complex formation.[39-41] Patients with dermatomyositis exhibit lymphocytic infiltration, ischemic necrosis, and loss of capillary beds in the perifascicular region of the involved muscles.[39-41] Cell-mediated autoimmunity and infectious agents also may play a mediating role in DM-PM.

Clinical Presentation

Progressive proximal muscle weakness is the primary systemic complaint and most often involves the upper and lower limbs.[39] Ocular involvement in dermatomyositis includes a lilac discoloration and edema of the eyelids, conjunctivitis, iritis, blepharoptosis, scleritis, uveitis, and extraocular muscle paralysis.[42] Cotton-wool spots, intraretinal hemorrhages, venous engorgement, and disc edema and optic atrophy have been observed primarily in childhood dermatomyositis.[43]

Diagnosis

The diagnosis is based on clinical findings.[39] Skeletal muscle enzymes, including creatinine kinase and aldolase, are elevated during active disease. Electromyography is abnormal. Muscle biopsy demonstrates the lymphocytic infiltration of the skeletal muscles.[39] Vasculitis is seen more commonly in childhood disease. Autoantibodies including ANA may be seen.

Differential Diagnosis

The differential diagnosis is large and includes multiple neurologic, muscular, and inflammatory disease, which can present with weakness and intraocular inflammation.[39] Included in the differential diagnosis are multiple sclerosis, SLE, polyarteritis nodosa, and sarcoidosis.

Treatment

Corticosteroids and immunosuppressive agents are helpful in managing these diseases but do not cure DM-PM.

Prognosis

The prognosis is better for childhood forms of the disease, with a 90% 5-year survival rate.[39] Patients with adult-onset disease fare worse, with a 30% to 60% mortality rate at 5 years. A major cause of mortality is muscle involvement.

Erythema Multiforme (Stevens-Johnson Syndrome)

Erythema multiforme (EM), or in its severest form, Stevens-Johnson syndrome, is an acute, self-limiting systemic vasculitis affecting the skin and mucous membranes.[40,41]

Etiology

The disease can be idiopathic or can occur after systemic infection or the ingestion of oral medications.[40,41] Herpes simplex virus and mycoplasmal infections have been noted in several reports and may precipitate the immune complex–mediated vasculitis. A hypersensitivity reaction to penicillin, sulfa drugs, and salicylates has been postulated.[40]

Epidemiology

The disease typically affects children and young adults.

Pathogenesis

Immune complex formation and deposition in the affected tissues may result in activation of complement and secondary vasculitis and perivasculitis.[42–49] C3d formation in this disease results in the recruitment of mononuclear cells and polymorphonuclear neutrophilic leukocytes. Secondary thrombosis and necrosis occur in affected tissues. The skin and mucous membranes are most often involved.

Clinical Presentation

Patients often have a viral-like prodrome of fever and malaise 1 to 14 days before the onset of erythema multiforme.[40,41] The onset is acute, with multiple polymorphous lesions involving the skin, nails, and mucous membranes. They begin as 1- to 2-cm round or oval macules or papules described as "target" lesions. The lesions are present on the trunk extremities and on the palms and soles. Bullae and hemorrhage can be noted and may progress to desquamation in severe cases.

With significant mucosal involvement, including the eyes, erythema multiforme is called the Stevens-Johnson (S-J) syndrome.[40,46] An acute conjunctivitis with bullae formation and ulceration is present in this form of the disease. Subepithelial conjunctival scarring, symblepharon, and epithelialization occur later in the disease course. Rarely, S-J syndrome may be recurrent with cycles of skin and mucous membrane inflammation.[50] Conjunctival biopsy can reveal an active vasculitis.

Diagnosis

The clinical picture is often diagnostic. The acute nature of the characteristic target lesions, constitutional complaints, and ocular findings should suggest S-J syndrome. Conjunctival biopsy can help in patients with episodic conjunctival inflammation following EM.[50]

Differential Diagnosis

Cicatricial pemphigoid can cause similar eye findings but is more chronic, with specific deposition of immunoreactants at the basement epithelium of the conjunctiva.

Treatment

Treatment is supportive during the acute phase of S-J syndrome. High-dose oral corticosteroids may be of some benefit.[40,41] Recurrent S-J syndrome may require systemic immunosuppression in severe cases. Topical lubricant and control of secondary cicatricial sequelae should be used after the acute phase of the disease.

Prognosis

S-J syndrome can be fulminant and carries a 20% mortality rate.[40,41] The cicatricial sequelae may compromise the ocular surface, and late complications including dry eye, ulceration, and entropion can occur.

Inflammatory Bowel Disease

Inflammatory bowel disease (IBD) includes Crohn's disease and ulcerative colitis.[51,52] These diseases are associated with several primary and secondary ocular findings.

Etiology

The etiology of Crohn's disease and ulcerative colitis is unknown.[47,48] There is a 50% to 70% association with HLA-B27 tissue type and the development of extraintestinal manifestations, including arteritis, sacroiliitis, and uveitis.

Epidemiology

Crohn's disease affects young adults. It is estimated that 2% to 10% of patients with IBD have uveitis and ocular manifestations.[53]

Pathogenesis

A granulomatous regional ileitis occurs in Crohn's disease, with full-thickness inflammation and fistula formation.[47,48] Ulcerative colitis causes a diffuse inflammation of the GI mucosa. Bacteria or circulating immune complexes are postulated to play a role in multisystemic involvement.[49]

Clinical Presentation

Patients with IBD experience chronic or relapsing abdominal pain, diarrhea, weight loss, and fever. The diarrhea may be bloody in ulcerative colitis. Psoriasis, arthritis with spondyloarthropathy distribution, and erythema nodosum can also be noted. Vascular complications, including thromboembolism, can be noted in 1% to 2% of patients.[54]

Ocular manifestations directly associated with IBD include a subepithelial keratopathy, episcleritis, and scleritis. The corneal infiltrates are small and white and are located at the peripheral cornea.[55] Episcleritis is the most common ocular findings.[5–58] Nongranulomatous iridocyclitis and granulomatous panuveitis can occur and may parallel intestinal symptoms.[49,57–59] Posterior segment manifestations include serous retinal detachment, retrobulbar neuritis, papillitis, and multifocal choroiditis.[60] Retinal vasculitis can develop and may be secondary to immune complex vasculitis or thromboembolic disease.[61,62]

Secondary eye findings include corticosteroid-induced cataracts and decreased night vision and Bitot's spots from vitamin A deficiency.[49]

Diagnosis

Tissue biopsy from colonoscopy establishes the diagnosis. The diagnosis can be supported by radiologic studies including barium enema and upper GI series.

Differential Diagnosis

Acute uveitis with GI complaints can be noted in Whipple's disease, giardiasis, and amoebiasis. Whipple's disease is associated with more constitutional symptoms, normal radiologic studies, and a characteristic small intestine biopsy. Stools for ova and parasite can help differentiate parasitic diseases.

Treatment

Surgical excision of the inflamed bowel may assist in controlling the extraintestinal symptoms, including eye disease in IBD.[47,48] Oral NSAIDs, corticosteroids, methotrexate, and cyclophosphamide are sometimes needed to control the disease in recalcitrant cases.

Ocular inflammation often responds to therapy for IBD.[49,55,56,62] In addition, topical and regional corticosteroids can be used adjunctly for keratopathy and uveitis.

Prognosis

The visual prognosis is generally good in this condition.

Juvenile Rheumatoid Arthritis

JRA is a multisystemic rheumatic childhood disease associated with a chronic arthritis and iridocyclitis.[63,64]

Etiology

The etiology of JRA is unknown but is thought to be a primary autoimmune disease. The chronic inflammatory disease is associated with autoantibody formation, which may be precipitated by a number of possible events, including trauma, infection, and stress.[63]

Epidemiology

JRA is much more common in girls (70%–75%) and onset is, by definition, before the age of 16 years.[63–65] Twenty percent of children with JRA develop uveitis.[66]

Pathogenesis

The synovium in JRA becomes hyperplastic, with subsynovial lymphocytic infiltration and edema.[63,67] Immune complexes have been found in the synovial fluid.[68]

Clinical Presentation

There are three forms of JRA. The acute, toxic form (Still's disease) accounts for 10% of cases.[63] This form presents with fever, hepatosplenomegaly, and arthritis in multiple large joints. Eye disease is rare. The polyarticular form of JRA (40%) is said to occur when five or more joints become involved within a 6-month period. The pauciarticluar form (50%) is associated with four or fewer affected joints over a 6-month period. Children with seronegative, ANA+ pauciarticular JRA are at the highest risk for developing eye disease and account for 95% of all cases.[66] Extra-articular manifestations may include pericarditis, pulmonary fibrosis, subcutaneous nodules, and a salmon-colored skin rash.

Chronic iridocyclitis develops in 5% to 20% of children with pauciarticular JRA.[69] Eye disease may precede the development of arthritis by several years. Ocular involvement may be insidious because of the absence of symptoms and signs early in the disease. JRA-associated iridocyclitis is typically chronic and bilateral (70%). The inflammation is nongranulomatous and primarily involves the iris and ciliary body. Chronic inflammation commonly results in band keratopathy (41%), posterior synechiae, glaucoma (19%), and cataract formation (42–92%)[70] (Fig. 17.2 and see Fig. 2.7).

JRA involves the anterior segment much more than the retina and choroid. Patients also may develop CME as a result of chronic iridocyclitis. Organization and fibrosis of the anterior vitreous may occur, resulting in further media opacification. Cyclitic membrane formation and ocular

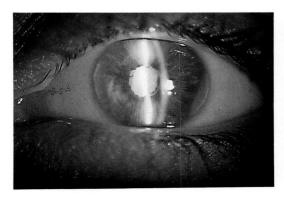

Figure 17.2. Type III hypersensitivity—juvenile rheumatoid arthritis. White, "quiet" eye with mild band keratopathy, chronic nongranulomatous anterior uveitis, posterior synechiae, and mature cataract in a patient with juvenile rheumatoid arthritis.

hypotony can develop in long-standing disease and after eye surgery in these children.

Diagnosis

JRA can be diagnosed in children with the characteristic arthritis and ocular findings.[63,64] The diagnosis can be further supported with a positive ANA (79%) and a negative rheumatoid factor.[71] Radiography of the involved joints and knee may also support the diagnosis.[63]

Differential Diagnosis

Juvenile onset arthritis and uveitis can be seen in SLE, polyarteritis nodosa, Reiter's disease, inflammatory bowel disease, and Lyme arthritis. Whereas younger boys may develop classic JRA, older boys more often develop an acute form of recurrent iridocyclitis associated with spondylitis and HLA-B27. Sarcoidosis can also cause a chronic uveitis in children with large-joint arthralgias. The uveitis is often granulomatous and frequently involves the retina and choroid as well.

Treatment

Treatment should be multidisciplinary. All children with JRA should undergo a thorough eye examination by an ophthalmologist.[67-75] If the eye is free of disease, children with pauciarticular disease should be evaluated every 2 to 3 months for the first 5 years. Routine examinations should be continued throughout childhood. Children with polyarticular forms should be examined every 6 months.

Children with evidence for uveitis require meticulous ophthalmic care to monitor disease course and response to therapy. JRA is often associated with a significant amount of persistent ocular flare, which represents a breakdown of the blood–eye barrier and is not an indication for therapy.[64] Intraocular inflammatory cells should be treated aggressively to prevent the blinding complications of chronic uveitis.

Topical corticosteroids and cycloplegics are the mainstay of therapy. The topical corticosteroid regimen should be determined by the clinical examination and response to therapy. Efforts should be made to find lowest dose required to control the iridocyclitis. The clinical course often changes and frequent visits to determine appropriate therapeutic modifications are needed every 2–4 weeks while active. Oral NSAIDs, antimalarial agents, and gold salts have been shown to help control both articular and ocular inflammation and can help decrease the amount of topical corticosteroid needed to control the uveitis.[63,72,73] Regional corticosteroids can be useful but are difficult to deliver in this age group and often require examination under general anesthesia.[64] Short courses of oral corticosteroids (1 mg/kg per day) can be used in severe cases and tapered according to the clinical response. Chronic oral corticosteroid use is often associated with multiple, severe side effects in children and should be used rarely.

Systemic immunosuppression should be considered in patients with steroid-resistant disease or steroid intolerance. Methotrexate is the most widely used second-generation immunosuppressive agent in this age group.[63] Although immunosuppressive therapy is safer than long-term corticosteroid therapy, side effects are nevertheless considerable. Therefore, these drugs should be prescribed cautiously and under the direction of physicians experienced with these medications.

Prognosis

The overall visual prognosis in JRA is guarded: 10% of children develop mild disease, 15% develop moderate uveitis, 50% have moderately severe disease, and 25% are unresponsive to therapy. Overall, 75% percent of children with JRA and moderate to severe uveitis experience visual loss due to band keratopathy, glaucoma, cataract, or phthisis.[69,75]

Removal of the band keratopathy can improve visual acuity. Lenticular and vitreous opacification should be treated with pars plana lensectomy/vitrectomy to afford better control of the inflammation and prevent cyclitic membrane formation and hypotony.[70,76,77] Standard anterior segment surgical approaches and the use of intraocular lenses are contraindicated.[64,66] Glaucoma surgery is challenging.[66,77,78] Trabeculodialysis has been successful in some children.[78]

Psoriatic Arthritis

Psoriasis is a chronic papulosquamous skin disorder associated with a seronegative, erosive arthritis and uveitis.[79]

Etiology

The etiology is unknown. An autosomal dominant inheritance pattern can be noted in some cases.[80] Whereas HLA-B13 and HLA-B17 have been associated with psoriasis, HLA-B27 has been associated with psoriatic arthritis and sacroiliitis (10%–60%).[79,81]

Epidemiology

The incidence of psoriasis is 1% to 2% of the general population; 5% to 20% may develop psoriatic arthritis.[79]

Pathogenesis

The skin develops hyperkeratosis with plaque formation and erythematous scales on the limbs and trunk.[79] Immune complex formation and low-grade vasculitis can be found on laboratory testing and skin biopsy.[82] The joints have synovial hypertrophy and lymphocytic infiltration.

Clinical Presentation

Discrete patches of papulosquamous dermatitis is the hallmark of psoriasis. Nail beds, when involved, are pitted. The distal interphalangeal joints, spine, and sacroiliac joints can develop seronegative arthritis.[79]

Ocular disease can be noted in patients with psoriatic arthritis.[83] An acute nongranulomatous iridocyclitis is the most common finding. The anterior uveitis may be associated with a posterior synechia and a mild vitritis. Secondary CME and mild retinal vasculitis have been reported.

Diagnosis

Psoriasis is a clinical diagnosis. The arthritis and uveitis are seronegative but can be associated with HLA-B27 positivity.[79] Elevated circulating immune complexes have been found in 50% of patients with psoriasis and associated arthritis.

Differential Diagnosis

Other HLA-B27–associated diseases can have a similar ocular presentation. These include ankylosing spondylitis, inflammatory bowel disease, and Reiter's syndrome.

Treatment

The arthritis and uveitis can be treated with oral NSAIDs. Topical, regional, and oral corticosteroids may be required to control the acute uveitis.[83] Methotrexate and cyclosporin have a beneficial effect in severe cases of psoriatic arthritis and uveitis.[84,85]

Prognosis

The ocular prognosis is good.

Reiter's Syndrome

Reiter's syndrome is a collagen vascular disorder associated with seronegative asymmetric arthropathy, urethritis, and ocular inflammation.[86,87]

Etiology

The etiology is unknown. Reiter's syndrome has a postvenereal and an epidemic enteric form.[86,87] Chlamydial urethritis or GI infection with *Salmonella*, *Shigella*, and *Yersinia* organisms have been associated with Reiter's syndrome.

Epidemiology

White men between the ages of 20 and 40 years are diagnosed most frequently with Reiter's syndrome.[86] The disease is uncommon in nonwhites and difficult to diagnose in women. Women do not typically present with the classic triad. Between 70% and 90% of patients with Reiter's syndrome have HLA-B27 tissue type.[88] Eye findings occur in 60% of cases.[86]

Pathogenesis

The primary site of articular inflammation in Reiter's syndrome is at the insertion of ligament to bone (enthesopathy).[86,87] This explains the commonly observed Achilles tendonitis, plantar fasciitis, and arthralgia pattern.

Clinical Presentation

Fever and malaise may precede the onset of Reiter's syndrome.[86,87] The major diagnostic criteria include large joint arthritis, urethritis, and ocular inflammation.[89] Achilles tendonitis, plantar fasciitis, sacroiliitis, prostatitis, diarrhea, and painless oral ulcer are also clinical features of the disease and are considered minor diagnostic criteria.

The most common ocular manifestation of Reiter's syndrome is papillary conjunctivitis, which may be acute with purulent discharge.[89] A recurrent, nongranulomatous iridocyclitis, often associated with hypopyon, can occur in 12% of patients (see Fig. 2.6). The midperipheral cornea can exhibit subepithelial infiltrates and disciform keratitis.[90,91] Retinal edema and retinitis have been reported rarely.

Diagnosis

The presence of three or more major criteria of polyarthritis, urethritis, and conjunctivitis/iritis and skin lesions defines the disorder.[86,89] Patients with two major and two minor criteria are said to have probable Reiter's syndrome. Two major and one minor finding constitute a possible diagnosis. During active stages of the disease, elevated ESR and white blood counts can occur. Positive HLA-B27 tissue typing adds to the clinical impression.

Differential Diagnosis

Hypopyon iridocyclitis, large-joint arthritis, and oral ulcers can occur in Behçet's disease. Ocular inflammation in Behçet's disease frequently involves the retina and choroid, and the oral ulcers are painful. Genital lesions are ulcerative in Behçet's disease. Other HLA-B27–associated diseases can also exhibit arthritis and hypopyon iridocyclitis. Ankylosing spondylitis, IBD, and psoriatic arthritis are associated with HLA-B27 and can be associated with

a severe, nongranulomatous anterior uveitis.

Treatment

Reiter's syndrome can be difficult to treat.[17,86] The systemic manifestations of Reiter's syndrome may respond to NSAIDs, especially indomethacin. A 4- to 6-week course of oral tetracycline to treat a possible chronic bacterial infection has been reported to be beneficial.[17]

Ocular manifestations should be treated with topical, regional, and oral corticosteroids.[17,89,90] Cycloplegia and mydriasis may be necessary. Steroid-resistant and intolerant patients and those with severe chronic disease benefit from low-dose, weekly methotrexate therapy.[17,92]

Prognosis

Cataract, glaucoma, and macular edema are sequelae of the recurrent inflammation in Reiter's syndrome. Because of continual disease activity and recurrences, intraocular lens implantation may be contraindicated.

Relapsing Polychondritis

Relapsing polychondritis is a collagen vascular disease that primarily affects the cartilaginous tissues.[93,94]

Etiology

The etiology is unknown but appears to be an autoimmune disease directed against type II collagen.[95]

Epidemiology

Relapsing polychondritis is a rare disease that may occur at all ages, but peaks in the fifth decade. It affects men and women equally.[93] There is an association with HLA-DR4.

Pathogenesis

Patients with polychondritis have circulating antitype II collagen antibodies.[95] Chondrocytic degeneration and granulation tissue formation may occur in cartilage throughout the body.[95-98] Both vitreous and cartilage are predominant tissues containing type II collagen. True vasculitis may be seen on conjunctival biopsy.[98] The presence of anticollagen antibodies in the tissues may suggest an arthus reaction or a type III hypersensitivity as well. These autoantibodies are thought to play a mediating role in the recurrent, granulomatous inflammation noted in this disease. Lymphocytic and macrophage infiltration causes a nongranulomatous chronic polychondritis.

Clinical Presentation

Systemically, patients are characterized by bilateral ear pinna inflammation and nasal cartilage destruction (72%).[93,94] Nasal septal damage typically results in a saddle-nose deformity. Secondary otitis, vertigo, tinnitus, and deafness may be noted. A nonerosive polyarthralgia may also bring

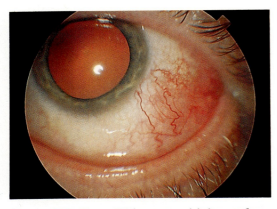

Figure 17.3. Type III hypersensitivity—relapsing polychondritis. Nodular scleritis and a mild nongranulomatous anterior uveitis in a patient with relapsing polychondritis and bilateral ear pinna inflammation.

the patient to medical attention. Laryngeal and tracheal ring cartilage may be involved and can cause acute respiratory distress as a result of upper airway collapse. Aortic ring involvement can cause severe cardiac manifestations.

Ocular involvement in relapsing polychondritis may occur in as many as 20% to 50% of cases[96-101] and is typically in the form of an episcleritis, scleritis, or conjunctivitis (Fig. 17.3). Corneal infiltrates, lid edema, and proptosis also have been reported. Anterior uveitis is observed in 20% of patients. Primary retinal or choroidal involvement is unusual. Retinal pigment epithelial and sensory retinal detachments, as well as choroidal thickening, can be noted as a result of localized posterior scleritis.[97]

Diagnosis

The diagnosis can be established by the pathognomonic bilateral ear pinna inflammation.[93,96] Biopsy of involved cartilage demonstrates the characteristic granulomatous chondritis.

Differential Diagnosis

Wegener's granulomatosis can cause uveitis and destruction of the nasal cartilage but rarely involves the ear.

Treatment

Prednisone, in combination with dapsone or cyclophosphamide, has proved to be the most effective in controlling this disease.[93,98,99] Dapsone does not appear to be as effective in patients with severe necrotizing forms of scleritis.[98] Destructive changes in the cartilage are not reversible, and the goal of therapy should be to limit further disease progression.

Prognosis

Relapsing polychondritis is a potentially fatal disease associated with a 30% mortality rate from pulmonary or cardiac complications.[93] Systemic immunosuppression appears to improve the prognosis.

Rheumatoid Arthritis

Rheumatoid arthritis (RA) is a chronic systemic inflammatory disease of unknown etiology that produces a distinct form of polyarticular and symmetric arthritis.[100]

Etiology

The etiology of RA is unknown. It is thought to have a strong autoimmune pathogenesis.

Epidemiology

The disease is more common in women (3:1) and typically begins between the ages of 30 and 40 years.[101] HLA-D4 has been found in 51% of patients with RA.[102]

Pathogenesis

An unknown antigenic stimulus is thought to promote autoantibody formation. Patients with RA have IgM, IgG, and IgA antibodies that are directed against the Fc portion of IgG.[100,103] The resulting immune complexes are postulated to play a role in both articular and extra-articular manifestations of the disease through activation of complement. Acute inflammation of the synovium results in pannus formation and destruction of cartilage in joints.

Clinical Presentation

Patients with RA report malaise, fatigue, weight loss, and arthralgia. Their joint disease is symmetric and often involves the small joints of the wrist and hand, excluding the distal interphalangeal joints.[101] Morning stiffness is characteristic. Extra-

articular involvement, including pleurisy, neuropathy, and ocular inflammation, is thought to be secondary to a systemic vasculitis and may represent a change from a local joint disease to a more serious systemic form of RA.[104,105]

Keratoconjunctivitis sicca, marginal keratitis, peripheral ulcerative keratopathy, and anterior scleritis comprise the most common anterior segment findings in RA.[8] Uveitis and direct involvement of the retina are rare. The retina can be involved secondarily with the development of posterior scleritis.

Posterior scleritis is less common than anterior forms of scleral inflammation. This condition is defined as scleritis posterior to the equator of the eye, and in one series it accounted for only 2% of all cases.[106,107] It is important to recognize, however, that posterior scleritis is much more difficult to detect. In one report of 30 eyes enucleated for ocular inflammation, 40% had previously undetected posterior scleritis.[108] Unlike anterior scleritis, posterior scleritis can be unilateral and is often associated with a profound decrease in visual acuity. There is pain and tenderness with motion or palpation. On biomicroscopic examination, the anterior segment is often normal or may exhibit only a narrow angle because of displacement by the posterior structures.

Fundus examination in posterior scleritis reveals choroidal thickening or choroidal nodules overlying the area of scleritis. Secondary choroidal folds and effusions may develop. The retina may demonstrate secondary striae and exudative retinal separations (Fig. 17.4A).[107] A venous stasis retinopathy may be noted with hyperviscosity secondary to a polyclonal gammopathy in RA.[109]

Diagnosis

Patients with the characteristic deforming arthritis associated with RA seldom present a diagnostic challenge.[101] Mild anemia, elevation of the ESR, and positive rheuma-

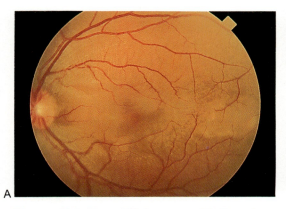
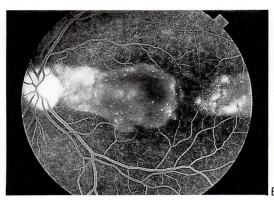

Figure 17.4. Type III hypersensitivity—rheumatoid arthritis. Posterior uveitis secondary to scleritis in a patient with RA. Ultrasound demonstrated posterior scleritis and fluid in Tenon's space. **A:** Visual acuity was reduced because of an exudative retinal detachment in the posterior pole. **B:** Fluorescein angiogram showed the punctate hyperfluorescent areas of choroiditis and RPE inflammation overlying the area of posterior scleritis.

toid factor (80%) may support the clinical diagnosis. In the absence of obvious systemic findings, scleritis may be the initial manifestation of occult rheumatic disease. Ultrasonography or computed tomography (CT) can document thickening of the sclera and choroid in posterior scleritis. There may be fluid in the contiguous Tenon's space. Fluorescein angiography illustrates the choroidal and retinal striae. A characteristic linear pattern of alternating hypofluorescent and hyperfluorescent streaks can be seen as a result of folds in the retinal pigment epithelial layer. Multifocal, punctate, hyperfluorescent choroidal lesions also can be noted, which may evolve into areas of exudative retinal detachment (Fig. 17.4B). The retinal circulation is typically unaffected.

Differential Diagnosis

Scleritis may be idiopathic or associated with other diseases such as SLE, polyarteritis nodosa, Wegener's granulomatosis, relapsing polychondritis, tuberculosis, syphilis, and herpes zoster infections.

Treatment

Artificial tears and lubricants can help with the complaints related to sicca. Therapy for rheumatoid scleritis should be directed at controlling the underlying systemic disease.[106,110–112] Local ocular therapy and regional steroids should be used with caution and only as adjuncts to systemic treatment. Regional steroids have been reported to cause scleral melting and ocular perforation and should be used only in extenuating circumstances. Mild cases can often be managed effectively by NSAIDs. Indomethacin (100–150 mg/day) has been reported to be effective for scleritis.[105,112] In more severe cases, oral corticosteroids, gold salts, and second-generation immunosuppressive drugs such as methotrexate, cyclophosphamide, and azathioprine should be considered.[111,113]

Prognosis

The prognosis depends in part on establishing the proper diagnosis and detecting the underlying rheumatic disease. The development of necrotizing anterior scleritis may indicate a more severe form of rheumatoid arthritis.[113] Patients with necrotizing disease have an 8-year mortality rate of 20%.

Polyarteritis Nodosa

Polyarteritis nodosa (PAN) is a multisystemic disease associated with a necrotizing vasculitis.[114]

Etiology

The etiology of PAN is unknown. An autoimmune mechanism is postulated to cause the vasculitis.

Epidemiology

PAN is a rare disease that affects 40- to 60-year-old adults. Men are affected more than women (2:1).[113]

Pathogenesis

Medium- to small-sized muscular vessels are characteristically affected with all stages of vasculitis noted in the involved tissues.[115] Mid-sized immune complexes can be found deposited within the vessel walls. Subsequent complement activation results in infiltration of the vessel wall and surrounding tissues with PMNs, lymphocytes, and eosinophils. These lesions frequently occur at bifurcations. Endothelial proliferation and fibrinoid necrosis result in thrombosis and tissue ischemia.

It has been reported that 30% to 70% of patients with PAN have antihepatitis B antibodies.[116] The significance of this observation has not been established.

Clinical Presentation

Patients with classic PAN may note fatigue, myalgia, weight loss, fever, arthralgia, and testicular pain.[114] The heart, kidneys, liver, GI tract, and CNS are commonly involved. Renal involvement is one of the more serious and potentially fatal complications. Abdominal pain due to intestinal infarction and headaches from CNS vasculitis are also serious and potentially life-threatening complications of this disease. A peripheral neuropathy with mononeuritis multiplex can be a presenting symptom. Pulmonary, spleen, and skin involvement are less commonly involved in classic PAN.

Ocular involvement is reported in 10% to 20% of patients with PAN.[11-120] Peripheral ulcerative keratitis, scleritis, and mild iritis are associated ocular manifestations. The iritis is acute and nongranulomatous. A mild vitritis may also be noted. The most common ocular findings in PAN are choroidal and retinal vasculitis.[120] Fundus examination reveals retinal vasculitis with associated intraretinal hemorrhages, cotton-wool spots, and retinal edema (see Fig. 2.27). Central retinal artery occlusion and optic atrophy have also been reported in PAN. Patients with PAN may also develop anterior or posterior scleritis. Posterior scleritis manifests with pain and chorioretinal folds similar to those seen in RA.

Chürg-Strauss (C-S) syndrome is a systemic necrotizing vasculitis subset of PAN. Patients with this syndrome, however, have pulmonary involvement and relapsing eosinophilia.[121] Immune complex deposition and an eosinophilic infiltration of the vessel and surrounding tissue are the hallmark of C-S syndrome. Both the upper and lower respiratory tracts are affected. Asthma (100%), rhinitis and nasal polyposis (70%), systemic vasculitis (100%), and an evanescent peripheral eosinophilia (100%) with total eosinophil counts to 1.5×10^9 eosinophils/L defines the clinical picture.[121] The kidney, skin, heart, and CNS also are affected. Optic neuritis, cranial nerve palsies, peripheral ulcerative keratitis, branch retinal artery occlusion, and panuveitis have been reported.[122-125] Laboratory testing demonstrates an elevated white blood count and ESR and an eosinophilia. Biopsy of involved tissue establishes the diagnosis. The disease is fatal without therapy and can be present for many years. C-S syndrome responds favorably to corticosteroid therapy and other second-generation immunosuppressive medications.[121–125]

Cogan's syndrome is a nonsyphilitic vasculitis that affects the vestibuloauditory system, causing an interstitial keratitis; 60% of patients have classic PAN.[126,127] In addition to symptoms from the systemic vasculitis, patients develop hearing loss, tinnitus, and vertigo. Patients report decreased vision and photophobia secondary to an interstitial keratitis.[128] Optic atrophy has also been reported. Serology for syphilis is negative, and evidence for a systemic vasculitis can be found on laboratory testing. Untreated patients have a 28% 5-year survival.[127] Cyclophosphamide and corticosteroids can help control the disease.

Diagnosis

Any patient with peripheral ulcerative keratitis, scleritis, or occlusive retinal vasculitis should be reviewed for systemic evidence of collagen vascular disease. Often, a biopsy of an involved artery or lesion demonstrates a hemorrhagic vasculitis and fibrinoid necrosis and establishes the diagnosis.[114] Testicular and skin biopsy can confirm the diagnosis in 50% to 80% of patients.[129,130] Laboratory tests may reveal elevated white blood cell and eosinophil count, decreased complement, elevated circulating immune complexes, and a negative rheumatoid factor (RF) and ANA. The ESR is markedly elevated and anti-neutrophilic cytoplasmic antibody (ANCA) may be positive. Hepatitis B surface antigen has been found in 10% to 50% of patients with classic PAN. Angiography in patients with abdominal pain may reveal aneurysmal dilation of the hepatic and renal arteries.

Differential Diagnosis

Overlap vasculitis syndromes and other forms of systemic vasculitis can cause multisystemic disease. The clinical features and tissue biopsy can help differentiate the PAN group of vasculitis from Wegener's granulomatosis, Behçet's disease, SLE, and others. Tuberculosis, syphilis, and sarcoidosis should also be considered in patients with ocular inflammation and widespread systemic disease.

Treatment

This group of diseases is potentially fatal.[114,119] Without therapy, classic PAN carries an 80% to 90% 5-year mortality rate. Corticosteroids reduce this rate to 50%.[131] The combination of corticosteroids with cyclophosphamide (1–2 mg/kg per day) results in an 80% 5-year survival rate. Patients may require high-dose intravenous steroids and cyclophosphamide early in the disease to gain control of severe forms.

Prognosis

Immunosuppressive therapy improves the overall prognosis and inflammatory sequela. The ophthalmologist often can help establish a diagnosis in these patients.

Systemic Sclerosis With or Without Scleroderma

Systemic sclerosis with or without scleroderma is a chronic autoimmune disorder that causes inflammation and fibrosis of the skin and other organs.[132]

Etiology

The etiology is unknown.

Epidemiology

Women in the fourth decade are affected more than men (4:1).[133]

Pathogenesis

The immune defect in progressive systemic scleroderma (PSS) is not completely understood, but autoantibody formation, circulating immune complex deposition, vasculitis, and secondary fibrosis of the vessels are thought to produce the clinical features of this disease.[132,134,135] Cell-mediated autoreactivity to collagen may also be a factor.

Clinical Presentation

Patients may present with either scleroderma or manifest other symptoms of the CREST syndrome (calcinosis, Raynaud's phenomenon, esophageal dysfunction, sclerodactyly, and telangiectasia). Taut skin on the back of hands is the most common finding.[132] Pulmonary fibrosis may be present at any stage of the disease. Many other organ systems can develop fibrosis including the heart, kidneys, colon, and lungs. Fatal complications occur as a result of organ failure.

Scleroderma commonly involves the eye. Keratoconjunctivitis sicca occurs in up to 70% of patients with PSS as a result of lacrimal gland fibrosis.[136] Filamentary keratitis, eyelid edema, and conjunctival shrinkage can also be noted. Patients with PSS may have fundus findings similar to patients with SLE. Intraretinal hemorrhages, cottonwool spots, retinal vasculitis, and choroidal infarctions have been observed.[137,138]

Diagnosis

The diagnosis can be established by the characteristic clinical picture of the scleroderma with or without the other CREST findings.[132] These systemic findings, in association with retinal microvascular infarctions and retinal vasculitis, support the clinical diagnosis. Laboratory testing may reveal a positive ANA with a speckled pattern. Fluorescein angiography can be used to document the cotton-wool spots and define the extent of choroidal nonperfusion. Skin biopsy demonstrates inflammation and fibrosis of the skin and dermal vessels.

Differential Diagnosis

Collagen vascular diseases in general should be considered; however, the dermatologic findings are characteristic. Chemical exposure may present with similar findings.

Treatment

Long-term systemic therapy has not been useful in controlling PSS and therapy is chiefly supportive.[139] Penicillamine and cyclosporin A have been used with some success. Artificial tears and lubrication are beneficial. Filamentary keratitis can be treated with bandage soft contact lenses.

Prognosis

Localized scleroderma has a relatively good prognosis. Systemic involvement has a worse prognosis with an 80% 10-year mortality rate.[132,139]

Sjögren's Syndrome

Sjögren's syndrome is a collagen vascular disease characterized by keratoconjunctivitis sicca, xerostomia.[139,140] Sjögren's syndrome has a primary form and a secondary form associated with a variety of connective tissue diseases.

Etiology

The etiology is unknown. HLA-Dw4 has been associated with RA and Sjögren's syndrome.[139]

Epidemiology

Sjögren's syndrome is the second most common autoimmune disorder after RA.[139,140] It can occur as a primary disease or be secondarily associated with other collagen vascular diseases such as RA, SLE, scleroderma, and polyarteritis nodosa. Approximately 10% to 25% of patients with RA have Sjögren's syndrome. The syndrome is more common in postmenopausal women, with a 9:1 female/male ratio.

Pathogenesis

Exocrine glands including the salivary and lacrimal glands demonstrate focal infiltration with lymphocytes and secondary fibrosis.[139,140] Most of the lymphocytes on immunohistochemistry are activated CD4, helper T cells. These patients develop antinucleoprotein antibodies, anti-SSA (anti-Ro), and anti-SSB (anti-La).[140] Antisalivary gland antibodies can be found in 10% to 68% of patients. Other antibodies, including ANA and elevated circulating immune complexes, may be found on laboratory testing.

Clinical Presentation

Patients with Sjögren's syndrome complain of dryness of the mouth and eyes. Salivary gland swelling may be noted. Other manifestations of primary Sjögren's syndrome include pneumonitis, renal tubular acidosis, polymyositis, gastritis, and CNS vasculitis.

Keratoconjunctivitis sicca is the most common eye finding.[141] The tear quantity and quality are poor. Schirmer's tear testing results in less than 5-mm wetting in a 5-minute period. Tear breakup time is rapid. Secondary filamentary keratitis can also be problematic. In one series, eight patients with Sjögren's syndrome developed anterior or intermediate uveitis.[142] In another report, two patients with progressive retinal vasculitis had anti-SSA antibodies, suggesting Sjögren's-like syndrome.[143] Their disease was unresponsive to corticosteroid, immunosuppressive, and panretinal photocoagulation therapy.

Diagnosis

Keratoconjunctivitis sicca, xerostomia, and salivary gland swelling with or without an underlying connective tissue disease establishes the diagnosis.[140] Rose Bengal staining documents the presence of superficial punctate keratitis. Laboratory testing may show a positive ANA, elevated ESR, and increased circulating immune complexes. Anti-SSI and anti-SSB antibodies can be detected.

Differential Diagnosis

KCS with filamentary keratitis can be found in cicatricial pemphigoid, neurotrophic keratitis.

Treatment

Artificial tears and ointment are the mainstay of therapy. Filamentary keratitis can be treated with a bandage soft contact lens. Punctal occlusion and moisture chambers can help preserve the ocular surface in advanced cases. Alternate day oral corticosteroid, 40 mg four times a day, was beneficial in one series of patients.[144]

Prognosis

Sjögren's syndrome is a chronic condition with no known cure. Systemic lymphoma may develop in these patients at a higher incidence than in the general population.

Systemic Lupus Erythematosus

SLE is a collagen vascular disease with protean and multisystemic manifestations.[145]

Etiology

The etiology of SLE is unknown.[145,146] It may be a common pathway of several initiating events in genetically predisposed persons. SLE is thought to be an autoimmune collagen vascular disorder.

Epidemiology

Ninety percent of patients with SLE are women at or around child-bearing ages.[21]

Pathogenesis

The pathogenesis of SLE is complex. A systemic necrotizing vasculitis may play a mediating role.[145,146] Patients with SLE have elevated ANA and circulating immune complexes.[145,147] These immune complexes are made up of autoantibodies and DNA and have been found in the walls of inflamed blood vessels and in the areas of fibrinoid necrosis.

The mechanism of primary lupus retinopathy may be secondary to capillary nonperfusion from immune complex damage and necrotizing vasculitis. Ten percent of patients with SLE also have lupus anticoagulant antibodies, which are known to increase the incidence of thrombosis. The relationship between this factor and lupus retinopathy is unclear but provocative.[148]

Clinical Presentation

Clinically, patients with SLE present with malaise, fatigue, anorexia, and low-grade fever. On examination they may have arthritis, facial rash, alopecia, and pleurisy.[149] Raynaud's phenomenon, oral ulcers, and CNS complaints are also common.

SLE may involve the eye in up to 50% of cases, depending on the series and the nature of the clinic reporting the findings.[150] Anterior segment findings include kerato-

conjunctivitis sicca, scleritis, and keratitis.[151] True uveitis is uncommon (0–16%). An optic neuropathy can occur with CNS involvement.[152] The retina and choroid may be primarily involved; however, it is important to separate lupus-associated retinal vasculitis from the secondary retinal and choroidal changes of SLE-mediated hypertension and anemia. Severe hypertension can occur in SLE as a result of nephritis. Arteriolar narrowing, intraretinal hemorrhages, exudate, and disc edema are characteristic of hypertensive retinopathy.

Three fundus presentations have been described in SLE.[151–156] The most common form is focal ischemia, which causes multiple cotton-wool spots. Intraretinal hemorrhages and mild disc edema can also be associated with this form of lupus retinopathy. A second form of retinopathy noted in SLE is a severe retinal vaso-occlusive disease without evidence of retinal vasculitis.[152,154,155] Retinal infarction and hemorrhage can result in severe and sudden loss of vision. The third form of retinopathy in SLE is proliferative lupus retinopathy (Fig. 17.5). Retinal vasculitis and secondary ischemia produce neovascularization of the optic nerve and elsewhere in the retina.[153]

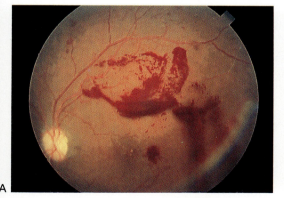
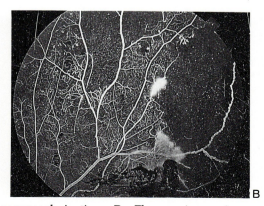

Figure 17.5. Type III hypersensitivity—systemic lupus erythematosus. A: Fundus photograph of a patient with active SLE showing vitreous hemorrhage, vascular sheathing, and retinal neovascularization. B: Fluorescein angiogram demonstrates peripheral capillary nonperfusion, retinal vasculitis, and retinal neovascularization.

This neovascularization can result in vitreous hemorrhage and even retinal detachment. The choroidal circulation may be involved in this process as well.[157] Choroidal infarction, exudative changes, and subretinal neovascular membranes have been reported in this form of SLE.

Diagnosis

SLE is a clinical diagnosis. The American Rheumatologic Association defines the disease by the presence of 4 of the 11 major symptoms and signs (Table 17.3). These include facial rash, discoid lupus, Raynaud's phenomenon, alopecia, photosensitivity, oral ulcers, arteritis, LE cells, false-positive Venereal Disease Research Laboratory test (VDRL), proteinemia, urinary casts, serositis, convulsions or psychosis, and leukopenia, anemia, or thrombocytopenia.[140] Laboratory testing may support the clinical diagnosis by revealing a positive ANA, anti-dsDNA antibodies, and elevated circulating immune complexes, in addition to the proteinuria, anemia, and false-positive VDRL. Fluorescein angiography may help define the extent of retinal involvement and may assist in differentiating secondary hypertensive retinopathy from the true retinal vasculitis noted in lupus retinopathy.

Table 17.3. Major diagnostic criteria for systemic lupus erythematosus.[a]

Macular rash
Discoid lupus
Photosensitivity
Oral or nasal ulcers
Arthritis
Serositis: pleurisy, pericarditis
Renal: proteinuria, urinary casts
Neurologic: psychosis, seizures
Hematologic: anemia, leukopenia, thrombocytopenia
Immunologic disorder: Anti-DNA antibody, LE prep,
    Anti-Sm, +VDRL
Antinuclear antibody

[a] Four of 11 required.
LE, lupus erythematosus; Anti-Sm, anti-Smith; +VDRL, positive Venereal Disease Research Laboratory test.

Differential Diagnosis

Other collagen vascular diseases can have multisystemic involvement and retinal vasculitis. Clinical features of polyarteritis nodosa, Wegener's granulomatosis, Behçet's disease, and Reiter's syndrome differentiate these disorders. Syphilis and sarcoidosis should be included in the differential diagnosis.

Treatment

Therapy for SLE varies according to the severity of symptoms. It is important to note that SLE may present in the eye 1 to 5 years before the onset of other systemic findings.[158] Lupus retinopathy may respond to systemic therapy including NSAIDs, corticosteroids, hydroxychloroquine sulfate (Plaquenil), gold, and immunosuppressants.[153–156] Proliferative lupus retinopathy can be treated with panretinal laser ablation to prevent the sequela of ocular neovascularization.[153]

Prognosis

The visual prognosis depends on the extent and location of the retinal ischemia. Systemic manifestations, if severe, can be fatal.

Temporal Arteritis or Giant Cell Arteritis

Temporal arteritis or giant cell arteritis (GCA) is a systemic vasculitis that involves medium-sized to large muscular arteries.[159] It is often seen in conjunction with polymyalgia rheumatica.

Etiology

The etiology is unknown, but GCA is thought to be an autoimmune collagen vascular disease.[159,160]

Epidemiology

Temporal arteritis affects those older than 50 years, with an average age of 70 years.[155,160]

Pathogenesis

The pathophysiology of this disease results in a panarteritis. Affected blood vessels have a mononuclear cell infiltration and giant cell formation within the vessel wall.[155,160] Subsequent destruction and fragmentation of the internal elastic membrane is noted.[161] Circulating immune complexes or local immune complex deposition may play a role in the disease.[162,163]

Clinical Presentation

Patients with GCA commonly present with fever, weight loss, malaise, and headaches.[159,160] Polymyalgia rheumatica (PMR) often coexists or predates CGA. Proximal muscle weakness and tenderness are hallmarks of PMR.

The most common ocular complication of GCA is ischemic optic neuropathy (ION).[164] The larger vessels supplying the optic nerve become inflamed and result in an infarction of the optic nerve. Rarely, the retinal vessels may be involved, producing a branch or central retinal artery occlusion.[165] Attenuation of the retinal arterioles, disc pallor, and optic atrophy may develop late. Primary uveitis or retinitis is uncommon. Choroidal nonperfusion and infarction may be noted.[166] Ocular ischemia may occur and results in a secondary inflammation with marked flare and mild cellular infiltration.

Diagnosis

The diagnosis can be made clinically in an older patient with malaise, fever, weight loss, headache, jaw claudication, and sudden loss of vision in one or both (65%) eyes as a result of ischemic optic neuropathy.[159,160,164] The diagnosis can be supported by the presence of a markedly elevated ESR and C-reactive protein. Temporal artery biopsy may demonstrate a granulomatous vasculitis and infiltration of the vessel wall with mononuclear cells, histiocytes, and giant cells and loss of the internal elastic membrane.[161]

Differential Diagnosis

Nonarteritic ischemic optic neuropathy can present with a sudden loss of vision, but will not exhibit the other clinical and laboratory features of GCA or PMR.

Treatment

Untreated, this disease has a poor prognosis, with irreversible loss of vision secondary to ION and death due to coronary or cerebral vasculitis.[167] Therapy should be initiated rapidly and temporal artery biopsy obtained when temporal arteritis is suspected to prevent bilateral optic nerve involvement. Prednisone, 1 mg/kg per day, is the treatment of choice in temporal arteritis.[168] A slow taper over months to years may be required.[168] Alternative day therapy is not as effective as low-dose daily regimens. The ESR can be used to guide steroid dosage. Second-generation immunosuppressive agents can be considered in corticosteroid-intolerant patients.

Prognosis

GCA and PMR results in blindness at the time of diagnosis in 7% to 25% of patients.[168]

Wegener's Granulomatosis

Wegener's granulomatosis is a multisystem disease associated with a necrotizing granulomatous vasculitis.[114,169]

Etiology

The etiology is unknown. Wegener's granulomatosis is thought to be an autoimmune necrotizing vasculitis.[114,169]

Epidemiology

The disease is uncommon and occurs between the ages of 8 and 80 years. Men are affected more than women (3:2).[114]

Pathogenesis

Immune complex formation and deposition within the small to medium-sized vessels is thought to mediate the vasculitis.[169] Acute and chronic lesions can be found simultaneously in the involved tissues and organs. The vascular lesions have a mononuclear cell infiltration with fibrinoid necrosis. Multinucleated giant cells can be found in the surrounding granulomas.

Clinical Presentation

Characteristically, Wegener's granulomatosis involves the upper and lower respiratory tracts.[114,169,170] Epistaxis, rhinorrhea, sinusitis, otitis, chronic cough, and saddle nose deformity are frequently observed. Chronic pulmonary infiltrates, nodules, and cavitary lesions are found in the lungs. Wegener's vasculitis commonly affects the kidneys and the CNS. A granulomatous glomerulitis can be found in 80% of patients.

Wegener's granulomatosis may involve the eye in 40% to 50% of cases.[171] The eye may precede other organ involvement. Proptosis and orbital pain from pseudotumor is the most common ocular finding (45%). Scleritis, peripheral ulcerative keratitis, conjunctivitis, and dacryocystitis are also frequently noted ocular manifestations of Wegener's vasculitis.[171] Posterior scleritis in Wegener's granulomatosis behaves similar to scleritis in other rheumatologic disorders and presents with decreased

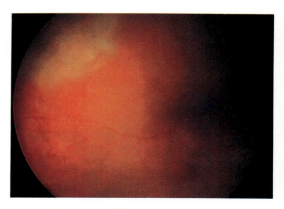

Figure 17.6. Type III hypersensitivity—Wegener's granulomatosis. Vitritis, retinal vasculitis, and peripheral geographic retinitis in a patient with Wegener's granulomatosis.

vision and pain. Secondary chorioretinal thickening and striae can be seen clinically and on fluorescein angiography. Uveitis, retinitis, and retinal vasculitis have been reported in 8% to 18% of cases (Fig. 17.6). Retinitis and retinal vasculitis in Wegener's granulomatosis may present as a geographic area of retinal edema and intraretinal hemorrhage, both of which can enlarge and be difficult to distinguish from a secondary opportunistic or viral retinitis.

Diagnosis

Wegener's granulomatosis should be suspected in patients with these ocular findings and respiratory, renal, or CNS involvement. The diagnosis can be supported by finding pneumonitis or cavitary lesions on chest radiograph.[114,169] Laboratory testing reveals an elevated white blood count, ESR, and serum IgA. Anti-neutrophilic cytoplasmic antibodies (ANCA) are present in this disease and are useful in advancing a diagnosis of Wegener's granulomatosis.[172,173] Biopsy of the involved tissue often establishes the diagnosis by revealing a granulomatous vasculitis.[174]

Differential Diagnosis

Lethal midline granuloma can involve the face but does not typically have pulmonary, renal, or ocular disease. Sarcoidosis can be characterized by chronic pulmonary disease and a granulomatous uveitis. Relapsing polychondritis may involve the nasal cartilage and cause a similar saddle-nose deformity.

Treatment

Wegener's granulomatosis is a serious and potentially fatal disease. Therapy should be designed to address both the ocular and systemic inflammation. Without therapy, the average survival is 5 months, with an 80% mortality rate by 1 year.[171,175] Corticosteroids prolong survival to 12.5 months. Cyclophosphamide (1–2 mg/kg per day), in combination with corticosteroids, is the treatment of choice, with a 90% remission rate. Maintenance therapy is required for 1 to 2 years and chronically for a subset of patients who relapse.

Prognosis

Immunosuppressive therapy is required to improve the prognosis for vision and life.

References

1. Opremcak EM. Collagen disorders: retinal manifestations of collagen vascular diseases. In: Albert DM, Jakobiec FA, eds. *Principles and Practice of Ophthalmology*. vol. 2. Philadelphia: WB Saunders; 1994:985.

2. Rodnan GP, Schumacher HR. The connective tissues: structure, function and metabolism. In: Rodnan GP, Schumacher RH, eds. *Primer on the Rheumatic Diseases*. 8th ed. Atlanta: Arthritis Foundation; 1983.

3. Hascall VC, Hascall GK. Proteoglycans. In: Hay ED, ed. *Proteoglycans, Cell Biology of Extracellular Matrix*. New York: Plenum Press; 1981.

4. Sanberg LB, Gray WR, Franzblau C, eds. *Elastin and Elastic Tissue*. New York: Plenum Press; 1977.

5. Friend J. Physiology of the cornea. In: Smolin G, Thoft RA, eds. *Cornea*. 2nd ed. Boston: Little, Brown; 1987.

6. Kelgren HJ. Epidemiology of rheumatoid arthritis. In: Dutker JJR, Alexander WRM, eds. *Rheumatic Diseases*. Baltimore: Williams & Wilkins; 1968

7. Calin A. Ankylosing spondylitis. In: Kelley WN, Harris ED Jr, Ruddy S, Sledge CB, eds. *Textbook of Rheumatology*. vol. 2, 2nd ed. Philadelphia: WB Saunders; 1985:993.

8. Brewerton DA, James DCO. The histocompatibility antigen (HLA-A27) and disease. *Semin Arthritis Rheum*. 1975;4:191.

9. Schlosstein L, Terasaki PI, Bluestone R, et al. High association of an HL-A antigen, W27 with ankylosing spondylitis. *N Engl J Med*. 1973;288:704.

10. Brewerton DA, Caffrey M, Hart FD, et al. Ankylosing spondylitis and HL-A27. *Lancet*. 1973;1:904.

11. Eastmond CJ, Calguneri M, Shinebaum R, et al. A sequential study of the relationship between fecal Klebsiella aerogenes and the common clinical manifestations of ankylosing spondylitis. *Ann Rheum Dis*. 1982;41:15.

12. Hare HF. Diagnosis of Marie-Strümpell arthritis with certain aspects of treatment. *N Engl J Med*. 1940;223:702.

13. Ball J. Enthesopathy of rheumatoid and ankylosing spondylitis. *Ann Rheum Dis*. 1971;30:213.

14. Brewerton DA, Chaffrey M, Nicholls A, et al. Acute anterior uveitis and HL-A27. *Lancet*. 1973;2:994.

15. Derhaag PJFM, de Waal LP, Linssen A, Feltkamp TEW. Acute anterior uveitis and HLA-B27 subtypes. *Invest Ophthalmol Vis Sci*. 1988;29:1137.

16. Tothova A, van Veenendaal WG, Lenssen A, et al. Clinical features of acute anterior uveitis. *Am J Ophthalmol*. 1987;103:137.

17. Iridocyclitis associated with arthritis syndromes (ankylosing spondylitis, Reiter's syndrome, juvenile rheumatoid arthritis). In: Smith RE, Nozik RA, eds. *Uveitis. A Clinical Approach to Diagnosis and Management*. 2nd ed. Baltimore: Williams & Wilkins; 1989:171.

18. Rosenbaum JT. Characterization of uveitis

associated with spondyloarthritis. *J Rheumatol.* 1989;16:792.

19. Belmont JB, Michelson JB. Vitrectomy in uveitis associated with ankylosing spondylitis. *Am J Ophthalmol.* 1982;94:300.

20. O'Duffy JD. Behçet's disease. In: Kelley WN, Harris ED Jr, Ruddy S, Sledge CB, eds. *Textbook of Rheumatology.* vol. 2, 2nd ed. Philadelphia: WB Saunders; 1985.

21. Numaga J, Kazumasas M, Mochizuki M, et al. An HLA-D region restriction fragment associated with refractory Behçet's disease. *Am J Ophthalmol.* 1988;105:528.

22. Mizuki N, Inoko H, Ando H, et al. Behçet's disease associated with one of the HLA-B51 subantigens, HLA-B 5101. *Am J Ophthalmol.* 1993;116:406.

23. Marquardt JL, Snyderman R, Oppenheim J. Depression of lymphocyte transformation and exacerbation of Behçet's syndrome by ingestion of English walnuts. *Cell Immunol.* 1973;9:263.

24. Aoki K, Fujioka K, Katsumata H, et al. Epidemiologic studies on Behçet's disease in Hokkaido district (Japanese). *J Clin Ophthalmol.* 1971;25:2239.

25. Michelson JB, Chisari VF. Behçet's disease. *Surv Ophthalmol.* 1982;26:190.

26. James DG, Spiteri MA. Behçet's disease. *Ophthalmology.* 1982;89:1279.

27. Chajek T, Fainaru M. Behçet's disease: report of 41 cases and a review of the literature. *Medicine.* 1975;54:179.

28. Colvard DM, Robertson DM, O'Duffy JD. The ocular manifestations of Behçet's disease. *Arch Ophthalmol.* 1977;95:1813.

29. Behçet's Disease Research Committee of Japan. Behçet's disease; guide to diagnosis of Behçet's disease. *Jpn J Ophthalmol.* 1974; 18:291.

30. Lehner T, Adinolfi M. Acute phase proteins, C9, factor B and lysozyme in recurrent oral ulceration and Behçet's syndrome. *J Clin Pathol.* 1980;33:269.

31. Hijakata K, Masuda K. Visual prognosis in Behçet's: effects of cyclophosphamide and colchicine. *Jpn J Ophthalmol.* 1978;22:506.

32. O'Duffy JD, Robertson DM, Goldstein NP. Chlorambucil in the treatment of uveitis and meningoencephalitis of Behçet's disease. *Am J Med.* 1984;76:75.

33. Tabbara KF. Chlorambucil in Behçet's disease. A reappraisal. *Ophthalmology.* 1983; 90:906.

34. Nussenblatt RB, Palestine AG, Chan CC. Effectiveness of cyclosporin therapy in Behçet's disease. *Arthritis Rheum.* 1985;28:671.

35. Assuman Ü, Müftüoglu H, Pazarli S, et al. Treatment of ocular involvement in Behçet's disease with ciclosporin A (preliminary report). In: Schindler R, ed. *Ciclosporin in Autoimmune Diseases.* Berlin: Springer-Verlag; 1985:147.

36. BenEzra D, Brodsky M, Peér J, et al. Ciclosporin (CyA) versus conventional therapy in Behçet's disease. Preliminary observations of a masked study. In: Schindler R, ed. *Ciclosporin in Autoimmune Diseases.* Berlin: Springer-Verlag; 1985:158.

37. Masuda K, Nakajima A. A double-masked study of ciclosporin treatment in Behçet's disease. In: Schindler R, ed. *Ciclosporin in Autoimmune Diseases.* Berlin: Springer-Verlag; 1985:162.

38. Pezzi PP, Gasparri V, de Liso P, Catarinelli G. Prognosis in Behçet's disease. *Ann Ophthalmol.* 1985;17:20.

39. Bradley WG. Inflammatory diseases of muscle. In: Kelley WN, Harris ED Jr, Ruddy S, Sledge CB, eds. *Textbook of Rheumatology.* vol. 2, 2nd ed. Philadelphia: WB Saunders; 1985.

40. Stevens AM, Johnson FC. A new eruptive fever associated with stomatitis and ophthalmia: report of two cases in children. *Am J Dis Child.* 1922;24:526.

41. Huff JC, Swinehart JM, Weston WL, et al. Immune complexes involving herpes antigen in erythema multiforme. *Clin Res.* 1979;27:242A.

42. Harrison SM, Frenkel M, Grossman BJ, et al. Retinopathy in childhood dermatomyositis. *Am J Ophthalmol.* 1973;76:786.

43. Bruce GM. Retinitis in dermatomyositis. *Trans Am Ophthalmol Soc.* 1938;36:282.

44. Stevens AM, Johnson FC. A new eruptive fever associated with stomatitis and ophthalmia: report of two cases in children. *Am J Dis Child.* 1922;24:526.

45. Lozada F, Silverman S Jr. Erythema multiforme: clinical characteristics and natural history in fifty patients. *Oral Surg Oral Med Oral Pathol.* 1978;46:628.

46. Kazmierowski JA, Wuepper KD. Erythema

multiforme: immune complex vasculitis of the superficial cutaneous microvasculature. *J Invest Dermatol.* 1978;71:366.

47. Imamura S, Yanase K, Taniguchi S, et al. Erythema multiforme: demonstration of immune complexes in the sera and skin lesions. *Br J Dermatol.* 1980;102:161.

48. Wuepper KD, Watson PA, Kazmiecrowski JA. Immune complexes in erythema multiforme and the Stevens-Johnson syndrome. *J Invest Dermatol.* 1980;74:368.

49. Huff JC, Swinehart JM, Weston WL, et al. Immune complexes involving herpes antigen in erythema multiforme. *Clin Res.* 1979;27:242A.

50. Foster CS, Fong LP, Azar D, Kenyon KR. Episodic conjunctival inflammation after Stevens-Johnson syndrome. *Ophthalmology.* 1988;95:453.

51. Farmer RG, Hawk WA, Turnbull RB Jr. Clinical patterns in Crohn's disease: a statistical study of 615 cases. *Gastroenterology.* 1975;68:627.

52. Good AE, Utsinger PD. Enteropathic arthritis. In: Kelley WN, Harris ED Jr, Rudd S, Sledge B, eds. *Textbook of Rheumatology.* Vol. 2, 2nd ed. Philadelphia: WB Saunders; 1987.

53. Knox DL, Schachat AP, Mustonen E. Primary, secondary and coincidental ocular complications of Crohn's disease. *Ophthalmology.* 1984;91:163.

54. Talbot RW, Heppell J, Dozois RR, Beart RW Jr. Vascular complications of inflammatory bowel disease. *Mayo Clin Proc.* 1986;61:140.

55. Schulman MF, Sugar A. Peripheral corneal infiltrates in inflammatory bowel disease. *Ann Ophthalmol.* 1981;15:109.

56. Salmon JF, Wright JP, Murray ADN. Ocular inflammation in Crohn's disease. *Ophthalmology.* 1991;98:480.

57. Petrelli EA, McKinley M, Troncale FJ. Ocular manifestations of inflammatory bowel disease. *Ann Ophthalmol.* 1982; 356.

58. Macoul KL. Ocular changes in granulomatous ileocolitis. *Arch Ophthalmol.* 1970;84:95.

59. Salmon JF, Wright JP, Bowen RM, Murray AD. Granulomatous uveitis in Crohn's disease. *Arch Ophthalmol.* 1989;107:718.

60. Ernst BB, Lowder CY, Meisler DM, Gutman FA. Posterior segment manifestations of inflammatory bowel disease. *Ophthalmology.* 1991;98:1272.

61. Ruby AJ, Jampol LM. Crohn's disease and retinal vascular disease. *Am J Ophthalmol.* 1990;110:349.

62. Duker JS, Brown GC, Brooks L. Retinal vasculitis in Crohn's disease. *Am J Ophthalmol.* 1987;103:664.

63. Cassidy JT. Juvenile rheumatoid arthritis. In: Kelley WN, Harris ED Jr, Ruddy S, Sledge CB, eds. *Textbook of Rheumatology.* vol. 2, 2nd ed. Philadelphia: WB Saunders; 1985.

64. Anterior uveitis. In: Nussenblatt RB, Palestine AG, eds. *Uveitis. Fundamentals and Clinical Practice.* Chicago: Year Book Medical Publishers; 1989:164.

65. Laaksonen A-L. A prognostic study of juvenile rheumatoid arthritis. Analysis of 544 cases. *Acta Paediatr Scand* 1966; (suppl 166).

66. Kanski JJ. Juvenile arthritis and uveitis. *Surv Ophthalmol.* 1990;34:253.

67. Bywaters EGL. Pathologic aspects of juvenile chronic polyarthritis. *Arthritis Rheum.* 1977;20:271.

68. Munthe E. Complexes of IgG and IgG rheumatoid factor in synovial tissues of juvenile rheumatoid arthritis. *Scand J Rheumatol.* 1972;1:153.

69. Kanski JJ, Shun-Shin GA. Systemic uveitis syndromes in childhood: an analysis of 340 cases. *Ophthalmology.* 1984;91:1247.

70. Giles CL. Uveitis in childhood: part I anterior. *Ann Ophthalmol.* 1989;21:13.

71. Kanski JJ. Anterior uveitis in juvenile rheumatoid arthritis. *Arch Ophthalmol.* 1977;95:1794.

72. Olson NY, Lindsley CB, Godfrey WA. Nonsteroidal anti-inflammatory drug therapy in chronic childhood iridocyclitis. *Am J Dis Child,* 1988;142:1289.

73. Lovell DJ, Giannini EW, Brewer EJ Jr. Time course of response to nonsteroidal antiinflammatory drugs in juvenile rheumatoid arthritis. *Arthritis Rheum.* 1984;27:1433.

74. Kanski JJ. Uveitis in juvenile rheumatoid arthritis: incidence, clinical features and prognosis. *Eye.* 1988;2:641.

75. Diamond JG, Kaplan HL. Lensectomy and vitrectomy for complicated cataract secondary to uveitis. *Arch Ophthalmol.* 1978; 96:1798.

76. Fox GM, Flynn HW Jr, Davis JL, Culbertson W. Causes of reduced visual acuity on long-term follow-up after cataract extraction in patients with uveitis and juvenile rheumatoid arthritis. *Am J Ophthalmol.* 1992;114:708.

77. Smiley WK. The eye in juvenile rheumatoid arthritis. *Trans Ophthalmol Soc UK.* 1974;94:817.

78. Kanski JJ, McAllister JA. Trabeculodialysis for inflammatory glaucoma in children and young adults. *Ophthalmology.* 1985;92:927.

79. Wright V. Psoriatic arthritis. In: Kelley WN, Harris ED Jr, Ruddy S, Sledge CB, eds. *Textbook of Rheumatology.* vol. 2, 2nd ed. Philadelphia: WB Saunders; 1985.

80. Lomholt G. Psoriasis: prevalence, spontaneous course and genetics. *Copenhagen Gad.* 1963.

81. McClusky OE, Cordon RE, Arnett FC Jr. HL-A27 in Reiter's syndrome and psoriatic arthritis: a genetic factor in disease susceptibility and expression. *J Rheumatol.* 1974;1:263.

82. Laurent MR, Panayi GS, Shepherd P. Circulating immune complexes, serum immunoglobulins, and acute phase proteins in psoriasis and psoriatic arthritis. *Ann Rheum Dis.* 1981;40:66.

83. Knox DL. Psoriasis and intraocular inflammation. *Trans Am Ophthalmol Soc.* 1979;127:210.

84. Black RL, O'Brien WM, Van Scott EJ, et al. Methotrexate therapy in psoriatic arthritis. *JAMA.* 1964;189:743.

85. Ellis CH, Gorsulowsky DC, Hamilton TA, et al. Cyclosporine improves psoriasis in a double-blind study. *JAMA.* 1986;256:3110.

86. Calin A. Reiter's syndrome. In: Kelley WN, Harris ED Jr, Ruddy S, Sledge CB, eds. *Textbook of Rheumatology.* vol. 2, 2nd ed. Philadelphia: WB Saunders; 1985.

87. Keat A. Reiter's syndrome and reactive arthritis in perspective. *N Engl J Med.* 1983;309:1606.

88. Brewerton K, Ahvonen PI, Alkio P, et al. Reiter's disease and HLA 27. *Lancet.* 1973;2:996.

89. Lee DA, Barker SM, Su WPD, et al. The clinical diagnosis of Reiter's syndrome. Ophthalmic and nonophthalmic aspects. *Ophthalmology.* 1986;93:350.

90. Luxenberg MN. Reiter's keratoconjunctivitis. *Arch Ophthalmol.* 1990;108:280.

91. Mark DB, McCulley JB. Reiter's keratitis. *Arch Ophthalmol.* 1982;100:781.

92. Farber GA, Forshner JG, O'Quinn SE. Reiter's syndrome treatment with methotrexate. *JAMA.* 1967;200:171.

93. Herman JH. Polychondritis. In: Kelley WN, Harris ED Jr, Ruddy S, Sledge CB, eds. *Textbook of Rheumatology.* vol. 2, 2nd ed. Philadelphia: WB Saunders; 1985.

94. McAdam LP, O'Hanllan MA, Bluestone R, et al. Relapsing polychondritis: prospective study of 23 patients and a review of the literature. *Medicine.* 1976;55:193.

95. Foidart J-M, Abe S, Marin GR, et al. Antibodies to type II collagen in relapsing polychondritis. *N Engl J Med.* 1978;299:1203.

96. Isaak BL, Liesang TJ, Michet CJ. Ocular and systemic findings in relapsing polychondritis. *Ophthalmology.* 1986;93:681.

97. Magargal LE, Donoso LA, Goldberg RE, et al. Ocular manifestations of relapsing polychondritis. *Retina.* 1981;1:96.

98. Hoang-Xuan Thanh, Foster CS, Rice BA. Scleritis in relapsing polychondritis: response to therapy. *Ophthalmology.* 1990;97:892.

99. Barranco VP, Minor DB, Solomon H. Treatment of relapsing polychondritis with dapsone. *Arch Dermatol.* 1976;112:1286.

100. Harris ED Jr. Rheumatoid arthritis: the clinical spectrum. In: Kelley WN, Harris ED Jr, Ruddy S, Sledge CB, eds. *Textbook of Rheumatology.* vol. 2, 2nd ed. Philadelphia: WB Saunders; 1985.

101. Kelgren HJ. Epidemiology of rheumatoid arthritis. In: Dutker JJR, Alexander WRM, eds. *Rheumatic Diseases.* Baltimore: Williams & Wilkins; 1968.

102. Stastny P. Mixed lymphocyte cultures in rheumatoid arthritis. *J Clin Invest.* 1976;57:1148.

103. Torrigiana G, Roitt IM. Antiglobulin factors in sera from patients with rheumatoid arthritis and normal subjects. *Ann Rheum Dis.* 1977;3:315.

104. Barr CC, Davis H, Culbertson WW. Rheumatoid scleritis. *Ophthalmology.* 1981;88:1269.

105. Watson PG, Hayreh SS. Scleritis and episcleritis. *Br J Ophthalmol.* 1976;60:163.

106. Benson WE, Shields JA, Tasman W, et al. Posterior scleritis: a cause of diagnostic confusion. *Arch Ophthalmol.* 1979;97:1482.

107. Singh G, Guthoff R, Foster CS. Observation on long-term follow-up of posterior scleritis. *Am J Ophthalmol.* 1986;101:570.

108. Fraunfelder FT, Watson PG. Evaluation of eyes enucleated for scleritis. *Br J Ophthalmol.* 1976;60:227.

109. Sarnat RL, Jampol LM. Hyperviscosity retinopathy secondary to polyclonal gammopathy in a patient with rheumatoid arthritis. *Ophthalmologyj.* 1986;93:124.

110. Watson PG. The diagnosis and management of scleritis. *Ophthalmology.* 1980;87:716.

111. Foster CS. Immunosuppressive therapy for external ocular inflammatory disease. *Ophthalmology.* 1980;8:148.

112. Mondino BJ, Phinney RB. Treatment of scleritis with combined oral prednisone and indomethacin therapy. *Am J Ophthalmol.* 1988;106:473.

113. Foster CS, Forstot SL, Wilson LA. Mortality rate in rheumatoid arthritis patients developing necrotizing scleritis or peripheral ulcerative keratitis. *Ophthalmology.* 1984;91:1253.

114. Conn DL, Hunder GG. Necrotizing vasculitis. In: Kelley WN, Harris ED Jr, Ruddy S, Sledge CB, eds. *Textbook of Rheumatology.* vol. 2, 2nd ed. Philadelphia: WB Saunders; 1985.

115. Christian CL, Sargent JS. Vasculitis syndromes, clinical and experimental models. *Am J Med.* 1976;61:385.

116. Gocke DJ, HSU K, Morgan C, et al. Association between polyarteritis and Australia antigen. *Lancet.* 1970;2:1149.

117. Stillerman ML. Ocular manifestations of diffuse collagen disease. *Arch Ophthalmol.* 1951;45:239.

118. Purcell JJ Jr, Birkenkamp R, Tsai CC. Conjunctival lesions in periarteritis nodosa. A clinical and immunopathologic study. *Arch Ophthalmol.* 1984;102:736.

119. Akova YA, Jabbur NS, Foster CS. Ocular presentation of polyarteritis nodosa. Clinical course and management with steroid and cytotoxic therapy. *Ophthalmology.* 1993;100:1775.

120. Goar EL, Smith LS. Polyarteritis nodosa of the eye. *Am J Ophthalmol.* 1952;35:1619.

121. Lanham JG, Elkon KB, Pusey CD, Hughes GR. Systemic vasculitis with asthma and eosinophilia: a clinical approach to the Churg-Strauss syndrome. *Medicine.* 1984;63:65.

122. Ashton N, Cook C. Allergic granulomatous nodules of the eyelid and conjunctiva. *Am J Ophthalmol.* 1978;87:1.

123. Shields CL, Shields JA, Rozanski TI. Conjunctival involvement in Churg-Strauss syndrome. *Am J Ophthalmol.* 1986;102:601.

124. Cury D, Breakey AS, Payne BF. Allergic granulomatous angiitis associated with uveoscleritis and papilledema. *Arch Ophthalmol.* 1955;261.

125. Weinstein JM, Chuy HC, Lane S, et al. Churg-Strauss syndrome (allergic granulomatous angiitis). *Arch Ophthalmol.* 1983;101:1217.

126. Cogan DG. Syndrome of nonsyphilitic interstitial keratitis and vestibuloauditory symptoms. *Arch Ophthalmol.* 1945;33:144.

127. Cheson BD, Bluming AZ, Alroy J. Cogan's syndrome: a systemic vasculitis. *Am J Med.* 1976;60:549.

128. Cobo LM, Haynes BF. Early corneal findings in Cogan's syndrome. *Ophthalmology.* 1984;91:903.

129. Maxeiner SR Jr, McDonald JR, Kirklin JW. Muscle biopsy in the diagnosis of periarteritis nodosa: an evaluation. *Surg Clin North Am.* 1952;10:1225.

130. Dahl EV, Baggenstoss AH, DeWeerd JH. Testicular lesions of periarteritis nodosa, with special reference to diagnosis. *Am J Med.* 1960;28:222.

131. Fauci AS, Doppman JL, Wolff SM. Cyclophosphamide-induced remissions in advanced polyarteritis nodosa. *Am J Med.* 1978;64:890.

132. LeRoy EC. Scleroderma (systemic sclerosis). In: Kelley WN, Harris ED Jr, Ruddy S, Sledge CB, eds. *Textbook of Rheumatology.* vol. 2, 2nd ed. Philadelphia: WB Saunders; 1985.

133. Maricq HR, LeRoy EC. Progressive systemic sclerosis: disorders of the microcirculation. *Clin Rheum Dis.* 1979;5:81.

134. Cohen S, Johnson AR, Hurd E. Cytotoxicity of sera from patients with scleroderma. *Arthritis Rheum.* 1975;18:525.

135. Stuart JM, Postlewaite AE, Kang AH. Evidence for cell-mediated immunity to col-

lagen in progressive systemic sclerosis. *J Lab Clin Med.* 1976;88:601.

136. Horan EC: Ophthalmic manifestations of progressive systemic sclerosis. *Br J Ophthalmol.* 1969;53:388.

137. Pollack IP, Becker B. Cystoid bodies of the retina in a patient with scleroderma. *Am J Ophthalmol.* 1962;54:655.

138. Farkas TG, Sylvester V, Archer D. The choroidopathy of progressive systemic sclerosis (scleroderma). *Am J Ophthalmol.* 1972;74:875.

139. Medsger TA, Masi AT, Rodnan GP, et al. Survival with systemic sclerosis (scleroderma): a life-table analysis of 309 patients. *Ann Intern Med.* 1971;75:369.

140. Whaley K, Alspaugh MA. Sjögren's syndrome. In: Kelley WN, Harris ED Jr, Ruddy S, Sledge CB, eds. *Textbook of Rheumatology.* vol. 2, 2nd ed. Philadelphia: WB Saunders; 1985.

141. Brown SI, Grayson M. Marginal furrows: a characteristic corneal lesion of rheumatoid arthritis. *Arch Ophthalmol.* 1968;79:563.

142. Rosenbaum JY, Bennett RM. Chronic anterior and posterior uveitis and primary Sjögren's syndrome. *Am J Ophthalmol.* 1987; 104:346.

143. Farmer SG, Kinyoun MD, Nelson JL, et al. Retinal vasculitis associated with autoantibodies to Sjögren's syndrome A antigen. *Am J Ophthalmol.* 1985;100:814.

144. Tabbara KF, Frayha RA. Alternate-day steroid therapy for patients with primary Sjögren's syndrome. *Ann Ophthalmol.* 1983; 15:358.

145. Zvaifler NJ, Woods VL Jr. Etiology and pathogenesis of systemic lupus erythematosus. In: Kelley WN, Harris ED Jr, Ruddy S, Sledge CB, eds. *Textbook of Rheumatology.* vol. 2, 2nd ed. Philadelphia: WB Saunders; 1985.

146. Decker JL, Steinberg AD, Gershwin ME, et al. Systemic lupus erythematosus: contrasts and comparisons. *Ann Intern Med.* 1975;82:391.

147. Mintz G, Fraga A. Arteritis in systemic lupus erythematosus. *Arch Intern Med.* 1965; 116:55.

148. Levine SR, Crofts JW, Lesse GR, et al. Visual symptoms associated with the presence of a lupus anticoagulant. *Ophthalmology.* 1988;95:686.

149. Estes D, Christian CL. The natural history of systemic lupus erythematosus by prospective analysis. *Medicine.* 1971;50:85.

150. Baehr G, Klemperer R, Schifrin A. A diffuse disease of the peripheral circulation (usually associated with lupus erythematosus and endocarditis). *Trans Assoc Am Phys.* 1935;50:139.

151. Gold DH, Morris DA, Henkind P. Ocular findings in systemic lupus erythematosus. *Br J Ophthalmol.* 1972;56:800.

152. Gold D, Feiner L, Henkind P. Retinal arterial occlusive disease in systemic lupus erythematosus. *Arch Ophthalmol.* 1977;95: 1580.

153. Vine AK, Barr CC. Proliferative Lupus retinopathy. *Arch Ophthalmol.* 1984;102:852.

154. Jabs DA, Fine SL, Hochberg MC, et al. Severe retinal vaso-occlusive disease in systemic lupus erythematosus. *Arch Ophthalmol.* 1986;104:558.

155. Gold D, Feiner L, Henkind P. Retinal arterial occlusive disease in systemic lupus erythematosus. *Arch Ophthalmol.* 1977;95: 1580.

156. Coppeto J, Lessell S. Retinopathy in systemic lupus erythematosus. *Arch Ophthalmol.* 1977;95:794.

157. Jabs DA, Hanneken AM, Schachat AP, et al. Choroidopathy in systemic lupus erythematosus. *Arch Ophthalmol.* 1988;106:230.

158. Wong K, Everett A, Jones JV, et al. Visual loss as the initial symptom of systemic lupus erythematosus. *Am J Ophthalmol.* 1981; 92:238.

159. Huston KA, Hunder GC, Lie JT, et al. Temporal arteritis. A 25 year epidemiological, clinical and pathological study. *Ann Intern Med.* 1978;88:162.

160. Hunder GG, Hazleman BL. Giant cell arteritis and polymyalgia rheumatica. In: Kelley WN, Harris ED Jr, Ruddy S, Sledge CB, eds. *Textbook of Rheumatology.* vol. 2, 2nd ed. Philadelphia: WB Saunders; 1985.

161. Albert DM, Searl SS, Craft JL. Histologic and ultrastructural characteristics of temporal arteritis. *Ophthalmology.* 1982;89:1111.

162. Papaioannou CC, Gupta RC, Hunder GG, McDuffie FC. Circulating immune complexes in giant cell arteritis polymyalgia rheumatica. *Arthritis Rheum.* 1980;23:1021.

163. Radda TM, Pehamberger H, Smolen J, Menzel J. Ocular manifestation of temporal

arteritis: immunologic studies. *Arch Ophthalmol.* 1981;99:487.

164. Keltner JL. Giant-cell arteritis. *Ophthalmology.* 1982;89:1101.

165. Whitfield JH, Bateman M, Cooke WT. Temporal arteritis. *Br J Ophthalmol.* 1963;47:555.

166. Quillen DA, Cantore WA, Schwartz SR, et al. Choroidal nonperfusion in giant cell arteritis. *Am J Ophthalmol.* 1993;116:171.

167. Cullen JF, Colier JA. Ophthalmic complications of giant cell arteritis. *Surv Ophthalmol.* 1976;20:247.

168. Aiello PD, Trautmann JC, McPhee TJ, et al. Visual prognosis in giant cell arteritis. *Ophthalmology.* 1993;100:550.

169. Goodman GC, Churg J. Wegener's granulomatosis: pathology and review of the literature. *Arch Pathol.* 1954;58:533.

170. Robin JB, Schanzlin DJ, Meisler DM, et al. Ocular involvement in the respiratory vasculitides. *Surv Ophthalmol.* 1985;30:127.

171. Bullen CL, Liesegang TJ, McDonald TJ, et al. Ocular complications of Wegener's granulomatosis. *Ophthalmology.* 1983;90:279.

172. Pulido JS, Goeken JA, Nerad JA, et al. Ocular manifestations of patients with circulating antineutrophilic cytoplasmic antibodies. *Arch Ophthalmol.* 1990;108:845.

173. Soukiasian SH, Foster CS, Niles JL, Raizman MB. Diagnostic value of antineutrophil cytoplasmic antibodies in scleritis associated with Wegener's granulomatosis. *Ophthalmology.* 1992;99:125.

174. Kalina PH, Lie JT, Campbell RJ, Garrity JA. Diagnostic value and limitations or orbital biopsy in Wegener's granulomatosis. *Ophthalmology.* 1992;99:120.

175. Fauci AS, Haynes BF, Katz P. The spectrum of vasculitis: clinical pathologic, immunologic and therapeutic considerations. *Ann Intern Med.* 1978;89:660.

18
Type IV Hypersensitivity

The diseases presented in this section are idiopathic or have a presumed type IV hypersensitivity mechanism. In certain diseases the evidence for a cell-mediated process is well supported. Histopathology, immunohistopathology, lymphocyte proliferation assays, animal models of diseases, and response to certain drugs that target T cells suggest such a pathogenesis.

In other disorders, the evidence for such a pathophysiologic mechanism is less compelling. Indeed, several disorders are included in this section because there is a lack of evidence to support an infectious etiology or type I, II, or III hypersensitivity reaction.

Skin Disorders

Contact Dermatitis—Lids

Contact dermatitis of the eyelids is an allergic, type IV hypersensitivity reaction in the skin.[1]

Etiology

Lipid-soluble, low-molecular weight haptens and other allergens form a covalent bond with the skin proteins. Ophthalmic preparations including atropine, neomycin, thimerosal, and other preservatives can cause this response.

Epidemiology

Contact dermatitis affects all ages, races, and both sexes.

Pathogenesis

The binding of chemicals to skin proteins results in an altered self-protein.[2] Antigen presentation by Langerhans' cells and regional lymph node processing causes a sensitization and proliferation of antigen-specific T-cell clones. These cells then home to the affected area of the skin. This disease can be studied in animal models in which the dermatitis can be adoptively transferred to a naive animal through T lymphocytes and not by humoral factor in serum. These findings support a true cell-mediated, type IV hypersensitivity mechanism.

Clinical Presentation

Contact dermatitis causes an irritation and itching. The skin becomes warm and edematous[1] (Fig. 18.1). Symptoms peak 24 to 48 hours after the contact. The reaction is often unilateral unless the drug or agent has been in contact with both eyelids.

Diagnosis

The history of exposure to drugs, antibiotics, or poison ivy and the development of a unilateral dermatitis can support the diagnosis, which can be confirmed by a patch test and skin testing.

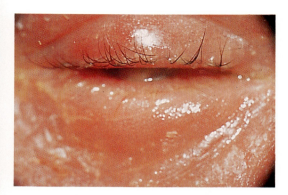

Figure 18.1. Type IV hypersensitivity—contact dermatitis. Lid edema and contact dermatitis from hypersensitivity to topical neomycin.

Differential Diagnosis

Atopic dermatitis may appear similar to contact dermatitis, but it is chronic and more generalized.

Treatment

Treatment involves avoiding the causative agent. The history of allergy should be noted on medical records to avoid similar reaction. Topical corticosteroid creams (hydrocortisone 1%) can be applied for local relief. In severe or widespread disease, such as caused by poison ivy, a short course of oral corticosteroids may be necessary.

Prognosis

The prognosis is good.

Sclera/Conjunctiva/Cornea

Phlyctenulosis

Phlyctenulosis is a type IV autoimmune hypersensitivity reaction that occurs in the conjunctiva and cornea.[3]

Etiology

The etiology of phlyctenulosis is frequently staphylococcal proteins from the eyelids.[3]

Historically, tuberculin proteins were thought to cause this condition as well.

Epidemiology

Phlyctenulosis can occur at any age and in all races. It is more common in males.

Pathogenesis

A local type IV hypersensitivity reaction occurs in the conjunctiva or cornea, often where the resting eyelid crosses the limbus. Lymphocytes and plasma cells are found on pathologic examination.

Clinical Presentation

Photophobia, blepharospasm, and mild itching are symptoms of phlyctenulosis.[3] Sectoral conjunctival hyperemia often surrounds a small, whitish foci or "microabscess." Lesions in the cornea may scar.

Diagnosis

The diagnosis can be made clinically.

Differential Diagnosis

Nodular episcleritis, foreign bodies, herpes simplex, and limbal vernal keratoconjunctivitis may all be considered.

Treatment

Treatment of an underlying blepharitis may be necessary. Lid scrubs and topical antibiotic ointment can eliminate the chronic infection. Short-term use of topical corticosteroid preparations may effect a rapid resolution.

Prognosis

The prognosis is good.

Iris and Ciliary Body

Idiopathic Iridocyclitis

Idiopathic iritis and iridocyclitis are inflammations involving the anterior structures of the uveal tract that are not associated with another specific systemic or ocular syndrome.[4,5]

Etiology

The etiology for most cases of idiopathic iritis and iridocyclitis is not known. No infectious agent has been routinely identified.

Epidemiology

Idiopathic anterior uveitis is the most common form of uveitis, occurring in 8 to 12/ 100,000 population.[4-6] There is a strong association (50% of patients) between human leukocyte antigen HLA-B27 and acute anterior uveitis.[7-9]

Pathogenesis

Immunohistochemical studies from iris biopsy specimens in idiopathic iritis have identified T lymphocytes predominantly, with no evidence for vasculitis or antibody deposition. Even quiet eyes with a history of iritis show a resident population of T cells, suggesting a T cell–associated immune mechanism.[10] Defects in T-cell regulation have been demonstrated in patients with idiopathic anterior uveitis.[11] Infectious microorganisms have not been seen. Other factors such as triggering infectious agents and trauma may play a role in a genetically susceptible patient.

Clinical Presentation

Patients with acute forms of uveitis present to the practitioner with ocular pain, photophobia, and mild tenderness.[4,5] Tearing and redness are common. More chronic forms, particularly in children, may be asymptomatic, and accurate diagnosis depends on biomicroscopic examination. Blurred vision may occur because of media opacity such as cataract or vitreous debris or secondary to cystoid macular edema (CME).

Ocular examination may reveal conjunctival hyperemia, characteristically at the limbus, creating a "limbal flush" (see Fig. 2.11). The hallmark of iritis, however, is the presence of inflammatory cells and aqueous flare in the anterior chamber (see Fig. 2.8). In iridocyclitis there may be some "spillover" cells into the anterior vitreous. These cells characteristically circulate in the anterior chamber because of the normal aqueous currents (see Fig. 2.9). When the iritis is severe, inflammatory cells may collect in the anterior chamber and form a hypopyon (see Fig. 2.10). The severity of the cellular reaction can be graded to assist in determining treatment response.

Inflammatory cells may precipitate on the corneal endothelium and form keratitic precipitates (KP) (see Fig. 2.3). In idiopathic iritis, the KPs are small and fine. The presence of granulomatous KPs often indicates an underlying systemic disorder.

The inflamed iris is typically miotic (see Fig. 2.11). If the inflammation is chronic or severe, the iris may adhere to the peripheral cornea or the anterior lens capsule, resulting in anterior and posterior synechiae, respectively.

Patients with HLA-B27–associated iridocyclitis appear to have a clinical course distinct from HLA-B27–negative patients.[12] Patients with B27 haplotype are younger, have a higher male/female ratio, more unilateral disease, more severe inflammation, and no granulomatous KPs. Ocular complications are also more common in this subgroup.

Diagnosis

It is common practice to view the first episode of a mild, anterior uveitis as an idiopathic, "garden variety" iritis. Other than a review of systems and a general physical examination to detect signs of an associated systemic disorder, attempts to establish an etiology for the inflammation are not typically rewarding. A differential diagnosis is generated and a laboratory evaluation designed, however, for those patients with recurrent, severe, medically unresponsive forms of iritis or those patients with evidence of an underlying systemic disease.

Differential Diagnosis

The differential diagnosis for iridocyclitis is provided earlier in Table 3.2. The history, review of systems, and physical and ocular examinations provide the information to manage a patient with iritis. It is important to note that several forms of uveitis may begin primarily as an anterior uveitis and evolve into a more posterior or diffuse form. Nongranulomatous forms of uveitis also may become granulomatous with time. Furthermore, patients without evidence for systemic involvement at the initial presentation may develop such evidence over the course of the illness.

Treatment

If a specific disease process can be identified, basic knowledge about the predominant pathophysiologic mechanism should be used to address the inflammation.[5] For example, if herpes simplex, herpes zoster, syphilis, tuberculosis, or toxoplasmosis is responsible for the iridocyclitis, then antiviral, antibacterial, or antiprotozoal agents should be administered by the most effective routes. Similarly, if the etiology of iritis is due to a poorly fit intraocular lens or to phacogenic uveitis, then surgical removal of the implant or any remaining lens antigens from the eye will effect a favorable response where medical therapy has failed. Finally, if a systemic disease is diagnosed, such as relapsing polychondritis, juvenile rheumatoid arthritis, Behçet's disease, or sarcoidosis, attention should be directed toward management of the systemic process. Often, with control of the underlying illness, the intraocular inflammation also subsides.

Because of the anterior nature of idiopathic iridocyclitis, the inflammation can be treated through the use of topically applied medications. Standard treatment regimens include the use of mydriatics, cycloplegics, and topical corticosteroid preparations. The rationale and principles of topical medical therapy are discussed in Chapter 5.

In general, therapy with corticosteroids should be initiated at a high dosing schedule. One drop every hour should be recommended, with a taper according to the clinical response. If the patient responds to the treatment with improvement in the intraocular cell, the medication can be tapered. On the other hand, if a patient demonstrates persistent or increased cellular reaction, the medications should be either maintained or increased. It is not uncommon for the patient to experience a flare-up while on a tapering course of medication. This information is helpful and can be used to determine a maintenance dose of drug required to control the disease. Intraocular pressures should be monitored while on topical corticosteroid drops to detect a steroid-induced glaucoma.

Topical, nonsteroidal anti-inflammatory drugs may play a role in sparing the amount of topical corticosteroids required to control the disease. Topical cyclosporin may prove beneficial in treating iridocyclitis.

Prognosis

The prognosis is good in idiopathic iridocyclitis if the inflammation is controlled in a timely fashion. Patients with the presence of HLA-B27 may have a higher complication rate, including cataract, glaucoma, and macular edema.[12]

Fuchs' Heterochromic Iridocyclitis (FHI)

Fuchs' heterochromic iridocyclitis (FHI) is an insidious, chronic anterior uveitis originally described by Fuchs at the turn of the century.[13]

Etiology

The etiology for FHI is unknown. Hereditary factors, toxic, sympathetic degeneration, vascular insufficiency, and infectious
and autoimmune mechanisms have all
been postulated. To date no one mechanism has proven to be present in patients
with FHI.[14–20]

Epidemiology

FHI may account for 2% to 5% of all cases
of uveitis.[21] It usually occurs in the third to
fourth decade of life. This disorder is typically unilateral but may be bilateral in 1%
to 15% of cases. There is no known HLA association. FHI has been reported in identical twins.[22]

Pathogenesis

Iris stromal atrophy and depigmentation
is noted on histology.[22] The iris sphincter
and dilator muscles become fibrotic. Fine
iris neovascularization is noted on the iris
surface. Lymphocytes and plasma cells
can be found within the remaining iris
stroma, suggesting a cell-mediated immune
response.[23] Recent studies have not demonstrated specific immune complex deposition or T-cell subsets in FHI.[17,18]
Histopathologic studies in FHI may be influenced by the stage of the disease at the
time of tissue sampling.

Clinical Presentation

The eye is most often white, "quiet," and
comfortable.[13,21] Early in the course of the
disease and in severe attacks, the eye may
rarely become hyperemic and painful.
More often, the disease is asymptomatic
and is picked up on routine examination.
Patients complain of floaters and blurred
vision. A change in the color of the iris
may also be noted.

On ocular examination the cornea has
fine, white stellate KPs distributed evenly
over the corneal endothelium (see Fig. 2.4).
On gonioscopy, fine radial vessels can be

seen crossing the trabecular meshwork.
Paracentesis and cataract surgery often in-
jure these vessels, resulting in hyphema.
The anterior chamber develops a mild to
moderate cellular reaction.

Iris findings can be pathognomonic. Iris
heterochromia may be dramatic but is
more often subtle[3,21,24] (see Fig. 2.15). Typically, the affected eye has a lighter colored
iris because of stromal depigmentation.
Lighter colored irides may experience little
color change until very late in the disease.
These eyes may develop a "reverse heterochromia" wherein the inflamed eye is the
darker, slate-blue color. The heterochromia
iridum is secondary to atrophy of the
stroma and subsequent baring of the underlying pigmented epithelium. Iris stromal
atrophy and marginal transillumination defects can be noted. Synechia formation is
uncommon.

Cataract and glaucoma can develop in
50% to 100% of patients. The chronic cyclitis will result in cells within the anterior
vitreous, often with "snowball" formation.
Pars plana neovascularization can occur
and may result in vitreous hemorrhage.

Diagnosis

The clinical picture is distinctive. FHI is a
commonly overlooked etiology for anterior
uveitis. A high degree of clinical suspicion
is helpful.

Differential Diagnosis

Any form of chronic uveitis may result in
iris stromal changes and atrophy. The
unique constellation of findings in FHI
facilitates distinction in most cases. Long-
standing, unilateral cases of pars planitis
can produce stromal atrophy and subtle
heterochromia.

Treatment

Inflammation in FHI is often recalcitrant to
therapy.[21,25] This condition is one of the
few forms of uveitis in which the clinician

may allow a mild persistent cellular reaction to go untreated. Fortunately, the inflammatory cells in FHI seem to be better tolerated than other forms of uveitis. In cases with pain or reduced vision due to severe vitritis or macular edema, topical or periocular corticosteroids can often improve the clinical picture.[25]

Prognosis

Cataracts occur in up to 50% of cases. Of all forms of uveitis, patients with FHI have the best outcomes with standard cataract surgery.[26] Intraocular lenses are generally well tolerated. These patients still have a higher incidence of postoperative capsular fibrosis, "cocooning," cyclitic membrane formation, and will develop inflammatory precipitates on the intraocular lens. Glaucoma can be very problematic: 25% to 50% of patients will develop elevated intraocular pressure.[27] Topical beta-blockers and oral carbonic anhydrase inhibitors are the mainstay of medical therapy. It is not uncommon for the glaucoma to progress and require filtration surgery, Seton implantation, or cyclodestructive procedures. Antimitotic agents may improve success rates with filtration surgery.

Vitreous Disorders

Pars Planitis

Idiopathic intermediate uveitis is called pars planitis. It has also been termed chronic cyclitis, peripheral uveitis, and angiohyalitis.[28-31]

Etiology

The etiology of pars planitis is unknown.[32] Type II collagen found in the vitreous is antigenic and in animal models is capable of inducing both ocular and joint inflammation.[33] Cell-mediated autoimmune responses to the autoantigens may play a role.

Epidemiology

The disease occurs in young adults, with a slight predilection for men over women. Pars planitis is one of the most common forms of uveitis seen in referral centers, accounting for 8% to 15% of patients.[34] An HLA association has not been established.

Pathogenesis

Retinal vasculitis with granulomatous inflammation of peripheral retina and vitreous base are found on pathologic examination.[35] Chronic mononuclear cell infiltration, astrocytic fibrous organization, neovascularization, and collapse of the vitreous base are also present. The nonpigmented ciliary epithelium becomes hyperplastic. True cyclitis or choroiditis on histopathologic examination is rarely found.[35]

Clinical Presentation

Patients with pars planitis have a chronic, bilateral (80%) blurring of vision and floaters.[28-31] Active disease can last many years. The eye is typically white and "quiet." Biomicroscopic examination reveals a mild, nongranulomatous cellular reaction in the anterior chamber. Most of the cells are noted in the anterior vitreous (see Fig. 2.20). Diffuse forms of pars planitis are characterized by inflammatory cells and vitreous snowball formation with no significant pars plana exudation or neovascularization[34] (see Fig. 2.22). The exudative form exhibits an inferior vitreous base and pars plana "snowbanking." This vitreous base exudate can best be observed by scleral depression. The active snowbank appears fuzzy and may have overlying snowballs. The extent of this exudate may be from a few clock hours to 360°. In "burned out" cases, the pars plana appears as a hard white "collagen band." The vitreous base can become vascularized, resulting in vitreous hemorrhage.

Perivasculitis, disc edema (50%), cataract (46%), synechia formation (25%), band keratopathy (9%), glaucoma (8%), retinal detachment (5%), and vitreous hemorrhage (3%) can all occur in patients with long-standing pars planitis.[28–31] CME is the primary reason for poor visual acuity (See Fig. 2.30). Untreated, permanent damage to the macula may occur with the formation of fixed, atrophic macular cysts with chronic CME.[36]

Diagnosis

Bilateral, intermediate uveitis, with or without pars plana exudation, in young healthy patients suggests pars planitis. Fluorescein angiography reveals a periphlebitis, perifoveal capillary leak, CME, and disc staining.[36] A massive leak from the peripheral retina can be seen with vitreous base neovascularization. Review of systems, general physical examination, and laboratory testing are unremarkable. Positive antiganglioside antibodies (44%), positive rheumatoid factor, and an elevated C-reactive protein have been reported in several series.

Differential Diagnosis

Syphilis, tuberculosis, sarcoidosis, FHI, demyelinating disease [multiple sclerosis (MS)], and Lyme disease may all present with an intermediate uveitis. Intermediate uveitis, periphlebitis, and retinal ischemia can be found in 8.5% to 27% of patients with chronic MS.[37–41] These patients often develop uveitis associated with a history of optic neuritis and other transient neurologic complaints secondary to the multifocal CNS demyelination. Reticulum cell sarcoma may also be characterized by vitritis. Patients with systemic complaints or medically unresponsive pars planitis should be evaluated for these disorders.

Treatment

Treatment protocols for patients with pars planitis are listed in Table 18.1. Patients who are asymptomatic with old, pigmented cells distributed unevenly through-

Table 18.1. Treatment protocols for pars planitis.

Level 1: Periocular corticosteroid and/or oral NSAIDs
Level 2: Oral corticosteroid regimens
Level 3: Pars plana cryopexy
Level 4: Unilateral disease—vitrectomy
Severe bilateral disease—vitrectomy or immunosuppression

NSAIDs, nonsteroidal anti-inflammatory drugs.

out the vitreous can be observed and do not require therapy.[32] Patients with active inflammatory cells should be treated. Oral nonsteroidal anti-inflammatory drugs (NSAIDs) often can reduce the cellular activity in these patients. Patients with a prominent vitritis and CME require more aggressive "stepladder" therapy. First-line treatment typically includes periocular corticosteroids (see Fig. 5.2). Triamcinolone (40 mg) given in the sub-Tenon's space often clears the vitreous and improves the CME over 4 to 6 weeks (see Fig. 5.3). This therapy may have to be repeated at 2- to 6-month intervals when in an active phase. Oral NSAIDs reduce the frequency and severity of attacks, as well as the need for frequent injections.

Patients who are unresponsive to periocular steroids or are intolerant can benefit from "pulses" of oral prednisone. Patients who fail this therapy are candidates for pars plana cryopexy, therapeutic vitrectomy, or immunosuppression with second-generation immunosuppressive agents.

Pars plana cryopexy carries the least risk and is often the next step in therapy. Two to three rows of a double "freeze-thaw" applied to areas of active pars plana exudation can be performed under indirect ophthalmoscopy. This procedure is achieved most comfortably with retrobulbar block and a following conjunctival incision.[42–44]

Pars plana cryopexy can be repeated two or three times in recalcitrant cases. It has been reported to "cure" the pars planitis or greatly reduce the need for medical therapy in most patients (65%). It is most effective for vitreous base neovascularization. Patients who fail this step in therapy are candidates for either therapeutic vitrectomy or systemic immunosuppression.[45-48] Patients with unilateral or asymmetric pars planitis should be offered therapeutic vitrectomy. Patients with active, sight-threatening, bilateral disease may benefit from systemic chemotherapy. Azathioprine, methotrexate, cyclophosphamide, and cyclosporin have all been used in the proper clinical setting. This therapy should be performed under the direct supervision of an experienced chemotherapist.

Pars plana lensectomy and vitrectomy can be performed in severe cases with cataract and marked vitreous opacification, medically unresponsive uveitis, and CME.[26] Patients with mild cases characterized by complete control of the inflammation can be considered for standard cataract extraction. Intraocular lens implantation should be considered only in eyes with complete disease remission. Even in quiet, "burned out cases," intraocular lens implantation has been associated with complicated postoperative courses.[26]

Prognosis

About 10% of patients experience a single self-limited episode of pars planitis; 30% experience a clinical course of multiple recurrent episodes of intermediate uveitis over several years; 60% of patients develop chronic disease. In up to 20% of patients, visual acuity is less than 20/200 due to permanent sequelae of the uveitis, primarily fixed macular cysts.

Idiopathic Vitritis or "Senile" Vitritis

Idiopathic "senile" vitritis is a mild, idiopathic inflammatory disorder of the vitreous in older patients.

Etiology

The etiology is unknown.[49-52]

Epidemiology

The disease is most common in white women between the ages of 40 and 70 years. It is thought to be more common than pars planitis as a cause of intermediate uveitis.[52]

Pathogenesis

The pathogenesis is unknown.

Clinical Presentation

Patients are otherwise healthy without evidence of underlying systemic disease.[52] The eye is white, "quiet," and comfortable. Blurring of vision and floaters are noted. Biomicroscopic examination reveals mild to moderate vitritis. A mild nongranulomatous anterior uveitis may be noted as well. The disease is typically bilateral. Pars plana exudation is absent. CME occurs in 27%.

Diagnosis

Idiopathic senile vitritis is a diagnosis of exclusion. It is made or clinical grounds.

Differential Diagnosis

Pars planitis occurs in a younger age group but may be related to senile vitritis. Large cell lymphoma or reticulum cell sarcoma should be considered in medically unresponsive cases of intermediate uveitis in an older population. CNS complaints are often present. Other causes of intermediate uveitis, such as sarcoidosis, Lyme disease, syphilis, and FHI, should be considered. Birdshot retinochoroidopathy can also occur in this age group. Early in the course of birdshot retinochoroidopathy, it can present with a bilateral vitritis and only subtle retinal lesions.

Treatment

Regional and oral corticosteroids can be used with variable responses.

Table 18.2. Inflammatory white dot syndromes of the fundus.

	VA	Age	Sex	Path	Lat	Size	Morph	Location
DUSN	↓	14	M > F (1.5:1)	RPE RET	Unilateral	1/4–1 dd	Evanescent crops	Post-pole and peripheral
Myiasis	↓↑	—	—	Subretinal	Unilateral	1/6 dd	Dotted tracks	Variable
ARPE	↓	29 (16–40)	=	RPE	75% Unilateral	Small	⊙	Macula
MEWDS	↓	26 (14–47)	F > M (4:1)	RPE RET	80% Unilateral	100–200 μm	Granular macula	Perifoveal
POHS	↓	41 (20–50)	=	C-R	62% Bilateral	200–700 μm	Punched out	Triad
PIC	↓	27	F	Choroid	Bilateral	100–300 μm	Discrete	Post-pole
MCP	↓	33	F > M (3:1)	Choroid RPE	80% Bilateral	50–350 μm	Punched out	Multifocal
SFU	↓	(14–34)	F 100%	Subretinal	Bilateral	Large Small	Stellate fibrous	Multifocal
Birdshot	↓	50 (35–70)	M:F (1:2)	Choroid RPE	Bilateral	100–300 μm	Ovoid	Post-equatorial
APMPPE	↓	29	=	RPE Choroid	Bilateral	Large	Placoid	Post-pole
Serpiginous	↓	45	=	Choroid RPE	Bilateral	Large	Serpiginous	Disc Macula
SO	↓	Young	M > F	Choroid	Bilateral	Small Drusen-like	Dalen-Fuchs nodules	Multifocal
VKH	↓	20–40	=	Choroid	96% Bilateral	Variable	Irregular	Multifocal

VA, visual acuity; Path, pathogenisis; Lat, laterality; Morph, morphology; A/C, anterior chamber; Vit, vitreous; FA, fluorescein angiography; EDG, electroomlogram; ERG, electroretinogram; Prog, Prognosis; DUSN, diffuse unilateral subacute neuroretinitis; ARPE, acute retinal pigment epitheliitis; MEWDS, multiple evanescent white dot syndrome; POHS, presumed ocular histoplasmosis syndrome; PIC, punctate inner choroiditis; MCP, multifocal choroiditis and panuveitis; SFU, subretinal fibrosis and uveitis; APMPPE, acute posterior multifocal placoid pigment epitheliopathy; SO, sympathetic ophthalmia; VKH, Vogt-Koyanagi-Harada syndrome; RPE, retinal pigment epithelium; RET, retina; C-R, chorioretinal; SRNVM, subretinal neovascular membrane; RD, retinal detachment; ON, optic nerve; EBV, Epstein-Barr virus; S-Ag, S Antigen; CNS, central nervous system.

Prognosis

The disease may wax and wane for several years. Epiretinal membrane formation occurs in 19% of patients.

Retina

This group of disorders primarily involves the retina. Many are considered the "white dot syndromes of the fundus", and have in common the presence of discrete, light-colored lesions in the fundus during at least one phase of the disease (Table 18.2). Several systemic diseases such as syphilis, tuberculosis, candidiasis, sarcoidosis, toxoplasmosis (PORT), acute retinal necrosis (ARN/BARN) syndrome, and large cell lymphoma may present with light-colored retinal or choroidal lesions and should be considered in the differential diagnosis of each of the "white dot diseases."

Acute Posterior Multifocal Placoid Pigment Epitheliopathy

Acute posterior multifocal placoid pigment epitheliopathy (APMPPE) is an inflammatory disorder of the fundus.[53,54]

Table 18.2. (*continued*)

Color	A/C	VIT	FA	EOG	ERG	Prog	Etiology	Rx
Gray-white	20%	100%	Block early Stain late	—	↓	Poor: ON and RPE toxicity	Nematode	Laser
Black	+	+	Contrasts with maggot	—	—	Variable	Maggot	Surgery
Black with halo	—	—	No leak ⊙	↓	↑	Good	Virus?	None
White	—	+	"Wreath" sign	↓	↓	Recover	Viral prodrome 50%	None
White-green	—	—	Stain SRNVM	OK	OK	Variable	Histoplasmosis	Laser, steroids
Yellow with pigment scar	—	−/+	Block stain	OK	OK	Poor if SRNVM	? Myopia	Steroids
Yellow	52%	98%	Early stain		↑↓	Poor	EBV?	Steroids, acyclovir?
White-yellow	−/+	+	Block stain	↓	↓	Poor	B Cells	Poor
Creamy, non pigmented	30%	100%	Vessel leak		↓	Chronic	S-Ag autoreactive	CSA
Whitish yellow	+	50%	Block stain	↓	↓	80% Good	50% Viral prodrome	None, steroids
Yellow gray	—	30%	Loss of choriocapillaris	↓	—	Poor	?	None
Yellow white	31%	+	Multiple choroidal leaks	—	—	88% with >20/70	Injury S-Ag autoreactive	Steroid, immunosuppressants
Depigmentation Pigment Scars	+	+	Choroiditis with exudative RD	—	—	25% Blind	CNS, ear, skin, eye	Immunosuppressants

Etiology

The etiology of APMPPE is unknown.[53,54] A viral-like prodrome consisting of upper respiratory tract symptoms, headache, and erythema nodosa may precede the onset of APMPPE in 50% of patients.

Epidemiology

The average age of onset is 29 years, with a range of 15 to 40 years.[53,54] The male/female ratio is equal. There may be an association with HLA-B7 (44%) and HLA-DR2 (57%).

Pathogenesis

Two mechanisms are suggested for the pathogenesis of APMPPE. One theory holds that the disease is a result of focal retinal pigment epithelium (RPE) inflammation as suggested by the irregular distribution of the APMPPE lesions within the posterior pole with little correspondence to underlying choroidal circulation patterns.[53,55] Transient inflammation of the RPE would also be compatible with a return of visual function, which is often noted in this disease. The electrooculogram (EOG) is impaired during the acute phases, supporting RPE dysfunction.[55] Choriocapillaris vasculitis and ischemia is another proposed mechanism for the APMPPE lesions.[56] Significant nonperfusion in the macula should result in more permanent loss of vision. Patients do have evidence for vasculitis involving the brain and possibly the kidneys. The disease has similarities to other uveomeningeal syndromes such as Vogt-Koyanagi-Harada (VKH) syndrome.

Clinical Presentation

A nonspecific viral-like prodrome can occur in 50% of patients.[53,54,57] Severe headache, upper respiratory tract complaints, and erythema nodosa are noted.[57–59] Urinary casts can be found on urinalysis. Headaches have been severe enough to require cerebral angiography, which was documented the presence of cerebral vasculitis. Meningeal signs, cerebrospinal fluid (CSF) pleocytosis, fixed neurologic defects, and deaths have been reported in APMPPE.[58,59]

Ocular symptoms include an acute, often bilateral but asymmetric loss of vision.[53–55] Multiple, large, yellowish white, plaque-like lesions are noted at the level of the RPE in the posterior pole (Fig. 18.2A,B). The acute lesions generally resolve in 10 days, with resultant RPE changes. APMPPE may be associated with anterior uveitis, vitritis (50%), episcleritis, subconjunctival hemorrhage, retinal perivasculitis, and papillitis.[60]

Diagnosis

The diagnosis can be made on clinical grounds. The characteristic fundus lesions can be seen on ophthalmoscopy. Fluorescein angiography supports the diagnosis, with the lesions blocking the dye early in the study and staining late[53] (Fig. 18.2C,D).

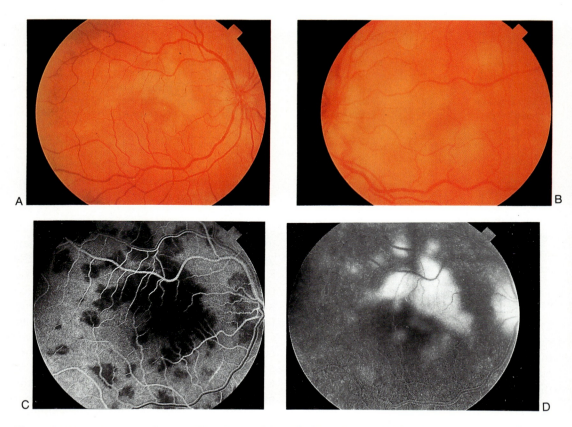

Figure 18.2. Acute posterior multifocal placoid epitheliopathy. A, B: Fundus photographs demonstrating bilateral, multifocal, deep, placoid lesions in posterior pole. **C:** Fluorescein angiogram shows the characteristic blocking early in the study, with **D**, late staining of the lesions.

Electrophysiologic studies demonstrate a decreased EOG and electroretinogram (ERG). Laboratory evaluation is unremarkable except for urinary casts and CSF pleocytosis.

Differential Diagnosis

Atypical cases of serpiginous chorioretinopathy can resemble APMPPE. Classic serpiginous chorioretinopathy occurs in a slightly older population; the disease is chronic and has a more serpentine appearance. The lesions are indolent and frequently originate from the optic disc. Visual loss is permanent in areas of the retina affected by serpiginous chorioretinopathy. Syphilis, tuberculosis, toxoplasmosis, candidiasis, sarcoidosis, and large cell lymphoma may also cause white dots of the fundus that can resemble APMPPE.

Treatment

In most cases, no treatment is indicated. In severe, bilateral disease with loss of central acuity due to macular lesions, regional or oral corticosteroids can be used without adverse effects.

Prognosis

APMPPE is rarely recurrent. The disease may have serious CNS involvement. Patients with severe headache and CNS findings should be evaluated by a neurologist. Visual prognosis can be good. Visual acuity will recover to 20/30 or better in 80% to 90% of patients.[61] Return of vision is frequently imperfect.[61] It should be noted that 20% of patients may have permanent visual impairment when the macula is involved.

Acute Retinal Pigment Epitheliitis

Acute retinal pigment epitheliitis (ARPE), also called Krill's disease, is an acute self-limiting inflammation of the retinal pigment epithelium.[62-64]

Etiology

The etiology for ARPE is unknown. Autoimmune and viral mechanisms have been postulated.[62-64]

Epidemiology

In contrast to age-related macular degeneration, patients with ARPE are generally younger, ranging between 16 to 40 years of age (average age, 29 years).[62-64] Men and women are affected equally.

Pathogenesis

The lesions appear to be at the level of the RPE on contact lens biomicroscopy.

Clinical Presentation

Otherwise healthy patients report a sudden, unilateral (75%) decrease in visual acuity.[62-64] On ocular examination, subtle, small, hyperpigmented lesions are noted in the RPE (Fig. 18.3). A hypopigmented "halo" can be seen surrounding these lesions. Two to four clusters of two to six "dots" are typically noted in the posterior pole. The overlying vitreous is quiet.

Diagnosis

The diagnosis is established by clinical examination.[62-64] Fluorescein angiography can assist by showing "target" lesions with small hypofluorescent dots with a surrounding hyperfluorescent halo. The lesions have a "honeycomb appearance" and can be associated with mild disc edema. CME and subretinal neovascularization are not typically found. Electrophysiologic testing shows a decreased EOG. The visual evoked response (VER) and ERG are normal.

Differential Diagnosis

Patients with age-related macular degeneration (ARMD) are typically older, have bilateral chronic disease, and develop subretinal neovascular membranes (SRNVMs).

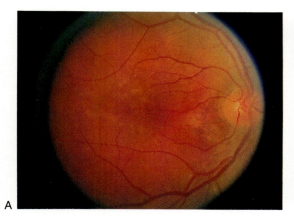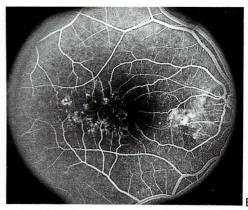

Figure 18.3. Acute retinal pigment epitheliitis. A: Fundus photograph of a patient with ARPE and sudden decrease of central acuity. Fundus examination revealed small, white lesions in the macula with hyperpigmented centers. **B:** Fluorescein angiogram shows a "honeycomb" appearance with hypofluorescent centers. Visual acuity returned to 20/20 without treatment.

Unlike with ARPE, macular degeneration is chronic. Central serous retinopathy is an acute disease of young adults but is not characterized by clusters of RPE lesions and is associated with subretinal fluid within the macula. Central serous retinopathy and ARPE may be related. Patients with ARPE can develop subretinal fluid similar to that seen in central serous retinopathy.

Treatment

No therapy is indicated in this self-limiting disease.

Prognosis

Complete recovery can be expected within 6 to 12 weeks, but the disease may be recurrent.[62-64]

Birdshot Retinochoroidopathy

Birdshot retinochoroiditis is a chronic inflammatory disease of the eye, with characteristic fundus findings.[65-68] The disorder was first described in 1980 by Ryan and Maumenee.[65] The term *birdshot chorioretinopathy* refers to the distinctive fundus lesions originally characterized as "multiple, small white spots that frequently have the pattern seen with birdshot in the scatter from a shotgun."[65] Gass[67] also described this condition and called it *vitiliginous choroiditis* because of the depigmented nature of the fundus lesions.

Etiology

The etiology of birdshot retinochoroidopathy is not known. The disease appears to have neither a strong familial association nor a recognizable mode of inheritance. It has a very strong major histocompatibility antigen (MHC) association. HLA-A29 phenotype is present in 80% to 96% of patients with this disease.[69,70] This is the strongest human class 1 MHC disease association reported with calculated relative risks between 50 and 224.[68,69] That is, persons with HLA-A29 have a 50 to 224 times greater chance of developing birdshot retinochoroidopathy than those with other HLA phenotypes.

Epidemiology

Unlike other forms of uveitis that typically occur in younger age groups, birdshot retinochoroidopathy occurs during middle age, the average age being 50 years, with a range of 35 to 70 years.[66-68,71] The reason for this age association is not clear. The disease also appears to have a gender preference—70% of reported cases are in women—and is relatively rare in heavily pigmented races.

Pathogenesis

Autoimmunity and specifically cell-mediated immune mechanisms are thought to play a mediating role in birdshot retinochoroidopathy. Patients exhibit lymphocyte proliferation responses to several retinal autoantigens.[72,73] S-Antigen (S-Ag) and interstitial retinoid binding protein (IRBP) are antigenic proteins found in the photoreceptor layer of the retina.[74,75] S-Ag is located in the cell wall of the photoreceptors, and IRBP is located in the intercellular matrix. S-Ag and IRBP are both immunogenic and can cause experimental uveitis in laboratory animals. Animals immunized with these autoantigens develop not only antibody and specific cellular immune responses to these proteins but also a severe ocular inflammation called experimental autoimmune uveitis (EAU).[74] The pineal gland develops a similar lymphocytic infiltration in this model. Adoptive transfer of lymphocytes that are specifically primed to these antigens into naive recipients also produce this experimental form of autoimmune uveitis.[76]

A strong cell-mediated immune response to S-Ag and IRBP occurs in 92% of patients with birdshot retinochoroidopathy.[72,73] In vitro lymphocyte proliferation to these autoantigens is rare in the normal population.

Few eyes with birdshot retinochoroidopathy have been available for pathologic and immunohistologic examination. In one report, an enucleated, phthisical eye from a patient with birdshot retinochoroidopathy in the other eye revealed a mild lymphocytic infiltration of the iris and ciliary body.[69] The retina had a diffuse, chronic granulomatous inflammation, with giant cells, epithelioid cells, and plasma cells in the outer retinal layers. The underlying choroid had a milder granulomatous infiltration, which was thought to be a secondary response.

Clinical Presentation

Patients with birdshot retinochoroidopathy are otherwise healthy[67] and typically present to the ophthalmologist complaining of a gradual, painless blurring of vision. They also note "floaters" or "cobwebs." Ocular symptoms are typically bilateral (85%) but may be asymmetric. Often, the disease begins on one side and over the course of the disease involves the contralateral eye. Besides diminished central acuity and "floaters," patients may also note a loss of color vision and difficulty with dark-light adaptation.[66,67]

On ocular examination, the eye appears "quiet" without hyperemia or limbal flush.[65] A mild, nongranulomatous iritis with fine keratic precipitates on the corneal endothelium may be present in 25% of patients. Synechiae are unusual.

Biomicroscopic examination of the eye reveals a diffuse vitritis. Inflammatory cells are present both in the anterior and posterior vitreous. This cellular reaction can be variable, however, ranging from trace to considerable numbers of discrete cells.[67] Fundus examination reveals the characteristic "birdshot" lesions. The lesions are typically bilateral and located in the postequatorial fundus. They are ovoid in shape, "cream-colored" in appearance,[65-67,75] usually symmetrically distributed, and often assume a radial orientation[67] (Fig. 18.4). The borders of these depigmented lesions are "soft" and ill-defined and are not "punched out."[3] The lesions are often easier to identify by using indirect rather than direct ophthalmoscopy. The size of the lesions can vary from small and discrete (50–100 μm) to quite large (500–1500 μm). The larger lesions may become confluent and result in geographic depigmenta-

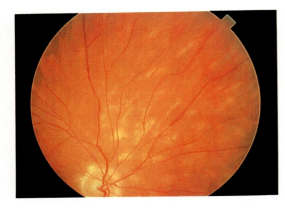

Figure 18.4.   Birdshot   retinochoroidopathy.
Ovoid, cream-colored fundus lesions of birdshot
retinochoroidopathy. The lesions are often radial
in orientation and occur in the postequatorial
retina.

tion or even produce a "blonde" appearance to the fundus.[65] It is unusual to find
many lesions within the posterior pole of
the fundus.[65] Importantly, lesions are not
usually associated with significant hyperpigmentation. A rare patient may develop
fine pigmentary changes in the fundus
or around retinal vessels.[65] Severe disc
edema and cystoid edema of the retina and
macula are common. Late in the disease,
the retinal vessels may become attenuated.[65,67] Optic nerve atrophy can develop.[66] Serous elevation of the sensory
retina (50%) and SRNVM formation have
also been reported.[77] These membranes
may hemorrhage and produce a disciform
scar, resulting in permanent loss of central
acuity.

Patients with birdshot retinochoroidopathy frequently complain of depression
and disruption of their sleep cycles, which
may result from trilateral inflammation involving the pineal gland. This gland possesses S-Ag and regulates both diurnal hormonal cycles and melatonin secretion. It is
interesting to correlate pineal dysfunction
as the cause of both the dysphoria and the
development of the "vitiliginous" lesions.

Diagnosis

The diagnosis is made clinically by identifying the characteristic fundus lesions.[65]
Bilateral, chronic blurring of vision and
floaters in a 50-year-old patient with a
"quiet eye," vitritis, and the presence of
ovoid, cream-colored lesions in the midperipheral retina establishes the diagnosis
of birdshot.

Laboratory studies are usually normal
and do not help establish the diagnosis.
Single-antigen haplotyping for HLA-A29
can be helpful in atypical presentations
or to confirm the diagnosis before the use
of second-generation immunosuppressive
agents. Lymphocyte proliferation assays to
S-Ag and IRBP are not widely available
but can be performed to support further
the clinical diagnosis.

Fluorescein angiography can be helpful
in supporting the diagnosis and in following the clinical course. The early phases of
the angiogram have been described as
"subnormal" or dark because of blockage
of choroidal fluorescence by retinal edema
and retinal vascular attenuation.[67] The
most prominent finding on angiography is
the profuse leakage of fluorescein dye from
the retinal vessels and capillaries[65] (see Fig.
2.28). Vascular incompetence results in
widespread retinal and macular edema.
The birdshot lesions, so distinctive on
ophthalmoscopy, are rather lackluster on
fluorescein angiography. They do not
typically block the underlying choroidal
phases of the angiogram and exhibit only
mild hyperfluorescence and staining in the
latter phases of the study. Electrophysiologic studies show a reduced ERG and
normal or reduced EOG responses.[66,69] Specifically, the ERG exhibits a reduced rod b-
wave amplitude and cone and rod b-wave/
implicit time ratios.

Differential Diagnosis

The differential diagnosis includes the other
"white dot syndromes," sarcoidosis, large

cell lymphoma, syphilis, and tuberculosis. The clinical picture is distinct and, in most cases, can be distinguished from that of other conditions. Many of these other diseases produce constitutional symptoms and physical findings to suggest an underlying systemic process. The fundus lesions of tuberculosis and lues are typically associated with RPE hyperpigmentation and are not necessarily ovoid.

Treatment

In the early stages of the disease, patients may be followed if they are relatively asymptomatic and the inflammation is mild. Most patients are symptomatic. Birdshot retinochoroidopathy characteristically responds poorly or incompletely to NSAIDs, corticosteroids, and most second-generation immunosuppressive agents.[65–67] Initial improvement can be seen with oral prednisone at relatively high doses (1 mg/kg per day) or periocular corticosteroid preparations. With tapering of the steroid dose, it is not unusual for patients to notice an exacerbation of their disease. Despite this historically poor response to corticosteroids, an initial trial on prednisone is indicated. Sub-Tenon's triamcinolone (40 mg/ml) can also help in patients with CME or severe inflammation.[65]

The disease appears to respond favorably to cyclosporine-A.[78] Doses ranging from 2 to 5 mg/kg/per day are often associated with a resolution of vitreous cells and restoration of the blood–eye barrier. Reduction in retinal edema improves visual function for many patients.

Prognosis

Birdshot retinochoroiditis is a chronic disease characterized by multiple clinical exacerbations and may persist over decades. It can result in the loss of useful vision in one or both eyes in 40% of patients.[65] Poor visual acuity is often a result of chronic CME or SRNVM formation.

Leber's Idiopathic Stellate Neuroretinitis

Leber's idiopathic stellate neuroretinitis (LISN) is an inflammatory disease, affecting the optic nerve and neurosensory retina. It was first described by Leber in 1916 as an acute loss of vision with disc edema and a macular star formation.[79–82]

Etiology

The etiology for LISN is unknown, with 50% of patients having a nonspecific, viral-like prodrome.[79–82]

Epidemiology

The average age for patients with LISN is 22 years, with a range of 8 to 48 years. There is an equal sex distribution.

Pathogenesis

The disease appears to affect the vessels of the optic disc. Peripapillary subretinal fluid and macular star formation are characteristic.

Clinical Presentation

The initial symptoms are a loss of vision and mild pain with eye movements.[79–82] An afferent pupillary defect can be detected on examination. Within a week, papillitis, peripapillary edema, and subretinal fluid develop, all of which can be associated with posterior vitreous inflammatory cell (90%), disc hemorrhage (35%), and an iritis (10%). After this acute phase with resolution of the inflammation, a lipid macular star develops (Fig. 18.5).

Diagnosis

The diagnosis is by exclusion and is established clinically. Papillitis, vitritis, and a macular star in a healthy patient should suggest LISN. Fluorescein angiography can help characterize the optic disc and vessel

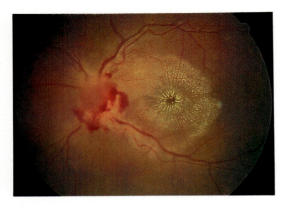

Figure 18.5. Leber's idiopathic stellate neuro-retinitis. Disc edema, mild hemorrhage, and lipid "macular star" formation in Leber's idiopathic stellate neuroretinitis. Visual acuity was reduced to 20/400.

leakage. The white blood cell count may be elevated and an increased ESR can be seen in some patients.

Differential Diagnosis

Neuroretinitis can be found in syphilis, tuberculosis, toxoplasmosis, and toxocariasis. Macular star formation is nonspecific and can be noted in anterior ischemic optic neuropathy, venous occlusions, diabetes, hypertension, and other vascular disease.

Treatment

In limited forms of LISN, no treatment is needed.[79-82] Oral and regional corticosteroids have been used in patients with LISN without adverse effects.

Prognosis

The prognosis is good, with 97% of patients achieving better than 20/40 acuity, and 66% have a return of 20/20 vision.[79-82] The papillitis resolves over 8 to 12 weeks, and complete resolution of the lipid macular star occurs over 1 to 12 months.

Multiple Evanescent White Dot Syndrome

Multiple evanescent white dot syndrome (MEWDS) is an idiopathic inflammatory disorder of the retina in healthy adults.[83,84]

Etiology

The etiology is unknown.[83,84] A viral-like prodrome precedes the onset of MEWDS in 50% of patients.

Epidemiology

MEWDS affects women more often than men at a ratio of between 4:1 and 10:1.[83,84] The average age is 26 years, with a range between 14 and 47 years.

Pathogenesis

Little is known about the pathogenesis of MEWDS. Clinical examination and fluorescein angiography support an inflammatory process involving the outer retina and the RPE.

Clinical Presentation

Patients with MEWDS note a sudden, unilateral (80%) decrease in vision.[83-85] On ocular examination, multiple, small (100–200 μm), outer retina/RPE white dots can be noted in the perifoveal and peripheral macula (Fig. 18.6A). A pathognomonic "granular" appearance to the macula can be observed in the acute phase of the disease. Mild vascular sheathing and vitritis can be seen on biomicroscopic examination. The anterior segment is not involved. Optic disc edema and decreased nerve function are also observed.

Diagnosis

The diagnosis is established by the history and fundus examination.[83-85] Fluorescein angiography can help demonstrate the deep retinal lesions and capillary leakage:

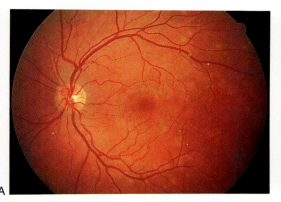 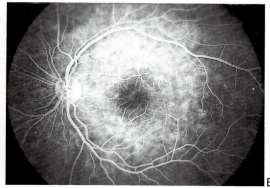

A   B

Figure 18.6. Multiple evanescent white dot syndrome. A: Fundus photograph in a patient with MEWDS showing the multiple white lesions in the posterior pole and the granular macula. **B:** Fluorescein angiogram demonstrates a "wreath sign" and mild hyperfluorescence to the "white dots."

The lesions demonstrate late staining; hyperfluorescence in the posterior pole distributed around the foveal has been called the "wreath sign"; peripheral lesions may have a characteristic "ring staining" (Fig. 18.6B). Electrophysiologic studies exhibit a decreased ERG and EOG.

MEWDS has been associated with the acute macular neuroretinopathy syndrome and the syndrome of prolonged enlargement of the blind spot.[86-89] Acute macular neuroretinopathy (AMN) is a rare disorder causing paracentral scotomata associated with a characteristic reddish brown, wedge-shaped retinal lesion.[86,87] Patients have developed AMN during the course of MEWDS.[86] Another rare disorder has been seen in patients with MEWDS—the syndrome of enlarged blind spot.[90] There may be a spectrum of disorders that can cause both enlargement of the blind spot and MEWDS.[88]

Differential Diagnosis

Other white dot syndromes of the retina should be considered in the differential diagnosis. These include APMPPE, ARPE, and punctate inner choroiditis.

Treatment

Treatment is not required in typical MEWDS.

Prognosis

Recovery can occur over a 7-week period. MEWDS can be recurrent in as many as 10% of patients.[85]

Subretinal Fibrosis and Uveitis Syndrome

Subretinal fibrosis and uveitis (SFU) syndrome has also been called the progressive subretinal fibrosis and uveitis syndrome. The most prominent feature of this disease is the development of stellate, subretinal fibrotic lesions.[91]

Etiology

The etiology for SFU is unknown.[91]

Epidemiology

SFU syndrome predominantly affects women.[91,92] In some series, 100% of patients were women.[91,92] The average age is between 14 and 34 years of age.

Pathogenesis

A granulomatous and nongranulomatous infiltration of the choroid can be seen on histopathology.[93,94] A chorioretinal biopsy from an active lesion demonstrated primarily B cells and plasma cells.[93] In another study, immunoperoxidase staining demonstrated a predominant T-helper cell subset in the infiltrates.[94] Complement and immunoglobulin G (IgG) were found beneath Bruch's membrane. Subretinal fibrosis is noted in involved areas. The cells appear to be derived from RPE. Viruses and other infectious agents were not identified.[93]

Clinical Presentation

Progressive inflammation results in a bilateral decrease of vision.[93–95] Early in the course, patients may develop a chronic iritis, episcleritis, and vitritis. A multifocal choroiditis can be noted.[92] These lesions are small (100–200 μm), yellow, and deep without significant hyperpigmentation. They may be found in the posterior pole and peripheral retina. Late in the disease, large stellate or angular subretinal fibrotic lesions develop, which are typically white and may have mild, secondary pigment changes (Fig. 18.7A). CME occurs in most

cases and is often the cause for decreased vision.

Diagnosis

SFU is a clinical diagnosis. On fluorescein angiography the stellate lesions block early and stain later[91,92] (Fig. 18.7B). SRNVMS can develop. Electrophysiologic studies show a diminished ERG and EOG.

Differential Diagnosis

Sympathetic ophthalmia, sarcoidosis, histoplasmosis, birdshot retinochoroidopathy, and APMPPE can all be characterized by white lesions and may resemble SFU at different stages of the disease. Multifocal choroiditis and panuveitis (MCP) syndrome can be identical early in the course of the disease and may represent a spectrum with SFU. Patients with MCP syndrome can progress over time and will develop the characteristic angular subretinal fibrotic lesion.

Treatment

SFU responds poorly to most forms of treatment.[91,92] Steroids and second-generation immunosuppressive agents have been used with little success. Serologic evidence for

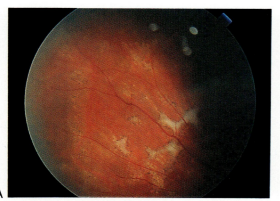
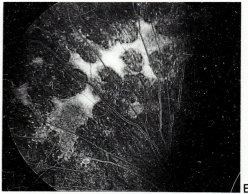

Figure 18.7. Subretinal fibrosis and uveitis syndrome. A: Bilateral diffuse uveitis and multifocal areas of white, subretinal fibrosis in a 34-year-old woman. **B:** Fluorescein angiogram demonstrates late staining in the fibrotic lesions.

Epstein-Barr virus (EBV) infection in patients with MCP and SFU is controversial. The presence of B cells on biopsy might support an infection with EBV. Acyclovir may have a beneficial effect in this regard.

Prognosis

The prognosis is poor: The disease is progressive and is medically unresponsive. Subretinal surgical removal of fibrotic tissue may improve the prognosis in selected cases.

Choroid

Multifocal Choroiditis and Panuveitis Syndrome

MCP is an idiopathic inflammation of the choroid and retina. It is also called the pseudohistoplasmosis syndrome.[96,97]

Etiology

The etiology of MCP is unknown. An association with elevated EBV serology has been reported in idiopathic MCP and is controversial.[98]

Epidemiology

The average age for patients with MCP is 36 years.[96–99] Women are affected more than men by a 3:1 ratio. MCP can occur in areas that are not endemic for histoplasmosis, and patients do not have a higher incidence of histoplasmin skin test positivity.

Pathogenesis

The pathogenesis for MCP is not well known. Both the RPE and choroid appear to be primarily involved with a secondary vitritis.

Clinical Presentation

The disease is typically bilateral (82%).[96–99] The multifocal lesions are small (50–350 μm) and yellowish when active. Peripapil-lary pigmentary scarring can be noted and resembles ocular histoplasmosis, but unlike in histoplasmosis, an anterior uveitis (52%) and vitritis (98%) are found associated with the multifocal lesions (see Fig. 2.34). SRNVMs (30%) and macular disciform scars can develop with disease progression.[97–99] Late in the disease the chorioretinal lesions develop pigment changes around the lesions, and subretinal fibrosis can be seen, which is similar to the lesions noted in SFU syndrome.[92]

Diagnosis

Idiopathic MCP is diagnosed clinically and by exclusion of other diseases than can present with multifocal chorioretinitis. Fluorescein angiography demonstrates early blocking with active choroidal infiltration and late hyperfluorescence. Electrophysiology has been variable.

Laboratory testing is not diagnostic. Positive EBV antibodies [EBV IgM and early antigen (EA) antibodies] were noted in one series of idiopathic MCP.[98] Other investigators have not noted this association in a more heterologous population of patients with multifocal choroiditis.

Differential Diagnosis

Syphilis, tuberculosis, and sarcoidosis should all be suspected in patients with an MCP-like picture. Other retinal white dot syndromes such as MEWDS, birdshot retinochoroidopathy, diffuse unilateral subacute neuroretinitis (DUSN), punctate inner choroiditis, and SFU should be included in the differential diagnosis. Histoplasmosis is not characterized by the panuveitis associated with the MCP syndrome, even though the fundus lesions may appear identical.[96–99]

Treatment

Oral or regional corticosteroids are the main treatment strategies.[96–99] Oral acyclovir 200mg PO 5 ×s day has also been used with variable results.

Prognosis

The prognosis is often poor, with medically unresponsive and progressive inflammation. Macular function may be compromised by the development of SRNVMs. Blind spot enlargement has been reported in patients with MCP.[100]

Punctate Inner Choroiditis

Punctate inner choroiditis (PIC) is an idiopathic, inflammatory disorder of the choroid.[101]

Etiology

The etiology for PIC is unknown.

Epidemiology

Women are affected more often than men.[101] The average age of onset is 27 years (range 18–37 years). All patients have had moderate myopia associated with the disorder.

Pathogenesis

The pathogenesis is unknown. Patients do not have histoplasmin skin sensitivity.[101]

Clinical Presentation

Patients note a bilateral decrease in visual acuity and a central scotoma.[101] Ocular examination demonstrates an absence of cell and flare in the anterior chamber or vitreous, which contrasts with MCP.[91] A mild peripapillary pigment change may be noted. Small, punctate, yellow, inner choroidal lesions (100–300 μm) are noted in the posterior pole with active choroiditis. RPE hyperpigmentation is noted late in the disease course. Serous detachment of the sensory retina (50%) and secondary SRNVM formation occur.

Diagnosis

The diagnosis is made clinically. Fluorescein angiography demonstrates early block-ing by the active choroidal infiltrates and late hyperfluorescence. Electrophysiologic studies have been normal.

Differential Diagnosis

Other idiopathic white dot syndromes of the retina should be considered. PIC, MCP, and SFU may be a spectrum of the same disease process. Small PIC lesions may evolve into larger lesions with more intraocular inflammation as described in MCP. In later stages, patients may develop characteristic stellate subretinal fibrosis as seen in SFU. High myopia can be associated with SRNVM and RPE scarring and should also be considered in the differential.

Treatment

Patients can be observed in mild cases. Oral and regional corticosteroids have been used without adverse effect. Laser photocoagulation to treat SRNVMs can be performed once the active inflammation has been treated or resolves.

Prognosis

Unlike the clinical course of progressive SFU and MCP, the disease is self-limiting, with spontaneous resolution in 1 month.[101] The development of a SRNVM may compromise macular function.

Serpiginous Chorioretinopathy

Serpiginous chorioretinopathy is a progressive idiopathic inflammatory disorder of the retinal pigment epithelium and choroid.[102–106] It has also been called geographic choroiditis and helicoid peripapillary choroiditis.

Etiology

The etiology of serpiginous chorioretinopathy is unknown.

Epidemiology

The disorder is rare and has an equal sex predilection.[102] It affects middle-aged adults between 40 and 60 years of age.

Pathogenesis

The pathogenesis is not well defined.[102-104] One report described a primary choroiditis with mononuclear cell infiltration and secondary loss of RPE and choriocapillaris.[105] Later in the disease, degeneration of the sensory retina occurs with secondary hyperpigmentation.

Clinical Presentation

Patients with serpiginous chorioretinopathy are otherwise healthy. Ocular symptoms include a progressive or recurrent bilateral decrease in vision.[102-106] Unlike with APMPPE, the process results in permanent scotoma. Ocular examination reveals large, peripapillary, pseudopodal, ill-defined, yellow-gray lesions at the level of the RPE (see Fig. 2.32). Rarely, a mild vitritis and retinal vasculitis has been reported.[107] Secondary RPE and choriocapillaris atrophy, SRNVM development, and hyperpigmentation are noted[106] (see Fig. 4.3). The disease is progressive with centripetal extension and recurrent attacks occurring over years.

Diagnosis

The characteristic fundus findings establish the diagnosis in most cases. Active lesions block the fluorescein angiogram early in the study and stain late[105] (see Fig. 2.32). Older lesions exhibit edge hyperfluorescence. Total loss of the underlying choriocapillaris is characteristic. Electrophysiologic studies show a diminished EOG.

Differential Diagnosis

Regional choroidal dystrophies can appear similar to serpiginous chorioretinopathy but do not typically progress in a "snake-like" fashion. Atypical cases of APMPPE can appear similar to serpiginous chorioretinopathy.

Treatment

Most forms of therapy have been ineffective.[107-109] Regional and oral corticosteroids can be used during acute episodes but do not have a significant impact on the long-term clinical course. Second-generation immunosuppressive regimens that combine prednisone, azathioprine, and cyclosporin have been used and have been reported to halt acute disease progression.[108] Anecdotal trials of oral acyclovir have also been used, with similar reports of improved clinical course.

Prognosis

The disease is progressive and medically unresponsive. Serpiginous chorioretinopathy results in permanent scotoma and, if the macula is involved, loss of central vision.

Sympathetic Ophthalmia

Sympathetic ophthalmia (SO) is a bilateral, non-necrotizing, diffuse, granulomatous panuveitis that occurs after ocular injury.[110-113]

Etiology

SO appears to be an autoimmune disease that is precipitated by ocular injury, typically resulting in uveal prolapse.[110-113] Disruption of blood–eye barrier, exposure to ocular autoantigens, and an adjuvant effect of contaminating bacteria (*Propionibacterium acnes*) may all play a role in the pathogenesis. Patients have evidence of immunologic education to several ocular autoantigens including S-Antigen, IRBP, and lens proteins.[114-116] A delayed-type hypersensitivity reaction toward these ocular antigens may play a mediating role in the

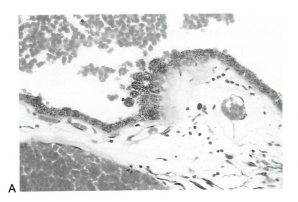

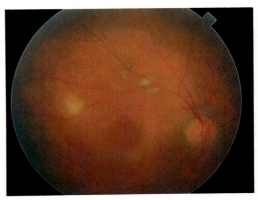

Figure 18.8. Sympathetic ophthalmia—Dalen-Fuchs nodules. A: Metaplastic RPE, epithelioid cell formation, and relative sparing of the choriocapillaris in a patient with sympathetic ophthalmia. **B:** Vitritis, cystoid macular edema, Dalen-Fuchs nodule, and a multifocal choroiditis in the contralateral eye.

chronic ocular inflammation.

Epidemiology

Because of occupational factors, men are affected more often than women.[111] Multiple studies have estimated the incidence of SO by using inpatient data, postoperative studies, post-trauma studies, histopathologic studies, and war statistics.[112] Although the incidence varies depending on the study, the most accepted incidence is thought to be 1.9/1000 nonsurgical penetrating injuries and 1/10,000 surgical cases.[111,112,117,118] There is an association (30%) with HLA-A11 in patients with SO.[119]

Pathogenesis

SO is a diffuse, non-necrotizing, granulomatous panuveitis.[118] The choroid shows a prominent epithelioid cell reaction with eosinophils and mild plasma cell infiltration.[118] The process characteristically "spares" the choriocapillaris. Dalen-Fuchs nodules are found in 35% of patients, representing a metaplasia of the RPE into epithelioid cells positioned on Bruch's mem-

brane[120] (Fig. 18.8A). Retinal inflammation and vasculitis are not common but can be observed.[118]

Immunohistochemical studies demonstrate activated T cells with surface markers for DR, and IL-2.[121–123] During active disease, CD4+ helper T cells predominate. Late in the disease process, CD8+ suppressor/cytotoxic T cells can be found in the choroidal infiltration. HLA-DR+ antigen-presenting cells can be seen in the uvea, postulated to be presenting autoantigen to immunologically primed T cells.[123]

Clinical Presentation

Patients with SO may note photophobia (67%), decreased accommodation (13%), and ocular pain.[111,113] Symptoms can occur between 5 days and 50 years after ocular injury. Most cases (70%) occur within 3 weeks to 3 months after the injury.[111]

On ocular examination, mild cases are characterized by a diffuse, nongranulomatous uveitis, Dalen-Fuchs nodules, and optic nerve involvement.[111,113] With disease progression or in severe cases, a granulomatous panuveitis with mutton fat KP, peripheral anterior synechiae, papillitis, and

Dalen-Fuchs nodules are noted. Multifocal areas of choroiditis and chorioretinal scarring can be noted in up to 25% of patients[111,113,118] (Fig. 19.8B). Lens-induced uveitis may occur in 23% to 46% of cases with SO.[118,124]

Diagnosis

The diagnosis is based on history and ocular examination. Fluorescein angiography demonstrates characteristic leakage from the optic nerve and Dalen-Fuchs nodules.[125] Multiple, punctate hyperfluorescent lesions in the choroid can be seen in active disease. The retinal vessels are not often affected. Chorioretinal biopsy or enucleation can confirm the clinical diagnosis if necessary in severe disease.

Differential Diagnosis

Post-traumatic uveitis and infectious endophthalmitis should be considered early in the course after ocular injury. True lens-induced uveitis can also occur after trauma to the lens or lens capsule. VKH syndrome can exhibit similar ocular findings but, typically, VKH is not associated with trauma and the patient has more systemic symptoms including vitiligo, hearing loss, alopecia, and CNS involvement.[126] In contrast to sympathetic ophthalmia, the choriocapillaris is involved in VKH syndrome.

Treatment

SO can be prevented by removing a potentially inciting eye after severe injury in cases where there is no hope of visual recovery, comfort, or a cosmetically normal eye.[113] In this setting, if the injured eye is removed within 2 weeks, the development of SO is unlikely; however, modern microscopic and vitreoretinal surgical techniques have made more difficult the decision to remove an injured eye so early.[127–129] Previously inoperable eyes can often be re-paired, with preservation of some useful vision. The decision to remove these eyes solely to prevent a rare disease should not be made without much deliberation. To prevent two cases of sympathetic ophthalmia, 998 eyes would have to be removed after ocular trauma. Anesthetic mortality for both local and general anesthesia in ophthalmology has been reported at a similar frequency, between 1.4/1000 and 1/5000 cases.[130] Anesthetic morbidity is even higher with myocardial infarction, pulmonary embolism, aspiration stroke, and hyperthermia.

Oral and regional corticosteroids have been the mainstay of therapy for SO during the acute and chronic phases of the disease.[113,131] Initial dose should be 1 to 1.5 mg/kg prednisone daily. Long-term anti-inflammatory therapy is often required. The prednisone can be slowly tapered over 1 year or more. Patients who are intolerant of the side effects of corticosteroids or who have medically resistant disease can be treated with second-generation immunosuppressive medications including azathioprine, cyclosporine A, cyclophosphamide, and methotrexate.[113,132,133]

Some evidence suggests that once SO has developed, the clinical course can be moderated by removing the inciting eye within 2 weeks of disease onset.[118,131] There is no clinical benefit if SO has been present more than 2 weeks. An inciting eye that has useful vision should not be enucleated, as it may turn out to be the eye with better vision.

Prognosis

With therapy, 64% of patients achieve at least 20/60 visual acuity.[134] With corticosteroid therapy and enucleation within 2 weeks, 88% achieve at least 20/100 visual acuity.[118,131] Disease recurrence and a chronic clinical course are common in most (60%) cases.

Vogt-Koyanagi-Harada Syndrome

VKH syndrome is a severe, diffuse granulomatous uveitis associated with CNS, vestibuloauditory, and cutaneous manifestations.[135–137] Components of the syndrome were described by Vogt in 1906, Koyanagi in 1929, and Harada in 1926.

Etiology

The etiology of VKH syndrome is unknown. Cell-mediated autoimmune mechanisms are thought to play a role.

Epidemiology

VKH syndrome affects young adults between 20 and 40 years of age of both sexes and all races.[138,139] The disease is more common in darker skinned individuals including those with Asian or American Indian ancestry.[138–140] In the United States, Asian-Americans account for the most cases (41%), followed by whites (29%), Hispanics (16%), and blacks (14%).[139] In Japan, VKH syndrome has been associated with HLA-MT3 (100%), HLA-Dr4 (88%), and HLA-Bw54 (40%).[139,141,142] HLA-DRw52 has been found in American Indians with VKH syndrome.[142]

Pathogenesis

VKH syndrome is a bilateral, granulomatous panuveitis.[138,139] Unlike sympathetic ophthalmia, the disease occurs without a history of injury or surgery. On histopathology, the choriocapillaris is infiltrated with macrophages, lymphocytes, and plasma cells. Dalen-Fuchs nodules can be seen. Exudative retinal detachment with widespread RPE disruption is characteristic. Immunohistology demonstrates a predominant T-cell infiltration of the choroid.[142–144] Early in the disease, T-helper cells (CD4+ cells) predominate.[142] Later in

the disease course and analogous to SO, CD8+ T cells are noted in the choroid.[143]

Patients with VKH syndrome have evidence of autoreactivity to retinal autoantigens.[145,146] Peripheral blood lymphocytes in these patients proliferate and secrete IL-2 in response to autologous presentation of ocular autoantigens, including S-antigen and IRBP.[116]

Clinical Presentation

Headaches and meningeal symptoms are common (61%).[138,147,148] The CSF contains activated T lymphocytes with CD8+ markers.[149] Vestibuloauditory complaints include high-range dysacousia, tinnitus, and vertigo. Hearing loss may be evanescent and is often unrecognized by the patient. Formal hearing testing may be needed to detect the high-end loss. The skin may be involved with poliosis, vitiligo, and alopecia (63–90% of patients).[150] Dermatologic findings may be subtle or dramatic, with complete cutaneous depigmentation and poliosis.

Ocular manifestations of VKH syndrome can be divided into anterior and posterior findings.[135,137] Vogt and Koyanagi described the anterior granulomatous uveitis associated with dermatologic and vestibuloauditory findings. Perilimbal vitiligo (Sugiura's sign), mutton fat KP, posterior synechiae, secondary glaucoma, and cataract formation are all common findings. They may occur without posterior uveitis and CNS involvement. Harada described the posterior segment and CNS symptoms and signs in VKH syndrome: headache, meningeal findings and vitritis, multifocal chorioretinitis, and disc edema.[137,138] With disease progression, a pathognomonic, bilateral exudative retinal detachment can be noted. With resolution of the detachment, marked RPE disruption and scarring develop[138] (see Figs. 2.33 and 2.35). Widespread depigmentation of the fundus results in the characteristic "sunset glow" appearance. Subretinal neovascularization can occur and may compromise macular function.

Diagnosis

The complete VKH syndrome is a distinct clinical picture. A patient with dermatologic, vestibuloauditory, CNS symptoms and bilateral panuveitis with exudative detachments presents in 12% of cases; this clinical presentation is pathognomonic. Incomplete forms of VKH have the characteristic ocular manifestations without dermatologic, auditory, or CNS involvement.

Fluorescein angiography reveals a unique multifocal punctate hyperfluoresce at the level of the RPE early in the study (see Fig. 4.2). The retinal vessels are not typically involved.[138,147-150] In severe cases, the choroiditis results in a breakdown of the RPE blood–eye barrier, and pooling of the dye in the subretinal space and exudative retinal detachment.

Ultrasonography can assist in the diagnosis.[151] Shifting, exudative retinal detachment and thickening of the choroid will be seen. Scleral thickening can also be seen.

Differential Diagnosis

Exudative retinal detachments and uveitis can be seen in syphilis, posterior scleritis, and the uveal effusion syndrome. Sympathetic ophthalmia may rarely develop exudative detachments.

Treatment

VKH syndrome responds to corticosteroids and second-generation immunosuppressive agents such as azathioprine (Imuran), cyclophosphamide (Cytoxan), and cyclosporin.[137,152] Steroids are the first line of therapy for active VKH syndrome. High doses at 1 to 1.5 mg/kg/per day should be initiated. Periocular injection of steroid can be useful to gain control of severe episodes. Therapy with both low-dose prednisone and cyclosporin may provide the greatest long-term control.[153,154] Even after disease

remission, however, the disease may recur years later. Retinal reattachment will occur with control of inflammation unless an underlying retinal break or vitreous traction develops. Vitreoretinal surgery may be required in nonresolving cases.

Prognosis

VKH syndrome causes loss of useful vision in 25% of patients. Vision loss is often due to retinal injury and macular scarring. Severe glaucoma appears to be prevalent, occurring in 38% of patients with this condition.[155]

Sarcoidosis

Sarcoidosis is a multisystem, noncaseating, granulomatous disease of unknown etiology that can incite many patterns of ocular inflammation.

Etiology

The etiology of sarcoidosis is unknown.

Epidemiology

Although all races can be affected, blacks are 10 times more likely to develop sarcoidosis than whites.[157-160] The disease affects young adults between the ages of 20 and 50 years and has a slightly increased prevalence in women. Ophthalmic manifestations can be found in 19% to 54% of patients with sarcoidosis.[157-160] Approximately 3% to 5% of all uveitis is thought to be secondary to sarcoidosis.

Pathogenesis

The disease is characterized by discrete noncaseating granuloma (see Fig. 4.5). Schaumann's bodies with acidophilic stars and basophilic spherules can be noted in the granulomas.[156-161] Immunohistopathologic examination demonstrates large numbers of T cells with CD4+ surface markers in the ocular granulomas. Very few B cells or cytotoxic/suppressor CD8+ T cells are seen. IL-2 receptors are present on the T cells, indicating a role for activated helper T cells in sarcoidosis. Despite the intense T-cell activity found in the end-organ, systemic anergy is noted during active stages of the disease. Patients may react to sarcoid-associated antigen in a Kveim skin test.

Clinical Presentation

The disease affects multiple organ systems. Patients may present with fever, weight loss, fatigue, and shortness of breath.[156,159] The upper and lower respiratory tracts are the most frequently involved structures (83%). Lymph nodes, (76%), skin (22%), liver, spleen (20%), and the CNS (8%) are also commonly involved. Large-joint arthralgias and arthritis can be noted in up to 37% of patients. On radiologic studies, the affected bones develop unique "punched out" lesions.

A specific form of sarcoidosis called Heerfordt's syndrome or uveoparotid fever will present with uveitis, parotid gland swelling, and cranial nerve VII involvement.

All parts of the eye can be involved. Sarcoid uveitis can begin as a nongranulomatous disease and evolve into the more classic granulomatous uveitis. The disease may be acute in onset, but is characteristically chronic. Table 18.3 lists the common ocular manifestations of sarcoidosis. These findings are present in 20% to 38% of patients with sarcoidosis. In one series, sarcoidosis was diagnosed in the eye 5 years before systemic manifestations appeared.

The anterior segment is affected more frequently than the retina and choroid.[156–160] A chronic granulomatous anterior uveitis with mutton fat KPs, Koeppe and Busaca nodules, and posterior synechiae are the most common ocular findings of sarcoid uveitis (see Fig. 2.12). The conjunctiva may have inflammatory nodules (see Fig. 2.2).

Table 18.3. Ocular manifestations of sarcoidosis.

Anterior segment (85%)
Conjunctival nodules (7%)
Band keratopathy
Iris nodules (Koeppe and Busacca) (35%)
Iritis (52%)
Cyclitis and ciliary body nodules (42%)
Angle granuloma (50%)
Glaucoma (11%)
Cataract

Posterior segment (30%)
Vitritis with snowballs (common)
Retinal granuloma (rare)
Retinitis (rare)
Retinal periphlebitis (20%)
Arteriolitis (rare)
Neovascularization of the disc/neovascularization elsewhere
Chorioretinitis (11%)
Choroidal granuloma (6%)

Orbital
Lacrimal gland swelling (16%)
Extraocular muscle (2%)
Optic disc edema and neuritis (7%)

Band keratopathy may be noted in chronic disease. Posterior segment disease includes vitritis, disc edema, periphlebitis, and choroidal nodules.[162–171] Peripheral retinal neovascularization and a primary sarcoid retinitis may occur rarely (see Fig. 2.26). The chronic nature of the inflammation will often result in cataract (17%), glaucoma (23%), and permanent retinal damage.

Diagnosis

The diagnosis of sarcoidosis can be made by tissue biopsy, which is confirmed by the presence of noncaseating granuloma in affected tissues. The chest radiograph will be positive with hilar adenopathy in 10% to 95% of patients[156,159] (see Fig. 4.11) Serum lysozyme, angiotensin-converting enzyme (ACE), and calcium are often elevated with pulmonary disease and may be used as screening tests.[172,173] Gallium scan can help determine the extent of systemic involvement but is not diagnostic.[156] Kveim skin testing is seldom performed in the United States. Skin testing may be unreactive and represents systemic anergy (to a panel of common antigens including *Candida* and mumps.)

Although the conjunctiva is often involved, blind biopsies yield positive results in only 8% to 50% of samples.[174] A directed biopsy of an inflammatory nodule in the conjunctiva, however, is often quite fruitful in establishing the diagnosis. The benign nature of this tissue sampling as compared with lung biopsy makes it a useful diagnostic test that should be performed when possible in patients suspected of having sarcoid uveitis.

Often a diagnosis of probable or possible sarcoid uveitis is made based on clinical grounds alone without tissue biopsy confirmation. Chronic, bilateral granulomatous uveitis, in the presence of hilar adenopathy, systemic anergy, and elevated serum lysozyme and ACE and a positive gallium scan is very suggestive of sarcoid uveitis.

Differential Diagnosis

Sarcoidosis should be considered in the differential diagnosis of many if not all forms of uveitis. Tuberculosis may cause a multisystem disease, protean ocular manifestations, pulmonary findings, and elevation of the ACE and lysozyme. A history of exposure to tuberculosis should be investigated and tuberculin skin testing and sputum cultures should be obtained to rule out tuberculosis in most cases of suspected sarcoid uveitis.

Treatment

Active sarcoid uveitis should be treated. In most cases the disease eventually "burns out," and the goals of therapy are to prevent permanent damage to any organ system including the eye. Sarcoidosis responds well to corticosteroid therapy.[156] Topical, regional, and oral corticosteroids are the mainstay of therapy. Initial doses of prednisone (1 mg/kg/per day) are usually successful in controlling ocular inflammation followed by a rapid taper. Often moderate or even very low doses of prednisone (5 mg orally, four times a day) are all that is needed to control the ocular inflammation. Treatment is usually extended.

Characteristically, sarcoidosis does not respond as well to NSAIDs or other immunosuppressive medications. Cyclosporine has helped some patients with steroid-resistant or intolerant cases of uveitis.[156]

Prognosis

The disease is chronic but typically remits over a 6- to 24-month period. One third of patients experience a mild clinical course, 33% a chronic course, and 33% a severe progressive form of the disease. Sarcoidosis may cause death in 5% to 10% of cases.

References

1. Fitzpatrick TB, Polano MK, Suurmond D. *Color Atlas and Synopsis of Clinical Dermatology*. New York: McGraw-Hill; 1983:6.
2. Roitt IM, Brostoff J, Male DK. *Immunology*. St. Louis: CV Mosby; 1987;22:1.
3. Grayson M. Immune and mucous membrane diseases. In: *Diseases of the Cornea*. St. Louis: CV Mosby; 1983:347.
4. Nussenblatt RB, Palestine. Anterior uveitis. In: *Uveitis: Fundamentals and Clinical Practice*. Chicago: Year Book Medical Publishers, 1989:164.
5. Opremcak EM. *Topical Therapy for Iritis. Clinical Modules for Ophthalmologists*. vol. 9, module 7. San Francisco: American Academy of Ophthalmology; 1991.
6. Vadot E, Barth E, Billet P. Epidemiology of uveitis. Preliminary results of a prospective study in Savoy. In: Saari KM, ed. *Uveitis*

Update. Amsterdam: Elsevier Science Publishers BV; 1984:13.

7. Brewerton DA, Caffrey M, Nicholls A, et al. Acute anterior uveitis and HL-A27. *Lancet.* 1973;2:994.

8. Linssen A. Acute anterior uveitis, ankylosing spondylitis and HLA-B27. Thesis, Amsterdam; 1987.

9. Mapstone R, Woodrow JC. HL-A27 and acute anterior uveitis. *Br J Ophthalmol.* 1975;59:270.

10. Stevens G Jr, Chan CC, Wetzig RP, et al. Iris lymphocytic infiltration in patients with clinically quiescent uveitis. *Am J Ophthalmol.* 1987;104:508.

11. Murray PI, Rahi AHS. New concepts in the control of ocular inflammation. *Trans Ophthalmol Soc UK.* 1985;104:152.

12. Rothova A, van Veenendaal WG, Linssen A, et al. Clinical features of acute anterior uveitis. *Am J Ophthalmol.* 1987;103:137.

13. Fuchs E. Uber komplikationen der heterchromie. *Z Augenheilkd.* 1906;15:191.

14. Makley TA. Heterochromic cyclitis in identical twins. *Am J Ophthalmol.* 1956;41:768.

15. Bistis J. La paralyse due sympathique dans l'etiologie de l'heterochromie. *Arch Ophthalmol.* 1912;9:631.

16. Schwab JR. The epidemiologic association of Fuchs' heterochromic iridocyclitis and ocular toxoplasmosis. *Am J Ophthalmol.* 1991;111:356.

17. Murray PI, Mooy CM, Visser-de Jong E, et al. Immunohistochemical analysis of iris biopsy specimens from patients with Fuchs' heterochromic cyclitis. *Am J Ophthalmol.* 1990;109:394.

18. La Hey E, Mooy CM, Baarsma GS, et al. Immune deposits in iris biopsy specimens from patients with Fuchs' heterochromic iridocyclitis. *Am J Ophthalmol.* 1992;113:75.

19. van der Gaag R, Broersma L, Rothova A, et al. Immunity to a corneal antigen in Fuchs' heterochromic cyclitis patients. *Invest Ophthalmol Vis Sci.* 1989;30:443.

20. Berger BB, Tessler HH, Kottow MH. Anterior segment ischemia in Fuchs' heterochromic cyclitis. *Arch Ophthalmol.* 1980;98:499.

21. Loewenfeld IE, Thompson HS. Fuchs's heterochromic cyclitis: a critical review of the literature. *Surv Ophthalmol.* 1973;17:394.

22. Saari M, Vourre I, Tilikainen A, Algvere P.

Genetic background of Fuchs' heterochromic cyclitis. *Can J Ophthalmol.* 1978;13:240.

23. Goldberg MF, Erozan YS, Duke JR, Frost JK. Cytopathologic and histopathologic aspects of Fuch's heterochromic iridocyclitis. *Arch Ophthalmol.* 1965;74:604.

24. Kimura SJ. Fuchs' syndrome of heterochromic cyclitis in brown-eyed patients. *Trans Am Ophthalmol Soc.* 1978;76:76.

25. Liesegang TJ. Clinical features and prognosis in Fuchs' uveitis syndrome. *Arch Ophthalmol.* 1982;100:1622.

26. Hooper PL, Rao NA, Smith RE. Cataract extraction in uveitis patients. *Surv Ophthalmol.* 1990;35:120.

27. Jones NP. Glaucoma in Fuchs' heterochromic uveitis: aetiology, management, and outcome. *Eye.* 1991;5:662.

28. Schepens CL. Examination of the ora serrata region: its clinical significance. In: *Acta XVI Concilium Ophthalmologicum, Britannia.* 1950, vol. 2. London: British Medical Association; 1951:1384.

29. Welch RB, Maumenee AE, Wahlen HE. Peripheral posterior segment inflammation vitreous opacities and edema of the posterior pole. *Arch Ophthalmol.* 1960;64:540.

30. Kimura SJ, Hogan MJ. Chronic cyclitis. *Arch Ophthalmol.* 1964;71:193.

31. Brockhurst RJ, Schepens CL, Okamura ID. Uveitis. II. Peripheral uveitis: clinical description, complications and differential diagnosis. *Am J Ophthalmol.* 1960;49:1257.

32. Intermediate uveitis and pars planitis. In: Nussenblatt RB, Palestine AG. *Uveitis: Fundamentals and Clinical Practice.* Chicago: Year Book Medical Publishers; 1989:32.

33. Stuart JM, Cremer MA, Dixit SN, et al. Collagen-induced arthritis rats. Comparison of vitreous and cartilage derived collagens. *Arthritis Rheum.* 1979;22:347.

34. Henderly DE, Haymond RS, Rao NA, Smith RE. The significance of the pars plana exudate in pars planitis. *Am J Ophthalmol.* 1987;103:669.

35. Pederson JE, Kenyon KR, Green WR, Maumenee AE. Pathology of pars planitis. *Am J Ophthalmol.* 1978;86:762.

36. Zenker H-J. Fluorescein angiography in inflammation of the peripheral fundus: involvement of the pars plana corporis ciliaris III. *Ophthalmologica.* 1985;190:205.

37. Arnold AC, Pepose JS, Hepler RS, Foos RY. Retinal periphlebitis and retinitis in multiple sclerosis. I. Pathologic characteristics. *Ophthalmology.* 1984;91:255.

38. Graham EM, Francis DA, Sanders MD, Rudge P. Ocular inflammatory changes in established multiple sclerosis. *J Neurol Neurosurg Psychiatry.* 1989;52:1360.

39. Vine AK. Severe periphlebitis, peripheral retinal ischemia, and preretinal neovascularization in patients with multiple sclerosis. *Am J Ophthalmol.* 1992;113:28.

40. Breger BC, Leopold IH. The incidence of uveitis in multiple sclerosis. *Am J Ophthalmol.* 1966;62:540.

41. Giles GL. Peripheral uveitis in patients with multiple sclerosis. *Am J Ophthalmol.* 1970;70:17.

42. Aaberg TM, Cesarz TJ, Flickinger RR. Treatment of peripheral uveoretinitis by cryotherapy. *Am J Ophthalmol.* 1973;75:685.

43. Devenyi RG, Mieler WF, Lambrou FH, et al. Cryopexy of the vitreous base in the management of peripheral uveitis. *Am J Ophthalmol.* 1988;196:135.

44. Waring GO III. Treatment of pars planitis. *Surv Ophthalmol.* 1977;22:120.

45. Steahly LP, Mader T. Vitrectomy and severe pars planitis. *J Ocular Ther Surg.* 1984; Jan/Feb:29.

46. Mieler WF, Will BR, Lewis H, Aaberg TM. Vitrectomy in the management of peripheral uveitis. *Ophthalmology.* 1988;95:859.

47. Gills JP, Buckley CE III. Oral cyclophosphamide in the treatment of uveitis. *Trans Am Acad Ophthalmol Otolaryngol.* 1970;74: 505.

48. Wong VG, Hersh EM. Methotrexate in the therapy of cyclitis. *Trans Am Acad Ophthalmol Otolaryngol.* 1965;March/April:279.

49. Gass JDM. Vitiliginous chorioretinitis. *Arch Ophthalmol.* 1981;99:178.

50. Gass JDM. Fluorescein angiography in endogenous intraocular inflammation. In: Aronson SM, Gable CN, Goodner EK, O'Connor GR, eds. *Clinical Methods in Uveitis. Fourth Sloan Symposium on Uveitis.* St. Louis: CV Mosby; 1968;202.

51. Gass JDM. Diffuse retinitis, vitritis and cystoid macular edema. In: *Stereoscopic Atlas of Macular Diseases. Diagnosis and Treatment.* 2nd ed. St. Louis: CV Mosby; 1977:306.

52. Brinton GS, Osher RH, Gass JD. Idiopathic vitritis. *Retina.* 1983;3:95.

53. Gass JD. Acute posterior multifocal placoid pigment epitheliopathy. *Arch Ophthalmol.* 1968;80:177.

54. Ryan SJ, Maumenee AE. Acute posterior placoid pigment epitheliopathy. *Am J Ophthalmol.* 1972;74:1066.

55. Smith VC, Porkorny J, Ernest JT, et al. Visual function in acute posterior multifocal placoid pigment epitheliopathy. *Am J Ophthalmol.* 1978;85:192.

56. Young NJA, Bird AC, Sehmi K. Pigment epithelial diseases with abnormal choroidal perfusion. *Am J Ophthalmol.* 1980;90: 607.

57. Deutman AF, Oosterhuis JA, Boen-tan TN, et al. Acute posterior multifocal placoid pigment epitheliopathy. *Br J Ophthalmol.* 1972;56:863.

58. Kerseten DH, Lessell S, Carlow TJ. Acute posterior multifocal placoid pigment epitheliopathy and late-onset meningo-encephalitis. *Ophthalmology.* 1987;94:393.

59. Smith CH, Savino PJ, Beck RW, et al. Acute posterior multifocal placoid pigment epitheliopathy and cerebral vasculitis. *Arch Neurol.* 1983;40:48.

60. Savino PJ, Weinberg RJ, Yassin JC, et al. Diverse manifestations of acute posterior multifocal placoid pigment epitheliopathy. *Am J Ophthalmol.* 1974;77:659.

61. Wolf MD, Alward WLM, Folk JC. Long-term visual function in acute posterior multifocal placoid pigment epitheliopathy. *Arch Ophthalmol.* 1991;109:800.

62. Krill AE, Deutman AF. Acute retinal pigment epitheliitis. *Am J Ophthalmol.* 1972;74: 193–205.

63. Deutman AF. Acute retinal pigment epitheliitis. *Am J Ophthalmol.* 1974;78:571–578.

64. Freiedman MW. Bilateral, recurrent acute retinal pigment epitheliitis. *Am J Ophthalmol.* 1975;79:567–570.

65. Ryan SJ, Maumenee AE. Birdshot retinochoroidopathy. *Am J Ophthalmol.* 1980;89: 31.

66. Kaplan HJ, Aaberg TM. Birdshot retinochoroidopathy. *Am J Ophthalmol.* 1980;90: 773.

67. Gass JDM. Vitiliginous chorioretinitis. *Arch Ophthalmol.* 1981;99:1778.

68. Opremcak EM. Birdshot retinochoroiditis. In: Albert DM, Jakobiec FA, eds. *Clinical Practice: Principles and Practice of Ophthalmology.* vol. 1. Philadelphia: WB Saunders; 1994:475.

69. Nussenblatt RB, Mittal KK, Ryan S, et al. Birdshot retinochoroidopathy associated with HLA-A29 antigen and immune responsiveness to Retinal S-Antigen. *Am J Ophthalmol.* 1982;94:147.

70. Priem HA, Kijlstra A, Noens L, et al. HLA typing in birdshot chorioretinopathy. *Am J Ophthalmol.* 1988;105:182.

71. Daussett J, Svejgaard A, eds. *HLA and Disease.* Copenhagen: Munksgaard; 1977.

72. Nussenblatt RB, Gery I, Ballintinee EJ, Wacker WB. Cellular immune responsiveness of patients to retinal S-antigen. *Am J Ophthalmol.* 1980;89:173.

73. de Smet MD, Yamamoto JH, Mochizuki M, et al. Cellular immune responses of patients with uveitis to retinal antigens and their fragments. *Am J Ophthalmol.* 1990;110:135.

74. Wacker WB, Donoso LA, Kalsow CM, et al. Experimental allergic uveitis. Isolation, characterization and localization of a soluble uveitopathogenic antigen from bovine retina. *J Immunol.* 1977;119:1949.

75. Donoso LA, Merryman CF, Sery T, et al. Human interstitial retinoid binding protein: a potent uveitopathogenic agent for the induction of experimental autoimmune uveitis. *J Immunol.* 1989;143:79.

76. Mochizuki M, Kuwabara T, McAllister C, et al. Adoptive transfer of experimental autoimmune uveoretinitis in rats: immunopathogenic mechanisms and histologic features. *Invest Ophthalmol Vis Sci.* 1985;26:1.

77. Soubrane G, Cosca G, Binaghi P, Bernard JA. Birdshot retinochoroidopathy and subretinal new vessels. *Br J Ophthalmol.* 1983;67:461.

78. Nussenblatt RB, Palestine AG, Chan CC, et al. Cyclosporin A therapy in treatment of intraocular inflammatory disease resistant to systemic corticosteroids and cytotoxic agents. *Am J Ophthalmol.* 1983;96:275.

79. Francois J, Verriest G, DeLaey JJ. Leber's idiopathic stellate retinopathy. *Am J Ophthalmol.* 1969;68:340.

80. Gass JD. Diseases of the optic nerve that may simulate macular disease. *Trans Am Acad Ophthalmol Otolaryngol.* 1977;83:766.

81. Dreyer RF, Hopen G, Gass JDM, Smith JL. Leber's idiopathic stellate neuroretinitis. *Arch Ophthalmol.* 1984;102:1140.

82. Maitland CG, Miller NR. Neuroretinitis. *Arch Ophthalmol.* 1984;102:1146.

83. Jampol LM, Sieving PA, Pugh D, et al. Multiple evanescent white dot syndrome. I. Clinical findings. *Arch Ophthalmol.* 1984;102:671–674.

84. Sieving PA, Fishman GA, Jampol LM, Pugh D. Multiple evanescent white dot syndrome. II. Electrophysiology of photoreceptors during retinal pigment epithelial disease. *Arch Ophthalmol.* 1984;102:675–679.

85. Aaberg TM, Campo RV, Joffe L. Recurrences and bilaterality in the multiple evanescent white-dot syndrome. *Am J Ophthalmol.* 1985;100:29–37.

86. Gass JDM, Hamed LM. Acute macular neuroretinopathy and multiple evanescent white dot syndrome occurring in the same patients. *Arch Ophthalmol.* 1989;107:189–193.

87. Miller MH, Spalton DJ, Fitzke FW, Bird AC. Acute macular neuroretinopathy. *Ophthalmology.* 1989;96:265.

88. Dodwell DG, Jampol LM, Rosenberg M, et al. Optic nerve involvement associated with the multiple evanescent white-dot syndrome. *Ophthalmology.* 1990;97:862.

89. Hamed LM, Glaser JS, Gass JDM, Schatz NJ. Protracted enlargement of the blind spot in multiple evanescent white dot syndrome. *Arch Ophthalmol.* 1989;107:194.

90. Palestine AG, Nussenblatt RB, Parver LM, Knox DL. Progressive subretinal fibrosis and uveitis. *Br J Ophthalmol.* 1984;68:667.

91. Singh K, de Frank MP, Shults WT, Watzke RC. Acute idiopathic blind spot enlargement. *Ophthalmology.* 1991;98:497.

92. Cantrill HL, Folk C. Multifocal choroiditis with progressive subretinal fibrosis. *Am J Ophthalmol.* 1986;101:107-180.

93. Palestine AG et al. Histopathology of the subretinal fibrosis and uveitis syndrome. *Ophthalmology.* 1985;92:838–844.

94. Kim MK, Chan C-C, Belfort R Jr, et al. Histopathologic and immunohistopathologic features of subretinal fibrosis and uveitis syndrome. *Am J Ophthalmol.* 1987;104:15.

95. Palestine AG, Nussenblatt RB, Parver LM, Knox DI. Progressive subretinal fibrosis and uveitis. *Br J Ophthalmol*. 1984;68:667.

96. Nozik RA, Dorsch W. A new chorioretinopathy associated with anterior uveitis. *Am J Ophthalmol*. 1973;76:758-762.

97. Dreyer RF, Gass JDM. Multifocal choroiditis and panuveitis: a syndrome that mimics ocular histoplasmosis. *Arch Ophthalmol*. 1984;102:1776-1784.

98. Tiedeman JS. Epstein-Barr viral antibodies in multifocal choroiditis and panuveitis. *Am J Ophthalmol*. 1987;103:659.

99. Morgan CM, Schatz H. Recurrent multifocal choroiditis. *Ophthalmology*. 1986;93:1138.

100. Khorram KD, Jampol LM, Rosenberg MA. Blind spot enlargement as a manifestation of multifocal choroiditis. *Arch Ophthalmol*. 1991;109:1403.

101. Watzke RC, Packer AJ, Folk JC, et al. Punctate inner choroidopathy. *Am J Ophthalmol*. 1984;98:572.

102. Laatikainen L, Erkkila H. Serpiginous choroiditis. *Br J Ophthalmol*. 1974;58:777.

103. Hamilton AM, bird AC. Geographical choroidopathy. *Br J Ophthalmol*. 1974;58:784.

104. Baarsma GS, Deutman AF. Serpiginous (geographic) choroiditis. *Doc Ophthalmol*. 1976;40:269.

105. Gass JDM. *Stereoscopic Atlas of Macular Diseases. Diagnosis and Treatment*. 2nd ed. St. Louis: CV Mosby; 1977:112.

106. Jampol LM, Orth D, Daily MJ, Raab MF. Subretinal neovascularization with geographic (serpiginous) choroiditis. *Am J Ophthalmol*. 1979;88:683.

107. Serpiginous choroidopathy (choroiditis). In: Nussenblatt RB, Palestine AG. *Uveitis: Fundamentals and Clinical Practice*. Chicago: Year Book Medical Publishers; 1989:309.

108. Hooper PL, Kaplan HJ. Triple agent immunosuppression in serpiginous choroiditis. *Ophthalmology*. 1991;98:944.

109. Laatikainen L, Tarkkanen A. Failure of cyclosporin A in serpiginous choroiditis. *J Ocular Therapy Surg*. 1984;3:280.

110. MacKenzie W. *A Practical Treatise on Disease of the Eye*. London: Longmans; 1830.

111. Marak GE Jr. Recent advances in sympathetic ophthalmia. *Surv Ophthalmol*. 1979;24:141.

112. Albert DM, Diaz-Rohena R. A historical review of sympathetic ophthalmia and its epidemiology. *Surv Ophthalmol*. 1989;34:1.

113. Nussenblatt RB, Palestine AG. Sympathetic ophthalmia. In: *Uveitis. Fundamentals and Clinical Practice*. Chicago: Year Book Medical Publishers; 1989:257.

114. Wong VG, Anderson R, O'Brien PJ. Sympathetic ophthalmia and lymphocyte transformation. *Am J Ophthalmol*. 1971;72:960.

115. Marak GE Jr, Font RL, Johnson MC, et al. Lymphocyte-stimulating activity of ocular tissues in sympathetic ophthalmia. *Invest Ophthalmol Vis Sci*. 1971;10:770.

116. Opremcak EM, Cowans AB. Enumeration of autoreactive helper T lymphocytes in uveitis. *Invest Ophthalmol Vis Sci*. 1991;32:2561.

117. Liddy N, Stuat J. Sympathetic ophthalmia in Canada. *Can J Ophthalmol*. 1972;7:157.

118. Lubin JR, Albert DM, Weinstein M. Sixty-five years of sympathetic ophthalmia. *Ophthalmology*. 1980;87:109.

119. Reynard M, Shulman IA, Azen SP, et al. Histocompatibility antigens in sympathetic ophthalmia. *Am J Ophthalmol*. 1983;95:216.

120. Font RL, Fine BS, Messmer E, Rowsey JF. Light and electron microscopic study of Dalén-Fuchs nodules in sympathetic ophthalmia. *Ophthalmology*. 1982;89:75.

121. Müller-Hermelink HK, Kraus-Mackiw E, Daus W. Early stages of human sympathetic ophthalmia. *Arch Ophthalmol*. 1984;102:1353.

122. Jakobiec FA, Marboe CC, Knowles DM II, et al. Human sympathetic ophthalmia. An analysis of the inflammatory infiltrate by hybridoma-monoclonal antibodies, immunochemistry, and correlative electron microscopy. *Ophthalmology*. 1983;90:76.

123. Kaplan HJ, Waldrep JC, Chan WC, et al. Human sympathetic ophthalmia: immunologic analysis of the vitreous and uvea. *Arch Ophthalmol*. 1986;104:240.

124. Blodi FC. Sympathetic uveitis as an allergic phenomenon. *Trans Am Acad Ophthalmol Otolaryngol*. 1959;63:642.

125. Spitznas M. Fluorescein angiography of sympathetic ophthalmia. *Klin Monatsbl Augenheilkd*. 1976;169:195.

126. Chan C-C. Relationship between sympathetic ophthalmia, phacoanaphylatic endo-

phthalmitis, and Vogt-Koyanagi-Harada disease. *Ophthalmology*. 1988;95:619.

127. Gass JDM. Sympathetic ophthalmia following vitrectomy. *Am J Ophthalmol*. 1982;93: 552.

128. Lewis ML, Gass JDM, Spencer WH. Sympathetic uveitis after trauma and vitrectomy. *Arch Ophthalmol*. 1978;96:263.

129. Maisel JM, Vorwerk PA. Sympathetic uveitis after giant tear repair. *Retina*. 1989;9: 122.

130. Lang DW. Morbidity and mortality in ophthalmology. In: Brice RA Jr, McGoldrick KE, Oppenheimer P, eds. *Anesthesia for Ophthalmology*. Birmingham: Aesculapius Publishing Co; 1982:195.

131. Reynard M, Riffenburgh RS, Maes EF. Effect of corticosteroid treatment and enucleation on the visual prognosis of sympathetic ophthalmia. *Am J Ophthalmol*. 1983; 96:290.

132. Moore CE. Sympathetic ophthalmitis treated with azathioprine. *Br J Ophthalmol*. 1968;52:688.

133. Wong VG, Hersh EM, McMaster RB. Treatment of a presumed case of sympathetic ophthalmia with methotrexate. *Arch Ophthalmol*. 1966;76:66.

134. Makley TA, Azar A. Sympathetic ophthalmia: a long-term follow-up. *Arch Ophthalmol*. 1978;96:257.

135. Vogt A. Frühzeitiges Ergrauen der Zilien und Bemerkungen üben den sogannten plözlichen Eintritt dieser Veränderung. *Klin Monatsbl Augenheilkd*. 1906;44:228.

136. Koyanagi Y. Dysakusis, Alopecia un Poliosis bei schwerer Uveitis nicht traumatischen Ursprungs. *Klin Monatsbl Augenheilkd*. 1929;82:194.

137. Harada E. Clinical observations of nonsuppurative choroiditis. *Acta Soc Ophthalmol Jpn*. 1926;30:356.

138. Nussenblatt RB, Palestine AG. The Vogt-Koyanagi-Harada syndrome. In: *Uveitis: Fundamentals and Clinical Practice*. Chicago: Year Book Medical Publishers; 1989:274.

139. Ohno S, Char DH, Kimura SJ, O'Connor GR. Vogt-Koyanagi-Harada syndrome. *Am J Ophthalmol*. 1977;83:735.

140. Davis JL, Mittal KK, Vreidlin V, et al. HLA associations and ancestry in Vogt-Koyanagi-Harada disease and sympathetic ophthalmia. *Ophthalmology*. 1990;97:1137.

141. Zhao M, Jhiang Y, Abrahams W. Association of HLA antigens with Vogt-Koyanagi-Harada syndrome in a Han Chinese population. *Arch Ophthalmol*. 1991;109:368.

142. Martinez JA, Lopez PF, Sternberg P Jr, et al. Vogt-Koyanagi-Harada syndrome in patients with Cherokee Indian ancestry. *Am J Ophthalmol*. 1992;114:615.

143. Inomata H, Sakamoto T. Immunohistochemical studies of Vogt-Koyanagi-Harada disease with sunset sky fundus. *Curr Eye Res*. 1990;9(suppl):35.

144. Kahn M, Pepose JS, Green WR, et al. Immunocytologic findings in a case of Vogt-Koyanagi-Harada syndrome. *Ophthalmology*. 1993;100:1191.

145. Hammer H. Cellular hypersensitivity to uveal pigment confirmed by leucocyte migration tests in sympathetic ophthalmitis and the Vogt-Koyanagi-Harada syndrome. *Br J Ophthalmol*. 1974;58:773.

146. Yokoyama MM, Matsui Y, Hamashiroya HM, et al. Humoral and cellular immunity studies in patients with Vogt-Koyanagi-Harada syndrome and pars planitis. *Invest Ophthalmol Vis Sci*. 1981;20:364.

147. Perry HD, Font RL. Clinical and histopathologic observations in severe Vogt-Koyanagi-Harada syndrome. *Am J Ophthalmol*. 1977;83:242.

148. Rubsamen PE, Gass JDM. Vogt-Koyanagi-Harada syndrome. Clinical course, therapy, and long-term visual outcome. *Arch Ophthalmol*. 1991;109:682.

149. Norose K, Yano A, Aosai F, Segawa K. Immunologic analysis of cerebrospinal fluid lymphocytes in Vogt-Koyanagi-Harada disease. *Invest Ophthalmol Vis Sci*. 1990;31: 1210.

150. Rosen E. Uveitis, with poliosis, vitiligo, alopecia and dysacousia (Vogt-Koyanagi syndrome). *Arch Ophthalmol*. 1945;33:281.

151. Forster DJ, Cano MR, Green RL, Rao NA. Echographic features of the Vogt-Koyanagi-Harada syndrome. *Arch Ophthalmol*. 1990;108:1421.

152. Moorthy RS, Chong LP, Smith RE, Rao NA. Subretinal neovascular membranes in Vogt-Koyanagi-Harada syndrome. *Am J Ophthalmol*. 1993;116:164.

153. Wakefield D, McCluskey P, Reece G. Cyclosporin therapy in Vogt-Koyanagi-Harada disease. *Aust NZ J Ophthalmol*. 1990;18:137.

154. Nussenblatt RB, Palestine AG, Chan CC. Cyclosporin A therapy in the treatment of intraocular inflammatory disease resistant to systemic corticosteroids and cytotoxic agents. *Am J Ophthalmol*. 1983;96:275.

155. Forster DJ, Rao NA, Hill RA, et al. Incidence and management of glaucoma in Vogt-Koyanagi-Harada syndrome. *Ophthalmology*. 1993;100:613.

156. Nussenblatt RB, Palestine AG. Sarcoidosis. In: *Uveitis: Fundamentals and Clinical Practice*. Chicago: Year Book Medical Publishers; 1989:274.

157. Crick RP, Hoyle C, Smellie H. The eyes in sarcoidosis. *Br J Ophthalmol*. 1961;45:461.

158. Jabs DA, Johns CJ. Ocular involvement in chronic sarcoidosis. *Am J Ophthalmol*. 1986;102:297.

159. Obenauf CD, Shaw HE, Sydnor CF, Klintworth GK. Sarcoidosis and its ophthalmic manifestations. *Am J Ophthalmol*. 1978;86:648.

160. James DG, Langley RA, Ainslie D. Ocular sarcoidosis. *Br J Ophthalmol*. 1964;48:461.

161. Chan C-C, Wetzig RP, Palestine AG, et al. Immunohistopathology of ocular sarcoidosis. *Arch Ophthalmol*. 1987;105:1398.

162. Letocha CE, Shields JA, Goldberg RE. Retinal changes in sarcoidosis. *Can J Ophthalmol*. 1975;10:184.

163. Denis P, Nordmann J-P, Laroche L, Saraux H. Branch retinal vein occlusion associated with a sarcoid choroidal granuloma. *Am J Ophthalmol*. 1992;13:333.

164. Spalton DJ, Sanders MD. Fundus changes in histologically confirmed sarcoidosis. *Br J Ophthalmol*. 1981;65:348.

165. Madigan JC Jr, Gragoudas ES, Schwartz PL, Lapus JV. Peripheral retinal neovascularization in sarcoidosis and sickle cell anemia. *Am J Ophthalmol*. 1977;83:387.

166. Chumbley LC, Kearns TP. Retinopathy of sarcoidosis. *Am J Ophthalmol*. 1972;73:124.

167. Duker JS, Brown GC, McNamara A. Proliferative sarcoid retinopathy. *Ophthalmology*. 1988;95:1680.

168. Gass JDM, Olson CL. Sarcoidosis with optic nerve and retinal involvement. *Arch Ophthalmol*. 1976;94:945.

169. Gould H, Kaufman HE. Sarcoid of the fundus. *Arch Ophthalmol*. 1961;65:161.

170. Marcus DF, Bovino JA, Burton TC. Sarcoid granuloma of the choroid. *Ophthalmology*. 1982;89:1326.

171. Campo RV, Aaberg TM. Choroidal granuloma in sarcoidosis. *Am J Ophthalmol*. 1984;97:419.

172. Weinreb RN, Kimura SJ. Uveitis associated with sarcoidosis and angiotensin converting enzyme. *Am J Ophthalmol*. 1986;89:180.

173. Baarsma GS, La Hey E, Glasius E, et al. The predictive value of serum angiotensin converting enzyme and lysozyme levels in the diagnosis of ocular sarcoidosis. *Am J Ophthalmol*. 1987;104:211.

174. Nichols CW, Eagle RC, Yanoff M, et al. Conjunctival biopsy as an aid in the evaluation of the patient with suspected sarcoidosis. *Ophthalmology*. 1980;87:287.

Ocular Inflammations Associated with Masquerade Syndromes

19
Neoplastic and Infectious Diseases Masquerading as Uveitis

Intraocular Lymphoma (Reticulum Cell Sarcoma)

Intraocular lymphoma has been termed reticulum cell sarcoma (RCS), histiocytic lymphoma, primary central nervous system (CNS) lymphoma, and non-Hodgkin's lymphoma of the CNS (NHL-CNS).[1-6] Although RCS is well ingrained in the ophthalmic literature, this disease is not a sarcoma, nor is it of histiocytic origin. RCS is the most inaccurate name for this disease; nevertheless, it is virtually interchangeable with intraocular large cell lymphoma in the literature.

Etiology

Intraocular lymphoma is a non-Hodgkin's large cell lymphoma that may originate in the eye or brain.[1-6] Spread outside the CNS is rare. If not diagnosed and treated, NHL-CNS is a fatal disease that can present as a uveitis.

Epidemiology

Men are slightly more affected than women. The average age of onset is 64 years; the youngest reported patient is 27 years of age.[6-8] NHL-CNS is a relatively rare neoplasm but has been increasingly observed over the past decade.[6]

Pathogenesis

The exact pathogenesis of this multifocal lymphoma is not known. It may begin in the eye, brain, or both. Involvement of these organs may be simultaneous or separated by years.[3] In the eye, neoplastic cells with large nuclei infiltrate the optic nerve, vitreous, and subretinal space.[2,3] The uveal tract has minimal involvement. The cells are typically polymorphic with scanty cytoplasm and eccentric nucleoli. Mitotic figures may be seen. Secondary, reactive inflammatory cells can be seen with the tumor cells.

Immunohistochemistry study reveals B-cell markers (CD19, 20, 22) with either kappa or lambda light chains.[6,9] It is interesting to note that the vitreous and retina are infiltrated with B cells, whereas the underlying choroid has a secondary T-cell response—perhaps a host response to contain the tumor.[9]

Clinical Presentation

Patients with NHL-CNS often have CNS signs and symptoms (56%). A visceral/lymphadenopathy form (16%) may have systemic involvement as well, but NHL-CNS may present solely within the eye without other organ involvement.[10] Untreated, these primary ocular forms spread outside the eye within 20 to 36 months.

Patients complain of bilateral (75%)

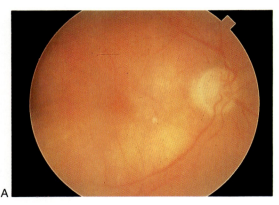
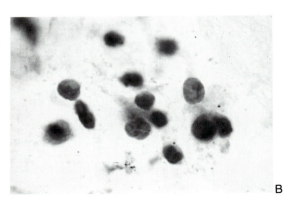

A   B

Figure 19.1. Masquerade syndrome—intraocular lymphoma. A: Medically unresponsive vitritis in a 73-year-old woman with multifocal subretinal infiltrates. **B:** Vitreous biopsy demonstrates the polymorphous neoplastic cells with large nuclei.

decreased vision with floaters.[1–10] The eye appears white and quiet. Biomicroscopic examination reveals cells without significant flare. These cells often appear clumped within the vitreous gel. Vitreous hemorrhage, hyphema, disc edema, vascular cuffing, vasculitis, and retinitis can all be noted.[11,12] Characteristic multifocal, solid, yellowish white retinal pigment epithelial detachments and subretinal infiltrates can be found in more advanced cases (Fig. 19.1A).[13–15]

Diagnosis

Chronic medically unresponsive uveitis, vitritis, and subretinal infiltrates in an elderly patient with CNS complaints should suggest NHL-CNS.[1–15] A high degree of clinical suspicion is required. A vitreous biopsy should be considered in this clinical setting to confirm the diagnosis.

Vitrectomy may be diagnostic.[16] It is not uncommon, however, to require several vitreous biopsies to establish the diagnosis, as many of the cells in the eye are reactive inflammatory cells.[4,6] The malignant cells are large and pleomorphic, with nuclear membranes ("reticulin"), mitotic figures, and scant cytoplasm (Fig. 19.1B).

Fluorescein angiography reveals early hypofluorescent lesions with late staining. Computed tomography (CT) or magnetic resonance imaging (MRI) studies may confirm CNS involvement with periventricular infiltration. Lumbar puncture may also demonstrate the tumor cells in the CNS forms of the disease. Cerebrospinal fluid analysis may be performed initially to establish the diagnosis prior to vitreous biopsy when CNS symptoms or radiologic findings are detected.

Differential Diagnosis

The differential diagnosis is large for diffuse uveitis, vitritis, and subretinal infiltration. In an elderly patient with CNS complaints and corticosteroid unresponsive disease, NHL-CNS should be considered. Other infectious forms of uveitis such as syphilis, tuberculosis, Lyme disease, sarcoidosis, birdshot retinochoroidopathy, and endogenous endophthalmitis are all in the differential diagnosis.

Treatment

Patients may experience a transient, beneficial response to a course of corticosteroids.[6]

Corticosteroids are lytic for lymphoma cells. Typically, the "uveitis" will return. Once the diagnosis has been established, consultation with a hematologist/oncologist will assist in the staging of the disease. Therapy can be designed predicated on the extent of disease and philosophy of the treatment center.[17,18] Ocular irradiation (3000 rads) is appropriate for localized disease. Radiation (4000 rads) to the brain and spinal cord and intrathecal methotrexate can be used with primary CNS large cell lymphoma. Systemic chemotherapy regimens have been added to radiation with increasing acceptance because of the poor prognosis associated with this disease.[19–22] Consensus as to the most effective chemotherapeutic regimen has not been reached, as all appear to improve the prognosis and natural history.

Prognosis

If untreated, RCS has a poor prognosis. The average survival after diagnosis is 21 to 35 months, with a 23% 5-year survival rate.[1–10] Chemotherapy can increase disease-free remission to a median of 41 months.[17]

Infectious Endophthalmitis

Endophthalmitis is a purulent inflammation of the intraocular contents.

Etiology

Most cases of endophthalmitis are associated with infectious agents.[23–25] Bacterial endophthalmitis is the most common form. Fungal infections account for 3% to 13% of all cases. The incidence of culture-negative, aseptic endophthalmitis is about 27%.

Epidemiology

Surgical or nonsurgical trauma accounts for 75% of all cases of endophthalmitis. The incidence of endophthalmitis after cataract surgery is 5 in 1000 cases; 7% to 10% of patients with nonsurgical trauma conditions also develop endophthalmitis.[26,27] Endogenous endophthalmitis accounts for the other 25% of reported cases of endophthalmitis.[28] Patients with endogenous endophthalmitis are typically immunocompromised. In contrast to exogenous forms, endogenous endophthalmitis is more commonly caused by fungal agents.

Pathogenesis

Contamination can occur in exogenous forms of endophthalmitis at the time of injury or as a result of poor healing after wound repair. Postoperative wound leaks, vitreous wick, or poor postoperative hygiene may also contribute to the development of endophthalmitis.

Endogenous endophthalmitis is a result of infectious emboli, metastatic to the uveal or retinal circulations.[28] Infection begins in the posterior structures and may cause widespread damage to the retina and choroid during the clinically silent phase of the disease. Immunocompromised patients on chemotherapy, patients with cancer, intravenous drug abusers, patients with severe diabetes, and patients on hemodialysis, hyperalimentation, or chronic antibiotic therapy are at higher risk for developing endogenous endophthalmitis.

Clinical Presentation

Endogenous, exogenous, bacterial, and fungal forms of endophthalmitis typically have disparate clinical presentations. Most patients with exogenous bacterial endophthalmitis report pain (73%) and decreased vision (57%).[23–25] Unlike true uveitis, endophthalmitis is associated with lid edema, conjunctival chemosis, corneal edema, and fibrin formation. Intraocular cell and flare, hypopyon, retinal vasculitis, hemorrhage, and edema may progress rapidly (Fig. 19.2). The vitritis may be severe and can obscure the fundus red reflex.

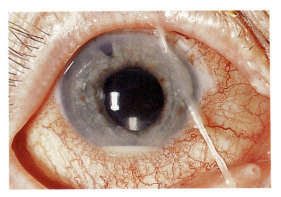

Figure 19.2. Masquerade syndrome—exogenous bacterial endophthalmitis. Decreased vision, pain, and redness 3 days after uneventful cataract operation. Note the fibrin and hypopyon in the anterior chamber. Cultures grew *Staphylococcus epidermidis*.

Endogenous fungal or even bacterial endophthalmitis in immunocompromised patients is more indolent, with a slower onset and a more chronic course.[28] Pain may be mild to absent. Vision may be good in fungal forms. The eye may be white and quiet (Fig. 19.3A,B). Bacterial forms have a more destructive course and can cause profound loss of vision.

Diagnosis

A high degree of clinical suspicion is necessary in the diagnosis of all forms of endophthalmitis. The clinical setting of recent trauma or surgery and an immunocompromised patient should suggest the possibility of infectious endophthalmitis. Aqueous and vitreous biopsy should be performed.[23-25] The specimen should be cultured for aerobic and anaerobic bacteria and fungus.

Differential Diagnosis

Surgical or nonsurgical trauma alone may cause noninfectious intraocular inflammation, which typically is mild and not associated with severe pain or significant loss of vision. The inflammation responds well to topical therapy.

Treatment

Exogenous, bacterial forms of endophthalmitis should be treated aggressively.[24,25,28-30] The prognosis has improved greatly in endophthalmitis as a result of the widespread use of intraocular antibiotic

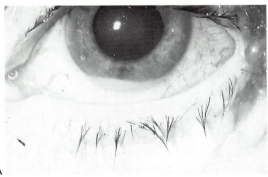
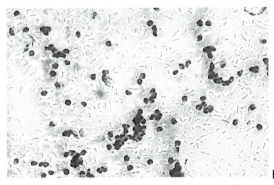

A   B

Figure 19.3. Masquerade syndrome—endogenous bacterial endophthalmitis. A: Comfortable, "quiet" eye in a debilitated patient with a liver abscess. Visual acuity was 20/100. Note the relatively quiet eye, absent limbal flush, and a prominent hypopyon. **B:** The smear from a direct vitreous aspirate showed innumerable gram-negative bacteria. Diagnosis was *Klebsiella pneumoniae*.

combinations. Amikacin (400 μg/0.1 ml) and vancomycin (1 mg/0.1 ml) are currently the antibiotics of choice of many vitreoretinal surgeons for postoperative endophthalmitis. Gentamicin (100 μg/0.1 ml), cefazolin (2.5 mg/0.1 ml), clindamycin (200 μg/0.1 ml) and ceftazidine 2–2.5 μg/ml are also widely used. Intravenous antibiotics such as cefazolin and gentamicin are often used adjunctly. The exact role for systemic, intraocular, and topical antibiotics is currently under investigation in the Endophthalmic Vitrectomy Study.[31]

The role of adjunctive vitrectomy is controversial.[32-35] The theoretical advantage of debriding the eye of bacteria, antigens, toxins, and inflammatory mediators must be weighed against the trauma of surgery. Severe inflammation, organized vitreous, inability to stabilize the eye, and the growth of virulent organisms are all relative indications for vitrectomy.

Adjunctive intraocular corticosteroid therapy (400 μg dexamethasone) has been used to treat endophthalmitis.[32,36] Animal studies and several small clinical series have demonstrated a beneficial effect.

Endogenous forms of endophthalmitis should be treated with systemic antifungal or antibacterial agents.[28] The breakdown of the blood–eye barrier allows good penetration of antibiotic in this disease. Intraocular antibiotics can also be used. Intraocular amphotericin B (4 μg/0.1 ml) can be given when fungal endophthalmitis is suspected or diagnosed.

Prognosis

Failure to diagnose infectious endophthalmitis or conservative therapy that does not include intraocular antibiotics results in loss of the eye. Enucleation will be required in as many as 60% of patients; in contrast, aggressive approaches can maintain useful vision in 50% of patients.[24,25,32-35] The prognosis is poor if virulent organisms are cultured.

Chronic Anaerobic Endophthalmitis

Chronic anaerobic endophthalmitis is a unique form of chronic intraocular infection secondary to anaerobic *Propionibacterium* species.

Etiology

Propionibacterium species are anaerobic, gram-positive, pleomorphic bacilli.[37-40] *P. acnes* and *P. granulosa* are normal skin flora and are found in 10% to 40% of skin cultures. The bacteria are characterized by low virulence and slow growth.

Epidemiology

P. acnes causes a granulomatous chronic skin disease.[38] Chronic postoperative and prosthetic infections can be secondary to contamination with this bacteria. Other anaerobic bacterial species (*Achromobacter*, *Clostridia*, *Bacteroides*) can cause infection that is typically more acute and fulminant.

Pathogenesis

P. acnes is a very low virulent organism. It resists polymorphonuclear (PMN) leukocyte ingestion and the lytic effects of lysozyme and peroxide.[41] The cell wall contains peptidoglycan-teichoic acid, which is a potent macrophage activator. Cell wall proteins from *Propionibacterium* species have been used as an adjuvant in certain cancer therapies due to this action.[41] In the eye, *P. acnes* is a replicating antigen and may combine with autoantigens such as lens proteins to promote a secondary autoimmune response as well as a low-grade infection.[37-40] Immunohistochemistry has demonstrated mostly PMNs (80–90%) with macrophages surrounding foci of infection.[42] Lymphocytes account for only 5% of the inflammatory cells. The lymphocytes present are all CD4 + helper T cells.

Clinical Presentation

Patients present with a history of an un-complicated cataract surgery and intraocu-lar lens implantation.[37,39] The initial post-operative period may be uneventful. One to nine months after surgery a mild, non-granulomatous anterior uveitis is noted. The inflammation may respond initially to topical steroids. Over time, the uveitis be-comes persistent. The eye develops a chronic, granulomatous (50%) uveitis with hypopyon (95%).[43] The posterior capsule often develops a whitish plaque.[43] The eye may have moderate pain and redness but typically good vision.

Diagnosis

The diagnosis is made by aqueous and vit-reous culture.[39] The smear reveals PMNs, "foamy" macrophages. Weakly staining, gram-positive pleomorphic rods can be seen on the smear.[37–40] Anaerobic culture demonstrates a slow-growing, fastidious, anaerobic bacilli. Cultures should be main-tained for 5 to 14 days.[39]

Differential Diagnosis

Postoperative inflammation, lens-induced uveitis, sympathetic ophthalmia, fungal endophthalmitis, and uveitis-glaucoma-hyphema (UGH) syndrome may all present as a chronic, postoperative inflammation. Preexisting uveitis may also be the cause of chronic postoperative inflammation.

Treatment

Vitrectomy may be both diagnostic and therapeutic.[39,43] Material is obtained from the flocculent areas surrounding the intra-ocular lens and lens capsule for culture. The involved capsule area of lens may be removed to debride the foci of infection. In-traocular cephalosporin or vancomycin (1 mg/0.1 ml) should be delivered when *P.*

acnes is suspected.[39,43] The organism is often resistant to aminoglycosides. In most cases, the intraocular lens can be left in position. If recurrent disease occurs, it may be necessary to remove the capsular bag and intraocular lens to sterilize the eye.

Prognosis

The prognosis for vision is often good for this form of bacterial endophthalmitis.

References

1. Nussenblatt RB, Palestine AG. Intraocular lymphoma and other malignancies. In: Nussenblatt RB, Palestine AG. *Uveitis: Fundamentals and Clinical Practice.* Chicago: Year Book Medical Publishers; 1989:315.
2. Barr CC, Green WR, Payne JW, et al. Intra-ocular reticulum-cell sarcoma: clinicopatho-logic study of four cases and review of the literature. *Surv Ophthalmol.* 1975;19:224.
3. Buettner H, Bolling JP. Intravitreal large-cell lymphoma. *Mayo Clin Proc.* 1993;68:1011.
4. Char DH, Ljung B-M, Miller T, Phillips T. Primary intraocular lymphoma (ocular retic-ulum cell sarcoma) diagnosis and manage-ment. *Ophthalmology.* 1988;95:625.
5. Sloas HA, Starling J, Harper DG, Cupples HP. Update of ocular reticulum cell sar-coma. *Arch Ophthalmol.* 1981;99:1048.
6. Whitcup SM, de Smet MD, Rubin BI, et al. Intraocular lymphoma: clinical and histo-pathologic diagnosis. *Ophthalmology.* 1993; 100:1399.
7. Hochberg FH, Miller DC. Primary central nervous system lymphoma. *J Neurosurg.* 1988;68:835.
8. DeAngelis LM, Yahalom J, Heinemann MH, et al. Primary CNS lymphoma: combined treatment with chemotherapy and radiother-apy. *Neurology.* 1990;40:80.
9. Lopez JS, Chan C-C, Burnier M, et al. Immu-nohistochemistry findings in primary intra-ocular lymphoma. *Am J Ophthalmol.* 1991; 112:472.
10. Freeman LN, Schachat AP, Knox DL, et al. Clinical features, laboratory investigations, and survival in ocular reticulum cell sar-coma. *Ophthalmology.* 1987;94:1631.
11. Ridley ME, McDonald HR, Sternberg P Jr, et

al. Retinal manifestations of ocular lymphoma (reticulum cell sarcoma). *Ophthalmology*. 1992;99:1153.

12. Gass JDM, Trattler HL. Retinal artery obstruction and atheromas associated with non-Hodgkin's large cell lymphoma (reticulum cell sarcoma). *Arch Ophthalmol*. 1991; 109:1134.

13. Jakobiec FA, Sacks E, Kronish JW, et al. Multifocal static creamy choroidal infiltrates. *Ophthalmology*. 1987;94:397.

14. Gass JDM, Sever RJ, Sanderson W, et al. Multifocal pigment epithelial detachments by reticulum cell sarcoma. *Retina*. 1984;4:135.

15. Lang GK, Surer JL, Green WR, et al. Ocular reticulum cell sarcoma: clinicopathologic correlation of a case with multifocal lesions. *Retina*. 1985;5:79.

16. Engel HM, Green WR, Michels RG, et al. Diagnostic vitrectomy. *Retina*. 1981;1:121.

17. DeAngelis LM, Yahalom J, Thaler HT, Kher U. Combined modality therapy for primary CNS lymphoma. *J Clin Oncol*. 1992;10:635.

18. Armitage JO. What is the best treatment for diffuse large cell lymphoma? *Hematol Oncol Ann*. 1993;1:15.

19. Longo DL, Duffey PL. Management of aggressive histology lymphoma: an approach based on data from the National Cancer Institute. *Hematol Oncol Ann*. 1993;1:19.

20. O'Reilly SE, Voss N, Connors JM. Primary treatment of patients with diffuse large cell lymphoma at the British Columbia Cancer Agency. *Hematol Oncol Ann*. 1993;1:31.

21. Chopra R, Linch DC, Goldstone AH. The University College and Middlesex Hospital's approach to primary treatment of diffuse large cell lymphomas. *Hematol Oncol Ann*. 1993;1:41.

22. Greer JP, Wolff SN, Stein RS. Therapy of large cell lymphoma at Vanderbilt University. *Hematol Oncol Ann*. 1993;1:51.

23. Forster RK. Etiology and diagnosis of bacterial postoperative endophthalmitis. *Ophthalmology*. 1978;85:320.

24. Puliafito CA, Baker AS, Haaf J, Foster CS. Infectious endophthalmitis: review of 36 cases. *Ophthalmology*. 1982;89:921.

25. Forster RK, Abbott RL, Gelender H. Management of infectious endophthalmitis. *Ophthalmology*. 1980;87:313.

26. Kattan H, Flynn HW Jr, Pflugfelder S, et al. Nosocomial endophthalmitis survey: current incidence of infection after surgery. *Ophthalmology*. 1991;98:227.

27. Javitt JC, Vitale S, Canner JK, et al. National outcomes of cataract surgery: endophthalmitis following inpatient surgery. *Arch Ophthalmol*. 1991;109:1085.

28. Greenwald MJ, Wohl LG, Sell CH. Metastatic bacterial endophthalmitis: a contemporary reappraisal. *Surv Ophthalmol*. 1986; 31:81.

29. Stern GA, Engel HM, Dreibe WR Jr. The treatment of postoperative endophthalmitis: results of differing approaches to treatment. *Ophthalmology*. 1989;96:62.

30. Olk RJ, Bohigian GM. The management of endophthalmitis: diagnostic and therapeutic guidelines including the use of vitrectomy. *Ophthalmic Surgj*. 1987;18:262.

31. Endophthalmitis Vitrectomy Study. *Arch Ophthalmol*. 1991;109:487.

32. Peyman GA, Rajchand M, Bennet TO. Management of endophthalmitis with pars plana vitrectomy. *Br J Ophthalmol*. 1980;64: 472.

33. Flicker LA, Meredith TA, Wilson LA, Kaplan HJ. Role of vitrectomy in *Staphylococcus epidermidis* endophthalmitis. *Br J Ophthalmol*. 1988;72:386.

34. Diamond JG. Intraocular management of endophthalmitis: a systematic approach. *Arch Ophthalmol*. 1981;99:96.

35. Chen C. Management of infectious endophthalmitis by combined vitrectomy and intraocular injection. *Ann Ophthalmol*. 1983; 15:968.

36. Maxwell DP Jr, Brent BD, Diamond JG, Wu L. Effect of intravitreal dexamethasone on ocular histopathology in a rabbit model of endophthalmitis. *Ophthalmology*. 1991;98: 1370.

37. Meisler DM, Palestine AG, Vastine DW, et al. Chronic *Propionibacterium* endophthalmitis after extracapsular cataract extraction and intraocular lens implantation. *Am J Ophthalmol*. 1986;102:733.

38. Ormerod LD, Paton BG, Haaf J, et al. Anaerobic bacterial endophthalmitis. *Ophthalmology*. 1987;94:799.

39. Meisler DM, Mandelbaum S. *Propionibacterium*-associated endophthalmitis after extracapsular cataract extraction. *Ophthalmology*. 1989;96:54.

40. Walker J, Dangel ME, Makley TA, Opremcak

EM. Postoperative *Propionibacterium granulosum* endophthalmitis. *Arch Ophthalmol*. 1990; 108:1073.

41. Roszkowski K, Roszkowski W, Ko HL, et al. Clinical experience in treatment of cancer by propionibacteria. In: Jeljaszewicz J, Pulverer G, Roszkowski K, eds. *Bacteria and Cancer*. Orlando: Academic Press; 1982:331.

42. Whitcup SM, Belfort R, deSmet MD, et al. Immunohistochemistry of the inflammatory response in *Propionibacterium acnes* endophthalmitis. *Arch Ophthalmol*. 1991;109:978.

43. Zambrano W, Flynn HW Jr, Pflugfelder SC, et al. Management options for *Propionibacterium acnes* endophthalmitis. *Ophthalmology*. 1989;96:1100.

Index